JUST MEDICARE:
WHAT'S IN, WHAT'S OUT, HOW WE DECIDE

EDITED BY COLLEEN M. FLOOD

Just Medicare

What's In, What's Out, How We Decide

UNIVERSITY OF TORONTO PRESS
Toronto Buffalo London

© University of Toronto Press Incorporated 2006
Toronto Buffalo London
Printed in Canada

ISBN-13: 978-0-8020-8002-8
ISBN-10: 0-8020-8002-2

∞

Printed on acid-free paper

Library and Archives Canada Cataloguing in Publication

Just medicare : what's in, what's out, how we decide/edited by
Colleen M. Flood.

ISBN-13: 978-0-8020-8002-8
ISBN-10: 0-8020-8002-2

1. Medical care – Law and legislation – Canada.   2. National health
insurance – Law and legislation – Canada.   3. Medical policy – Canada.
I. Flood, Colleen M. (Colleen Marion), 1966–

KE3404.J88 2006   344.7104'1   C2005-906471-4   KF3605.J88 2006

University of Toronto Press acknowledges the financial assistance
to its publishing program of the Canada Council for the Arts and the
Ontario Arts Council.

University of Toronto Press acknowledges the financial support for
its publishing activities of the Government of Canada through the
Book Publishing Industry Development Program (BPIDP).

Contents

**Part Three: Access for the Vulnerable: Case Studies
from Aboriginal Health and Mental Health**

Part Four: Rationing Access: The Role of the Physician Gatekeeper

**Part Five: Free Trade Agreements: Strengthening or Undermining
Access to Health Care?**

Acknowledgments

First and foremost I would like to thank the contributors to this book and my health law colleagues across the country. They are always a joy to work with and it is a privilege to be part of this community.

This book would not have been possible without the financial support of the Canadian Health Services Research Foundation through the auspices of the Medicare Basket Grant of which I am one of the principal investigators, along with my colleagues Carolyn Tuohy and Mark Stabile. This book would also not have been possible without the generous financial support of the Ontario Ministry of Health and Long-Term Care.

I would also like to thank our research manager, Greig Hinds, for his superb work in organizing the 2004 National Health Law Conference in Toronto at which all the chapters herein were presented and for his help in preparing this manuscript. I would also like to thank our talented research assistants Mona Awad, Andrew Botterell, and Lisa Minuk. Thanks also to Bernadette Mount, who cheerfully and efficiently deals with all administrative crises. The Faculty of Law at the University of Toronto and Dean Ron Daniels have been unflagging in their support of the health law and policy group of which I am privileged to be a member.

More personally, love and thanks to my family, Tony, Rosie, James, and Ali, who make every day a wonderful day.

And finally, I would like to dedicate this book to the memory of my father, Robert Michael Flood, who is never far from my thoughts.

JUST MEDICARE:
WHAT'S IN, WHAT'S OUT, HOW WE DECIDE

Introduction

COLLEEN M. FLOOD

The most important issue facing Canadian health care today is access to care – what services should be available to Canadians and how these services are best managed. Newspaper headlines bemoan increasing waiting times, the aging population, and ever-increasing demands for expensive new treatments. Costs are portrayed as spiralling. The solution to these problems is not obvious. Growing distrust of the ability of governments to manage health care systems effectively, coupled with a heightened scepticism regarding the authority and judgment of physicians, have led increasing numbers of citizens to demand a greater role in deciding how their own health care system is managed. So what is to be done? Who should decide what services will be publicly funded, and how should they decide? The essays in this volume address these crucial questions. They explore the diverse means by which law influences what should (and should not) be covered by publicly funded Medicare in Canada and provide insightful points of comparison by considering how other countries address the question. Together, the contributors to this volume demonstrate the multi-faceted role of law in shaping the boundaries of Canadian Medicare. They illuminate the challenges we face in ensuring a just, fair, and equitable health care system from both a Canadian and an international perspective.

Part One begins by exploring the explicit legal challenges patients have made to restrictions on access. Mark Stabile, Carolyn Tuohy, and I document the various layers of decision-making that cumulatively determine what is covered by Medicare – what is in and what is out. The principles that guide these decision-makers are not properly articulated, and consequently they are difficult to identify without reforms to improve the transparency of the process and make the

decision-makers accountable. Nevertheless, when patients go to court
to challenge governmental limits on publicly funded Medicare the courts
have responded very deferentially. We ask, is such deference appropriate, given these weaknesses in the decision-making processes? Donna
Greschner also addresses the deference that courts have shown to governments in her discussion of the recent Supreme Court decision of
Auton.[1] In that case parents sought funding for Lovas therapy, which
they believed helped their autistic children. Since this kind of therapy
is provided outside of hospitals, a court order requiring governments
to fund the therapy would alter significantly Medicare's boundaries.
The plaintiffs were successful in the British Columbia Court of Appeal
but the Supreme Court overturned this decision, showing strong deference to the difficult policy choices that governments must make. Professor Greschner argues strongly in favour of evidence-based
decision-making as a principle for determining what is in and out of
publicly funded Medicare. Because of the lack of evidence about the
efficacy of Lovas therapy she thus does not contend the justice of the
Supreme Court's decision in *Auton*. However, the court's decision here
raises starkly the extent to which courts should defer to the black-box
of government decision-making. There is a danger that decisions are
made on the basis of what serves the short-term political interests of
governments and major stakeholders, such as the medical and nursing
associations. The court in *Auton* had a golden opportunity, which it
failed to take, to send a strong signal to decision-makers that they must
articulate clear and fair principles when determining what services
attract public funding.

Just after this manuscript was completed the Supreme Court released
the *Chaoulli* decision.[2] *Chaoulli* is a constitutional challenge to laws in
the province of Quebec prohibiting private health insurance for 'medically necessary' hospital and physician services given what are portrayed to be long and unacceptable waiting times. In a narrow and
bitter four to three decision the Supreme Court of Canada in *Chaoulli*
struck down Quebec laws prohibiting the sale of private health insurance on the basis that they violate Quebec's *Charter of Human Rights and
Freedoms*. Three of the four judges in the majority also found the provisions, in light of wait times in the public sector, violate section 7 of the
Canada's *Charter of Rights and Freedoms*, which protects the life, liberty,
and security of the person. But three other judges in a blistering dissent
found that the insurance restrictions violated neither the Quebec nor
the Canadian *Charters*. Thus, the court was split on the issue of whether

similar laws in other provinces should also be overturned, although it seems likely that Justice Dechamps, who ruled on the Quebec *Charter* alone, would, if required, come to a similar conclusion on the Canadian *Charter*.

The significance of this decision cannot be underplayed. Medicare is the only universal program of entitlements in Canada which rich and poor alike are treated on the same basis and those with means cannot 'exit' to the private sector. The *Chaoulli* decision portends the fall of Medicare, the most cherished social program in Canadian history and abandonment of the principle that access to care should be allocated on the basis of need and not ability to pay. The contributions to this manuscript were finalized before the *Chaoulli* decision was available but their relevance survives the decision. Martha Jackman, who appeared as counsel for the Charter Committee on Poverty Issues and the Canadian Health Coalition in *Chaoulli* takes issue with the plaintiffs and interveners who argue that there is a fundamental right under Canada's *Charter of Rights and Freedoms* to purchase private insurance but there is no right to publicly funded health care. She describes how such a narrow interpretation of the *Charter* undermines access by the poor.

The majority in *Chaoulli* were very clear in pointing out that the applicants were not seeking publicly funded care but rather the right to purchase private insurance and that given long waiting times in the public sector their rights to life and security, guaranteed by section 7 of the *Charter* were violated. But this does raise the very interesting question of whether or not in a future case an applicant affected by long waiting times in the public sector but without the means to buy private insurance could seek as a remedy the right to *public funding* for more timely treatment and/or fairer and more just processes for determining priorities on waiting lists. After all, not to do so would result in two-tier *Charter* rights – only those with the means to purchase private insurance would be able to avail themselves of their section 7 rights in the face of long wait times causing death or suffering. Lisa Forman illustrates the potential outcome if Canadian courts were to find a positive right to publicly funded health care and explores the power of a constitutional right to publicly funded health care. Such a right sliced through the ideology of South African officials who, in the face of overwhelming evidence to the contrary, persistently denied the efficacy and safety of antiretroviral medications in the treatment of HIV/AIDS. This leaves some hope that law can indeed insure access to health care for those most in need.

Part Two shifts the focus to women's access to health services, particularly abortion and reproductive health care. The chapters illustrate that securing legal entitlements is but one battle in the larger struggle to ensure that those rights continue to mean something in practice. Sanda Rodgers reflects on the illusion that *Morgentaler*,[3] and subsequent decisions striking down provincial barriers to access, have secured Canadian women meaningful access to abortion services. Many Canadian women are either not able to get abortions at all or are able only to obtain them with delays or costs that they cannot afford. Joanna Erdman and Rebecca Cook look into the heart of the process of creating law and critique the paternalistic assumptions driving recent federal regulation of emergency contraception. Referring back to the discussion of evidence-based decision-making by Donna Greschner, they argue that the evidence clearly indicates that women can safely self-diagnose, self-select, and self-administer emergency contraception. Notwithstanding this, in Canada, women must be subjected to questioning and counselling from a pharmacist, and they cannot buy this safe form of contraception over the counter. Barriers to access can flow from the law itself particularly where laws trying to improve access do not take account of financial, social, and cultural factors. Finally, in this section Robert Kouri focuses on the province of Quebec to discuss laws affecting access to emergency oral contraception and abortion. He points out the tensions and contradictions in government policy that simultaneously wish to recognize women's reproductive freedom, yet wish also to ensure the growth of a francophone population. These tensions are reflected in the Quebec government's choice of policy and laws which, on the one hand, attempt to facilitate reproductive choice and, on the other, do nothing to dismantle the many socio-economic and geographic barriers to meaningful access.

The challenges that vulnerable and disadvantaged groups face, in particular the Aboriginal peoples of Canada and the seriously mentally ill, are the focus of Part Three. At first glance redistribution and ensuring that vulnerable groups get access to care appear to be the main issues, but the three essays in this part each demonstrate the complexity of the challenge. The kind of care that vulnerable populations need or value does not necessarily equate to the care needed or valued by the mainstream population. The media are replete with stories of under-provision of care, growing waiting times and lists, and the need for new technologies. Sheila Wildeman's critique of the compulsory treatment of psychiatric patients contrasts with this view. She writes that 'not all treatment is experienced as a benefit, and [that] the discourse on access may at least in this context mask a deeper orientation toward ensuring compliance as opposed to enabling choice.' Professor Wildeman seeks to shift the focus of policies on serious mental illness away from questions of cost-effectiveness and/or beneficent promotion of the patient's well-being towards reconsideration of the implications of the legal and moral obligation to respect individual autonomy.

Mainstream values and expectations cannot be neatly superimposed on other, different, populations and that complicates the process of developing uniform legal rights to care. Constance MacIntosh provides many stories of how, in the case of Aboriginal peoples, the complex problem of catering for their very different needs is compounded by the failure of any one level of government to be accountable for the delivery of health services and for the achievement of better health outcomes for and by Aboriginals. There is a long Canadian tradition of subjecting difficult issues to examination by a commission. The health status of Aboriginals has already been the subject of a study by the Royal Commission on Aboriginal Peoples in 1996. Continuing this tradition, the Romanow Commission on the Future of Health Care in Canada put forward a series of recommendations for overhauling governance of Aboriginal health in its report published in 2002. Janesca Kydd tests these recommendations and finds some merit in the proposals to improve the health of rural Canadians, with spillover effects for a large proportion of Aboriginal people who live in rural areas. However, with regard to Aboriginal health she finds Romanow's recommendations, although noble in intention, too vague and lacking the specifics needed for implementation. True to history, Aboriginal health, and to a large extent Romanow's recommendations for reform of rural care, have been ignored in the more recent rounds of federal-provincial negotiations over the future of Medicare. Jurisdictional quagmires and avoidance of accountability for Aboriginal health seem destined to stall any hope of improvement in the shameful results Canada has seen in Aboriginal health. There are some lessons here from the South African experience, discussed by Lisa Forman, which demonstrated the potential power of a positive constitutional right to health care. To cut through government intransigence, legal scholars in Canada will need to return to the Constitution and various treaties signed with Aboriginal peoples to argue more forcefully for a positive right to health care.

Shifting from an examination of the law as directly impeding or enabling access, Part Four explores the role of law in regulating physicians. As gatekeepers to the rest of the health care system, physicians diagnose a patient's health need, and then they facilitate what treatments a patient will receive, for example, by writing a prescription, making a referral to a specialist, sending the patient for an x-ray, or admitting a patient to hospital. Regulations affecting the interaction between patients and physicians thus have the potential to affect decision-making about who receives what care and when. This issue has taken on much more momentum in Canada as the realm of care delivered privately by physicians has expanded, and there are increased calls for a greater role for private for-profit clinics and hospitals.[4] The worry is that introducing a profit incentive for physicians will undermine the delivery of care. In this regard, Sujit Choudhry, Niteesh Choudhry, and Adalsteinn Brown caution that Canada's existing regulatory regimes are not up to the challenge. They advocate stricter regulation of the conflicts of interests that arise when physicians are allowed to own or have interests in private for-profit facilities. In apparent contradiction to calls for explicit regulatory bans is the contribution from Richard Saver, who reflects on the U.S. experience. Although the U.S. system has very different values underpinning it, and although it fails to provide coverage for all, it nonetheless can serve Canadian policy-makers as a giant laboratory of some 280 million people. Professor Saver discusses how regulation banning 'gain-sharing,' which occurs when hospitals give financial rewards to doctors who successfully implement productivity improvements, has had unintended and negative consequences. He notes that 'sometimes a zero-tolerance approach, with heavy-handed efforts to ban physician conflicts of interest in healthcare allocation decisions, can end up doing more harm than good.' This experience from south of the border suggests that we should be careful with heavy-handed prohibitions against the use of financial incentives. The goal should be to ensure access for those who most need it; if well-targeted financial incentives can achieve this goal then policy-makers should be open to the idea. However, the two contributions in this section do not wholly contradict each other; indeed, they are far more in accord than discord. Saver is careful to distinguish gain-sharing activity from the kickbacks and self-referral practices discussed by Choudhry and colleagues. Each practice is different and must be viewed in its proper context; gain-sharing poses the problem of underutilization of services while kickbacks and self-referral practices pose the problem of excess utilization of services. The clearest lesson is that not all conflicts of interest are the same and that the regulatory response should be calibrated to these differences.

Moving from the local to the international stage, Part Five explores the capacity of free trade agreements in strengthening or undermining access to health care. Roxanne Mykitiuk and Michelle Dagnino find that international trade agreements, like the Agreement on Trade-Related Intellectual Property Rights (TRIPs), have become a context for informing the fair allocation and distribution of health benefits. The most frequent example cited of the inequality caused by intellectual property rights agreements such as TRIPs is the inordinate costs of some pharmaceuticals – costs that are completely out of reach for most citizens of developing countries. But the experience from Europe, as reported by André den Exter, puts a different spin on free trade agreements. There the mobility and portability provisions of the European Communities (EC) Treaty are being used by citizens to achieve access by compelling social insurance funds (akin to our Medicare) to pay for out-of-country treatments. In this case a free-trade agreement seems to be facilitating rather than impeding access, in contradistinction to the claims of Mykitiuk and Dagnino. But den Exter argues that this apparent benefit is actually problematic. In the short term individuals may gain access to the latest technology, treatment, and faster service but there are longer-term sustainability issues. In the long run, as social insurance schemes come under intense financial pressure, access for many more people could become jeopardized.

Finally, we explore how demand or 'need' for health care is manufactured. Obviously, the future sustainability of any public insurance plan, particularly one like Canada's that seeks to serve all of its population and prohibits two-tier insurance, will pivot on the range and the cost of services characterized as 'needed' or 'medically necessary.' And in this regard, Canada suffers from its proximity to its enormous neighbour to the south where demand (or 'need') is fuelled and met by private markets and propped up by enormous public subsidies. In this last part of the book Timothy Caulfield and Patricia Peppin critically examine the role, respectively, of the media and advertising in generating demand and manufacturing 'need.' Peppin focuses on the sophisticated means that drug advertisers use to create product identification and desire for particular products in order to enhance the drug manufacturers' profits and how direct advertising to consumers provides consumers with the illusion, as opposed to the reality, of power. Advertising of drugs, she argues, impedes access to the full range of available treatments and fair allocation through distorted perceptions, skewed prescribing patterns, and vastly increased expenditures. She also discusses the pernicious effects of advertising directed at physicians to influence their treatment decisions (harking back to the discussion of Choudhry and colleagues and Saver in their discussion of regulation of physicians as gatekeepers to the rest of the system).

Caulfield further explores the theme of commercialization of those who are trusted to make judgments about need. He argues that, for a variety of reasons related to the impact of commercial interests on researchers, media portrayals of biomedical research results are consistently positive. This optimism constitutes an insidious form of advertising because it appears to be legitimate, based as it is on the public's trust in university researchers. Trudo Lemmens, in turn, examines the increased commercialization of university research – including concerns about the integrity of the scientific literature arising out of non-disclosure, ghost-writing of articles, and inadequate disclosure to the public and regulatory agencies of connections between researchers and commercial endeavours. The information that we need to assess the effectiveness of health care so that we can make principled decisions about what to fund publicly may be tainted at its source. Elaborating on these concerns in different contexts, Jocelyn Downie discusses competing interests and obligations as they apply to research regulators, research funders, patient advocacy groups, and much closer to home, health care ethics and health law experts – all of whom have a significant role in making research policy. In this latter regard she notes how experts in both ethics and law are increasingly connected to industry as consultants, through industry support for research projects and institutes, and through personal membership on industry committees or boards. Industry may use the credibility of experts in ethics and law to bolster general trust in their products. The links between the kind of research conducted and endorsed and the kinds of products and services that inevitably are put forward for consideration for public funding are indirect yet obvious.

I am delighted with the contributions of my health law colleagues in Canada and internationally to this volume. Each has made a unique contribution to filling the scholarship vacuum in this important area, and I thank them for their magnificent efforts. Economists and political scientists have long dominated the debate about the future of health care policy in Canada. Until fairly recently legal scholars have not had much input. The role of law is usually underestimated by those in health policy, but as demonstrated in these essays, law can both exacerbate and ameliorate unfair or unprincipled allocation decisions in a myriad of ways throughout the system. The role of law in shaping and configuring the boundaries of Medicare is as complex as the interlocking decisions that cumulatively determine what health care is funded and for whom. Health law and policy scholarship is needed to help us understand how our health care system works and how law affects decision-making about what and who attract public funding. Apart from helping to achieve a better understanding of how the system works at present, legal scholars can also contribute to making it better. First, lawyers can contribute to the debate about what fairness means when it comes to allocating scare health resources. Second, legal scholars have much to contribute to what constitutes fair processes for decision-making. Finally, in the face of unprincipled or unfair decision-making, legal scholars can use challenges in constitutional or administrative law or actions in tort to seek justice in health care.

NOTES

1 *Auton (Guardian ad litem of) v. British Columbia (Attorney General)*, [2004] 3 S.C.R. 657.
2 *Chauolli v. Quebec (Attorney General)*, [2005] S.C.R. 35. A copy of the judgments of the trial judge, the Court of Appeal, and the Supreme Court of Quebec, and copies of briefs and related materials are available at http://www.utoronto.ca/healthlaw/ (accessed 23 September 2005). See also Colleen M. Flood, Kent Roach, and Lorne Sossin, *Access to Care, Access to Justice: The Legal Debate over Private Health Insurance in Canada* (Toronto: University of Toronto Press, 2005).
3 *R. v. Morgentaler*, [1988] 1 S.C.R. 30.
4 Michael J. Kirby and Wilbert Keon, 'Why Competition Is Essential in the Delivery of Publicly Funded Health Care Services' (2004) 5:8 Policy Matters 1 at 4.

PART ONE

Constitutional and Administrative Law Challenges to the Boundaries of Medicare

1 What Is In and Out of Medicare? Who Decides?

COLLEEN M. FLOOD, MARK STABILE, AND CAROLYN TUOHY

In recent years five bodies[1] have independently investigated and issued reports on the sustainability of publicly funded Medicare in Canada. In spite of the different ideologies of the governments that commissioned them, all confirmed certain fundamental principles. The last, the Romanow Commission on the Future of Health Care in Canada, came to the 'overriding conclusion that there is no need to abandon the principles or values underpinning Canada's health care system.'[2]

That system rests on two bedrock principles. First, access to important medical care is distributed on the basis of need, rather than ability to pay. Second, the services covered under Medicare are financed almost exclusively through general taxation revenues. Notwithstanding their repeated endorsement, profound questions about the application of these principles linger long after the many volumes of commission reports have gathered dust. Specifically:

- What health care services should be publicly funded in full?
- Who decides what services should be publicly funded?
- What are the processes by which these decisions are made?

These questions are made pressing by the Health Accord of 2003 in which the prime minister and all provincial and territorial premiers agreed that the core of publicly funded Medicare should be expanded beyond hospital and physician services to include home care and prescription drugs. As the *categories* of services eligible for full public funding increase, it becomes even more crucial to determine who decides, or should decide, what particular services within those categories are eligible for public funding and what principles and processes guide the decision-making.

With respect to the question of 'what' services to fund, it is impossible to generalize across nations, given their different resource constraints and values. The International Convention on Economic, Social and Cultural Rights adopted a human rights perspective to determine a basic minimum of access to health care.[3] Beyond that, however, much greater uncertainty ensues in developed countries over what health care services should be publicly funded and what services should be left to the private sector.

Take health care delivery options created by technological advancements. How does one decide which delivery option to choose – on cost alone? Should a treatment that costs $150,000 but offers only a 5 per cent chance of success be publicly funded? Or should a new drug that is equally effective but with fewer side effects be funded as opposed to an existing drug that costs 20 per cent less? In theory, the choices should be made on the basis of a combination of information about *relative* costs and health benefits, the values that we hold about preventing and/or curing specific illnesses or disabilities, the values that we have with regard to equality and fairness (as set out in the Constitution through the *Canadian Charter of Rights and Freedoms*[4]), the resources available, and, of course, opportunity costs. Money spent on one thing cannot be spent on another; trade-offs (investing in health care versus eduction, for example) must always be made. A decision-maker must be entrusted to make the necessary trade-offs between competing sets of values and competing claims.[5]

A Decision-Making Framework Grounded in the Canadian System

There have been many models put forward to guide decision-making about what should and should not be publicly funded both in Canada and internationally.[6] However, these theoretical models have not been implemented in Canada or particularly successfully in any jurisdiction. In our view they suffer from being too general, too abstract, and divorced from messy local details. In particular, the existing models fail to take into account the political economy of particular systems. In any system of decision-making considerations of values, resources, and information about costs and benefits are filtered through local structures and processes. As we discuss further below, in Canada, these structures and processes are characterized by accidents of history and by long-held accommodations between governments and the medical profession, inflexible and inadequate regulations and law, and the interaction of different stakeholders and interest groups.

Thus, before we can theorize about what processes and principles should be adopted we must understand how decisions are made now. The existing system will constrain what reforms are possible. For example, starting from the top, the overarching normative framework that governs it, the *Canada Health Act* (CHA),[7] drives decision-making about what is in and what is out of Canadian Medicare. The CHA requires that provinces publicly fund all 'medically necessary' hospital services and 'medically required' physician services in order to receive federal funding. But, the CHA does not provide definitions of 'medically necessary' or 'medically required.'[8] Nor, in turn, does provincial legislation provide such definitions. How, then, do provinces determine which particular health care services to fund?

In general, decision-making about what is in and out of publicly funded Medicare reflects the different silos of funding that support different sectors of the health care system. Thus, as we will describe further below, there are significantly different approaches to funding depending on what sector we are dealing with, whether physician services, hospital services, new technologies, pharmaceuticals, or home-care, say. For example, which physician services are publicly funded is largely a matter of negotiation between a provincial government and its respective medical association. By comparison, the process of determining which prescription drugs to include in provincial formularies (and thus those that are publicly funded) involves a much more technocratic evaluation of the costs and benefits of the drugs. In this chapter, we report our research to date on how decisions are made in Ontario regarding which physician services are publicly funded, but we will refer to other sectors by way of comparison. More specifically we look at the extent to which decision-makers and the decision-making process weigh the relative costs and benefits of particular treatments vis-à-vis all other possibilities (cost-effectiveness analysis). We also explore the extent and nature of public participation in decision-making as a proxy for exploring the extent to which decision-makers are being held accountable for their decisions and also the extent to which public values are being incorporated in the decision-making process.

Decision-Making in Ontario

At least four bodies or institutions in Ontario are involved in determining what physician services are included in the publicly funded basket of services. These are: (1) the Physician Services Committee, which is a joint committee comprising officials from the Ministry of Health and

Long-Term Care (the Ministry) and the Ontario Medical Association (OMA); (2) Medical Directors, who are salaried physicians within the Ministry and may determine claims for public funding; (3) the Health Services Appeal and Review Board; and (4) the courts. We discuss each of these decision-making bodies in turn. By exploring the existing processes in depth we hope eventually to make more meaningful prescriptions for reform of decisions regarding what is in and what is out of publicly funded Medicare.

Physician Services Committee

Long-held accommodations between the medical profession and Canadian governments are fundamental to Canadian Medicare.[9] Not surprisingly, then, decision-making regarding which physician services are to be publicly funded is driven by the process of fee negotiations between the Ministry and the OMA, the latter being the bargaining agent for physicians in Ontario.[10] Negotiations between the OMA and the Ministry effectively determine the *range* of physician services to be publicly funded. By default these services are deemed 'medically necessary.' Thus, the phrase 'medically necessary'[11] does not derive from an explicit application of principle. Rather it is a label applied ex post to negotiations between specialties within the OMA and between the OMA and the Ministry.

The Physician Services Committee (PSC) is a key forum for the relationship between the OMA and the Ontario government. It was created pursuant to the 1997 Agreement between the OMA and the Ministry[12] and continues to operate pursuant to the 2000 Agreement.[13] The PSC has ten members, five appointed by the OMA and five by the Ministry, and it is chaired by a professional facilitator. This committee is an important vehicle for negotiating governmental and professional relations, and there is general concurrence that the PSC has greatly contributed to the improvement of these relations. In addition, however, the PSC performs an important public role in reviewing the utilization of resources and recommending the listing or delisting of particular services in order to meet certain financial targets.[14]

Determining what principles or criteria should guide decision-making about what is funded is a problem with which all health care systems must grapple. As Rudolph Klein has noted, '[t]he challenge everywhere is about how to organize and orchestrate what, for the foreseeable future, will be a continuing dialogue between politicians, professionals, and the public about the principles that should be invoked in making decisions about rationing and about how best to reconcile conflicting values and competing claims.'[15] Given that the PSC is the body that effectively decides what physician services are publicly funded for the 12.4 million people who live in Ontario,[16] it is relevant to ask what principles or values inform the PSC's decision-making process. Our research shows that there is little or no transparency about what these guiding principles are, thus allowing the possibility that self-interest or irrelevant considerations guide the PSC's decision-making. Both the 1997 agreement and the 2000 agreement stipulate that the review of and changes to the Schedule of Benefits are to be accomplished using a mix of 'tightening' and 'modernization.' Neither agreement defines these terms. Indeed our research has revealed little evidence of a systematic approach to the listing or delisting processes.[17] The overall effect of the negotiation process is largely to perpetuate the status quo. Fee increases are spread among existing services, and there is little movement off the Schedule of Benefits of services covered. In other words, it is extremely difficult for services to be delisted. The difficulty of delisting services limits the potential funding of new services and technologies; funding for these must come from what resources remain after increases to existing services have been made. The end result is little flexibility to allow new and more beneficial services or treatments to replace older, less beneficial services or treatments. This process contrasts sharply with processes used to determine whether to fund prescription drugs, where cost-effectiveness studies are more regularly employed before a new drug is listed.[18] Thus, across two sectors that are equally important we have two very different *approaches* to the use of technical evidence in decision-making, although the ultimate *impact* of these different approaches has yet to be measured.

Many of the PSC's decisions must necessarily involve more than technocratic assessment of the clinical benefits of a treatment. For example, the delisting of particular health care services can have profound access effects on often very vulnerable groups. Values are clearly important in listing and delisting decisions. One important way of ensuring that a full scope of public values is canvassed is to provide a level playing field for participation by a wide range of groups and individuals. However, the respective roles for public participation and procedural fairness in the PSC process are minimal. Appendix A of the 1997 Agreement provides the only indication of procedural fairness: the

PSC 'is committed to giving appropriate opportunity to affected parties to provide timely input to the PSC before making recommendations to the Ministry and the OMA.'

Different groups have complained that they have been given inadequate opportunity for input into the decision-making process. Not surprisingly, most of these complaints come from groups of health care providers who have a particular stake in the outcome. For example, the Ontario Association of Speech-Language Pathologists and Audiologists (OSLA) has challenged the openness of the PSC's decision-making process.[19] OSLA's concerns arose from a PSC recommendation to the Minister that hearing aid evaluations be delisted and that coverage of diagnostic hearing tests be restricted. Essentially this delisting affects audiologists, who formerly practised on their own but are now limited to working within a physician's office if they are to receive public funding for the provision of diagnostic hearing tests.

OSLA's account of the PSC's decision-making process is troubling, even allowing for its own self-interest in the proceedings. Participation is limited to invitation by either the Ministry or the OMA. The membership of subcommittees whose recommendations are often extremely influential is no more diverse than is the PSC itself. Both the Ministry and the OMA have agendas that may not necessarily align with the public interest: the Ministry's agenda presumably is often one of restraining increases in government spending, and the OMA's agenda presumably is primarily that of furthering the interests of its members through fee increases.

Of course, the argument against greater public participation in this process is that sustainability would be threatened as government restrictions on spending increases may be more difficult to enforce. But this assumes public participation within the context of the present negotiation processes as opposed to first rethinking the accommodations reached between physicians and provincial and territorial governments. If the process of determining what is in and what is out of Medicare could be unbuckled from determinations of which physician services to fund, then it may become possible to establish a more rigorous and principled process, infused with public participation, that would allow relatively high benefit services and technologies to be funded in place of lower benefit services and technologies. The argument also assumes that greater public spending on health care is *politically* unsustainable whereas, arguably, with greater public participation in determining what is in and out of publicly funded Medicare, there may be a greater appetite for the necessary tax levels to sustain growth in publicly funded Medicare.

Thus, the PSC plays an important yet hidden role in determining the boundaries of publicly funded Medicare in Ontario. The PSC and its various subcommittees and related working groups are almost completely populated by representatives from the OMA and the Ministry. The result is closed decision-making with no processes in which the interests of other parties are explicitly incorporated. There is no opportunity for any form of public participation in the PSC's decision-making. The public must rely on the Ministry to represent the larger public interest in its negotiations with the OMA over what is in and out of publicly funded Medicare. There have been a variety of complaints made by those affected by the PSC's decision-making process because they have not been able to participate in the process. Complaints are to be expected at any point where a decision is made to remove a service from the list of publicly funded services. Nevertheless, there are obvious concerns regarding conflicts of interest when decisions are made by physicians' groups to delist services that are not 'physician' services (for example, services provided by independent audiologists).

A further concern about the PSC's decision-making process is the lack of any meaningful principles according to which decisions are made to exclude or include services in the publicly funded basket (other than 'tightening' and 'modernization'). On the positive side, the PSC has been an innovative development from a labour relations perspective: significantly improving the working relationship between the provincial government and the OMA. However, if decision-making is to remain closed within the world of negotiations between the OMA and the Ministry, they should account to the general public for the principles upon which their decisions rest.

Medical Directors

Where do patients go if they are unhappy that a particular treatment has been delisted or they want a new treatment covered or they find they are waiting too long? Surprisingly, given the importance of Medicare and issues of access in the minds of Canadians almost nothing is written of the measures that dissatisfied citizens can take to challenge resource allocation decisions.

The first recourse of patients in Ontario is to appeal to the Ministry of

Health and Long-Term Care. In that case, our investigations indicate that a Medical Director may often play a pivotal part in the decision of whether to deny or allow funding. Medical Directors are salaried physicians employed by the Ministry (and indeed every province employs several Medical Directors). A Freedom of Information and Protection of Privacy Act[20] application revealed that the Medical Directors from different provinces meet biannually through the auspices of the Interprovincial Health Insurance Agreements Coordinating Committee.[21] The transcript of one of the meetings obtained suggests that provinces may pressure each other not to list new procedures and technologies because of the pressure such action places on other provinces to fund similar treatments. Applications for access to more information about these meetings have been made, to date with no success.[22]

Our research indicates that Medical Directors are important decision-makers, deeply embedded within the provincial health ministries.[23] We have identified and interviewed Medical Directors in each province, hoping to discover what values and principles drive their decisions on applications for public funding. Interviews with the Medical Directors indicate that the following three considerations are weighed with respect to discussions in an interprovincial meeting: (1) the medical effectiveness of the treatment; (2) the cost-effectiveness of the treatment; and (3) the approach of other provinces to the treatment. When asked to order the importance of these considerations, most Medical Directors polled put either medical evidence or cross-provincial comparisons first, followed by economic considerations. This hierarchy suggests that Medical Directors are primarily concerned with discussing matters relevant to medical efficacy and cross-provincial uniformity than with conducting any kind of cost-effectiveness analysis. When queried about whether the size of an affected subpopulation was a consideration, most Medical Directors interviewed reacted with some chagrin, suggesting that the threshold for funding is medical necessity, and the relatively small size of an affected group is a more or less immaterial consideration.

Thus, although the good news is that Medical Directors may have actualized the values of universality and portability into their decision-making processes (such values being expressly adopted as criteria into the *Canada Health Act*), the bad news is the more or less uniform agreement among Medical Directors about the relative unimportance of public opinion. Most Medical Directors seemed to indicate that they never considered public opinion directly. Reasons Medical Directors cited for avoiding this consideration involved concern about the public's lack of expertise in the medical aspects of these issues, including the concern that public opinion might be somewhat volatile, reflecting interest in a treatment because of its relative newness rather than because of the medical evidence behind it.

The views of the Medical Directors reflect in turn a wider view that it is better not to be explicit or transparent about how decisions are made regarding what to fund or not to fund. A spokesperson for former Health Minister Tony Clement is reported to have said that discussions regarding what is in and out of Medicare should remain behind closed doors: 'Let's be frank, there will always be somebody saying, "Don't do that,"' he said, referring to patients who will lobby to protect coverage of particular items.[24] The fear is that if decisions are transparent, it will be more difficult to ration services and control costs.[25] But, in contrast to this stance, many have recognized transparency as a fundamental condition for a fair process for decision-making about entitlements. For example, Norman Daniels and James Sabin in their seminal work on 'accountability for reasonableness' argue that 'decisions regarding coverage for new technologies (and other limit-setting decisions) and their rationales must be publicly accessible.'[26] In our work on Medical Directors we have considered whether a lack of meaningful interaction with the public and a lack of transparency are acceptable given the nature and content of the discussion that occurs at these interprovincial meetings. There is a strong argument for greater transparency, as opposed to more formal participatory processes, so that citizens, patients, and taxpayers can be assured of the basis upon which decisions are made or policy is formulated and to provide a check to ensure that the principles followed in decision-making are those that reflect the larger public interest and values, as opposed to political or other interests.

The Health Services Appeal and Review Board

In addition to transparency, Daniels and Sabin argue that fairness and legitimacy requires that there be a 'mechanism for challenge and dispute resolution regarding limit-setting decisions, including the opportunity for revising decisions in light of further evidence or arguments.'[27] But in most provinces, the only recourse from a decision not to fund a particular treatment or service is to seek relief in the general courts, either through judicial review or through a *Charter* challenge. Some relief may be obtained from appeal to an Ombudsman in the case of decisions made by the government or government-owned institutions (i.e., some psychiatric hospitals).[28] The Ombudsman, however, intervenes as a last recourse; complainants have to first use all other complaints processes or means of appeal available to them before the Ombudsman will conduct an investigation.[29] Quebec has a more generous system in that there is a Patient Ombudsman, charged with specifically investigating health complaints.[30]

Three provinces (Ontario, Alberta, and British Columbia) have administrative tribunals to which the citizens thereof can bring (on limited grounds) an application to review a decision not to publicly fund a service or treatment. In Quebec, the Tribunal administrative du Québec hears appeals concerning health treatment or service coverage in Quebec as well as appeals from all administrative bodies in the province. [31] Of all the specific tribunals Ontario's is the most active and has a broader mandate to review decisions but, as we discuss below, its discretion nonetheless remains limited.

The Ontario Health Service Appeal and Review Board (the Board)[32] is composed of at least twelve members, who are appointed by the Lieutenant-Governor in Council on the recommendation of the Minister of Health and Long-Term Care.[33] Members of the Board are appointed for three years and work on a part-time basis. No more than three members can be physicians, and no member can be employed in the public service or otherwise by the Crown. Most of the members of the Board are lawyers, which as we discuss further below is problematic given that while some legal expertise is needed for determinations of what to publicly fund, there are other skill-sets that should be included. Most of the work of the Board involves conducting appeals from decisions made by the General Manager of the Ontario Health Insurance Plan (OHIP) under *Ontario's Health Insurance Act*[34] and its regulations.

The ability to seek relief before an administrative tribunal rather than having to apply to the general courts offers the prospect of quicker, easier, and cheaper recourse to justice. However, many who do appeal to the Ontario Board are disappointed to find that its discretion to review delisting or failure to list decisions is significantly constrained by the terms of the act and the regulations. For example, section 24 of the relevant regulations[35] lists medical services that are specifically excluded from OHIP coverage. These include: in subsection 24(1), services solely for the purposes of altering or restoring appearance (para. 10), treatment for a medical condition that is generally considered experimental (para. 17); in vitro fertilization, except in limited circumstances (para. 23); reversal of sterilization (para. 22); and the fitting and evalua- tion of hearing aids (para. 27). These services are not insured services (and thus, by a process of reverse engineering, are considered not 'medi- cally necessary' under the *Canada Health Act*). The Board has almost no discretion to reverse a decision not to publicly fund these services.

The Board does have some discretion with respect to access to out-of- country services. This occurs in two circumstances: when a citizen of Ontario requires unanticipated, emergency treatment while travelling, and/or when a citizen of Ontario secures prior approval to obtain treatment that is unavailable, or unavailable without significant delay, in the province. Most of the Board's discretion, and the most interesting decisions, revolve around the issue of pre-approved treatment. The relevant subsection states:[36]

> Services that are part of a treatment and that are rendered outside Canada at a hospital or health facility are prescribed as insured services if,
> (a) the treatment is generally accepted in Ontario as appropriate for a person in the same medical circumstances as the insured person; and
> (b) either,
>> i. that kind of treatment is not performed in Ontario by an identical or equivalent procedure; or
>> ii. that kind of treatment is performed in Ontario but it is necessary that the insured person travel out of Canada to avoid a delay that would result in death or medically irreversible tissue damage.

To qualify for coverage an applicant must receive approval first from the General Manager of OHIP before leaving the country.[37] Moreover, the total costs reimbursed are capped in a schedule and are significantly less than the actual costs incurred by most people who would travel to the United States, for example. These issues tend to cluster around two sets of questions or considerations: (1) whether treatment is 'generally accepted as appropriate' in Ontario for a person in the same medical circumstances as the appellant, and (2) if so, whether it is (a) unavail- able ('not performed') in the province or (b) whether a delay in treat- ment would result in death or irreversible tissue damage.

Thus, the Board must first determine that the treatment is generally accepted in Ontario as acceptable for a patient in the same medical circumstances, and then it must *also* determine that the treatment is not performed in Ontario, either as an objective or practical matter. This presents a Catch-22 for most patients, as the Board seems to use evidence that a particular treatment is *not* performed in Ontario to indicate that treatment is not generally accepted in Ontario. When the treatment in question is new it is, of course, not surprising that it is difficult to surmount the first part of the test. The limits of the Ontario system in this regard are in sharp contrast to the much more generous approach of the European Court of Justice (discussed by André Den Exter in this volume) to claims by European citizens for new and innovative treatments in other countries within the European Community.

The other main issue is the determination of what constitutes a sufficiently serious delay to merit seeking out-of-country health care services. The statute is clear: the delay at issue must be such that to deny treatment any longer would result in death or medically irreversible tissue damage. For the Board to find that there has been or would be a sufficiently significant delay, it generally requires evidence from a 'physician who *practices medicine in Ontario*' that delay *would*, and not *could*, result in death or medically significant irreversible tissue damage.[38] Our review of the Board's decisions indicates that this definition often frustrates appellants who bring appeals before the Board in hopes that it will be compassionate with respect to the psychological effects of delay, only to have the Board reiterate its limited jurisdiction.

Apart from the substantive issue that the Board's discretion is constrained through the Act, there are also significant issues of access to the Board and transparency in decision-making. The Board's judgments are not online and appointments must be made to view the judgments in Toronto – clearly, this has a disproportionate impact on anyone living outside of Toronto but particularly on applicants in northern and remote areas. Moreover, the judgments are not indexed and one needs to know the name of the case in order to locate the decision.

Fettering appeal routes is tempting for any government wishing to avoid the ire of public judgment for the inevitable choices that have to be made in defining health care benefits. However, the long-term consequences of doing so are insidious, resulting in mounting frustration and disillusionment on the part of those whom Medicare is meant to serve and undermining political support for it.

The Courts

The role of the courts in determining the boundaries of Medicare is often overstated in the media and/or assumed to be much more significant than is actually the case. There are two main mechanisms by which the courts play a role in determining what is in and what is out of Medicare: judicial review through general administrative law and through *Charter* challenges. In general, plaintiffs are unsuccessful.[39]

Faced with a challenge in administrative law, courts demonstrate their deference for determining what is in and out of Medicare, by reviewing decisions on the standard of 'patent unreasonableness.' This is the most deferential standard of review possible in administrative law, with the other possibilities being 'reasonableness simpliciter' and 'correctness' (the latter being the least deferential). For example, the only successful judicial review claim before the courts with regard to waiting times has been *Stein v. Québec (Régie de l'Assurance-maladie)*.[40] In this case Mr Stein waited months for surgery, even though his doctors warned that his life was in danger if he was not operated on within four to eight weeks. He was successful before the Quebec Superior Court in overturning the Quebec health insurance board officials' refusal to pay for his treatment in a New York hospital on the grounds that, given the facts of the case, the decision was patently unreasonable. Thus, the court was prepared to be very deferential to the Board's decision-making; however, even allowing for this very high standard of deference the court felt compelled to overturn the Board's decision. The courts will check the *rationality* of governmental decisions about what is in and out of Medicare, but to date have not held the government or other institutions to any higher standard.

Another example of the court's deferential stance towards the decision-making processes is the 2001 case of *Shulman v. College of Audiologists and Speech-Language Pathologists of Ontario*.[41] In that case, the College of Audiologists and Speech-Language Pathologists of Ontario (CASLPO) was unsuccessful in its application to review a decision to delist audiology services not provided under the direct supervision of a physician.

Notwithstanding that this case was unsuccessful, the mere possibility of legal challenge has in the view of some cast a chill over the prospects for further delisting. Perversely, decision-makers may welcome the excuse of a fear of litigation in order to avoid having to make tough choices attracting the ire of different groups. For example, one of the most commonly cited candidates for delisting is the annual general check-up. Family doctors, however, would undoubtedly be upset if annual check-ups were delisted given the potential impact on their incomes, and they will undoubtedly rail against such a move (and against the Ontario Medical Association should it support such an initiative). So there is the prospect that the mere *threat* of judicial review, and the political heat that accompanies a judicial challenge, even an unsuccessful one, will help to perpetuate the status quo and reinforce rigidities in the system.

With respect to Charter challenges, applicants have met with a similar lack of success. For example, the courts to date (with one exception) have not found that section 7 of the *Charter*, which guarantees life, liberty, and security of the person, entitles Canadians to publicly funded health care.[42] Indeed, as Martha Jackman discusses further in this volume, the Supreme Court in the *Chuoulli* case[43] heard a claim that Section 7, rather than guaranteeing a right to publicly funded care, instead guarantees a right to buy, if one is able, private insurance covering 'medically necessary' services.

Most of the *Charter* challenges to limits on publicly funded health care are brought arguing Section 15, the equality provision. Despite the absence of a *Charter* right to publicly funded health care, once a government elects to provide some publicly funded health care services, it must do so in compliance with the equality provisions of the *Charter*. Section 15(1) provides that '[E]very individual is equal before and under the law and has the right to the equal protection and equal benefit of the law without discrimination and, in particular, without discrimination based on race, national or ethnic origin, colour, religion, sex, age or mental or physical disability.' However, even if discrimination is found under section 15(1), it may be 'saved' by section 1 of the *Charter*, which provides that 'the *Canadian Charter of Rights and Freedoms* guarantees the rights and freedoms set out in it subject only to such reasonable limits prescribed by law as can be demonstrably justified in a free and democratic society.' Thus, a government may defend a finding that a particular policy or decision is discriminatory by pointing to the principles and processes that were followed in making it and arguing that although the needs of those discriminated against were considered, there were other countervailing needs or considerations that outweighed these concerns.

There have been a number of section 15 challenges that have grabbed attention.[44] But between 1985 and 2002 of the thirty-three cases that have challenged health care policy, only eleven have been successful.[45] More specifically, of the cases that have challenged policies limiting insured medical services only one has been upheld at the Supreme Court level. The successful case was in 1997, *Eldridge v. British Colum-*

bia,[46] which was a claim by a deaf couple that they were discriminated against in contravention of their section 15 rights by the failure of the British Columbian government (and more specifically a hospital) to fund interpretation services. The facts of this case were very compelling. The deaf woman was giving birth to twins and there were problems at the time of delivery. A nurse communicated to the mother through gestures that the heart rate of one of the babies had gone down. The twins were whisked away from the distressed women who did not know what was going on apart from a note being flashed at her with the word 'fine' written thereon.

In the wake of *Eldridge* there were two ways to interpret the decision. The first one is that its effect should be limited to the extent that the applicants were not seeking any new health treatments per se but the right to communicate and receive information about the *same* health treatments as those enjoyed by people without hearing loss. The Supreme Court strongly emphasized that effective communication is an indispensable component of the delivery of a medical service. This interpretation would significantly narrow the scope for future *Charter* challenges. The second interpretation is that the decision represented an opening of the floodgates to the use of the *Charter* by those unhappy with government restrictions on public financing. In the recent decision of *Auton*, discussed more fully by Donna Greschner in this volume, the Supreme Court of Canada made it very clear that the correct reading of *Eldridge* was the first interpretation above.[47]

There are many issues that are raised by the court's review on *Charter* grounds of decisions not to publicly fund treatments. The first point to note is that only a very few patients have been successful. The expense and delay inherent in *Charter* litigation means that recourse to the *Charter* remains an unsatisfactory way to deal with *most* grievances and concerns that citizens have regarding access to health care services. Also, although the *Charter* can, in certain circumstances, address explicit rationing decisions by governments (for example, failing to fund a particular service or delisting a particular service), it has far less capacity to challenge the multitude of resource allocation decisions that are made in the health care system every day. In other words, although the *Charter* can protect against explicit governmental decisions that openly deny or prevent access to a particular treatment, most decisions are not explicit and have an indirect effect on access. Governments can eviscerate a health care system through underfunding so that services are available in theory although not in practice, and it is much harder to launch legal challenge against such methods of dilution. Second, it is important to note that *Charter* challenges are a one-way street, and they do nothing to counter the difficulty of *delisting* treatments and may, indeed, exacerbate the existing reluctance of decision-makers to formally delist treatments that are of relatively less benefit. However, given that the *Charter* as part of the *Constitution* is as clear a statement of agreed-upon public values as one is likely to find, the courts play a critical role in checking governmental decision-making, which increasingly emphasizes cost-effectiveness analysis and the objective of restraining government spending, that may unlawfully discriminate against marginalized and vulnerable groups of people. To eliminate, then, the prospect of successful *Charter* challenges and to ensure decision-making that respects public values, *Charter* issues should be taken into account at the time decisions are made to list or delist, that is, *Charter* considerations and values need to be adopted by local decision-makers and included in local decision-making processes.

Discussion

In this concluding section we reflect on what our research has revealed to date and focus on four themes for discussion and further research: the extent to which our present system is designed to focus on outputs rather than inputs; the role of physicians and other interest groups in impeding and enabling reform; the role for public values and public participation in decision-making; and, finally, the role for law and legal institutions.

Focus on Outputs Rather Than Inputs

What is the result of the layers of decision-making and the processes that we have described? The cumulative effect is stagnation and maintenance of the status quo, that is, services are rarely delisted, thus limiting the possibility of new services being added to the range of services that are publicly funded. There are few systematic reviews of older technologies and treatments to determine whether they remain cost-effective. Furthermore, there is enormous resistance to changing the range and types of services that we publicly fund, primarily by individuals with vested interests in maintaining public funding for certain procedures. Also governments and medical associations are wary of being exposed to either judicial review or *Charter* challenge, even when the courts have indicated that they will be extremely deferential to decision-making in this regard and even given the relatively low number of successful administrative and *Charter* challenges. The net result is that newer treatments and technologies are looked at with a much more sceptical eye and are more frequently scrutinized for cost-effectiveness. New drugs must not only prove cost-effectiveness, they must also prove that they outperform existing drugs on the market if they are more expensive. New home care services must wait for additional funding before they replace existing in-hospital care. New hospital technologies are frequently delayed only because of cost until long after they have diffused into other medical markets.

We have significant concerns about this approach. Undoubtedly, there are quagmires and irresolvable tensions in attempting to articulate and operationalize a set of principles guiding determinations of what is publicly funded. But, at a minimum, the treatment should be effective, that is, the treatment must provide a reasonable chance of achieving a particular health state (such as recovery or the alleviation of pain). Yet studies in evidence-based medicine in the developed world demonstrate little or no evidence of effectiveness for up to 30 to 40 per cent of the health care services that physicians recommend.[48] That there is much to be done to improve the processes of decision-making in Canada is illustrated by that fact that there is full funding for routine annual general check-ups despite the consensus of expert medical panels – since 1979 – that they have little effect on the detection of disease, while there is not full funding for life-saving drugs, for example, insulin, for all Canadians.

Much of the reluctance to fund new technologies comes from the fact that they are relatively untested and usually quite expensive. In a system that has no formal mechanism to remove an expensive and ineffective technology, it is quite understandable that policy-makers would be reluctant to introduce new treatments. However, many newer treatments may indeed be cost-effective and superior to existing treatments. Enhancing the flexibility to fund new treatments of relatively greater benefit and replace older treatments would allow us to improve the health care available to Canadians and dispel the long-standing criticism that our system lags behind other developed countries in technology adoption.

A useful way of thinking about health care technologies has been suggested by David Cutler.[49] Figure 1.1 shows a dichotomy of technologies divided into high and low cost along the Y-axis and into high and low effectiveness along the X-axis. The most successful technologies

Figure 1.1 Cost and Effectiveness Dichotomy

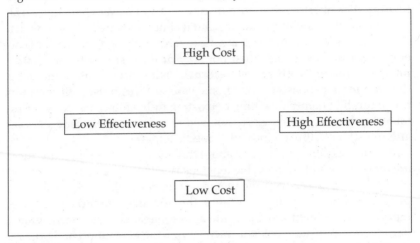

Note: Adapted from David Cutler, *Your Money or Your Life* (New York: Oxford University Press, 2004).

will be those that are both highly effective and low in cost (represented by the bottom right box). However, some technologies will be highly effective and expensive, and successful health care systems will also adopt these technologies (the upper right corner) if the benefits exceed the costs. Unfortunately, many technologies fall into neither of these categories, but rather into the left-hand side of the box representing relatively ineffective technologies. Systematic review of existing technologies would allow our system to remove those technologies that over time do not show themselves to belong on the right-hand side. Cutler argues that many innovative and costly technologies may require more time to demonstrate their cost-effectiveness. While universal systems such as those in Canada may need to exercise more caution when adopting new technology than health care insurers in a more private setting, flexibility in technology adoption coupled with rigorous review – and removal – processes might broaden the number of cost-effective and beneficial technologies that are available to Canadians. There are enormous barriers to making this transition, but we must ask why we do not allocate resources to more high-benefit procedures. The likely answer is that under the current framework, once a technology is adopted, it is here for good, or at least until it becomes obsolete.

The History of Political Accountability and Interest Groups

There is enormous resistance to change in the health care system, and to a large extent this resistance is attributable to those who work within and are paid by it. Part of the problem is that a change in the breadth and nature of services that are publicly funded, in a fee-for-service system, correlates with changes in the ability of physicians (and to a lesser extent other health care providers) to maintain or improve on their incomes.

We must review the basis of long-held accommodations between governments and the medical profession and explore the basis for a new deal that would increasingly reward physicians for performance rather than through inputs. Partly the problem is a lack of incentives and the need to align them. Can we reward physicians for the improvements in health outcomes that they achieve as opposed to the services they provide, regardless of quality or effectiveness? What is the appropriate level (patient/practice/region) at which to measure physician outcomes? As physician remuneration is central to the ongoing redefinition of the Medicare basket, extraneous factors shape its definition rather than technical evidence and public values. Is it possible to incorporate technical evidence and public values into the present process? What are the prospects of requiring an ex ante evaluation of cost-effectiveness for physician services as is required for publicly funded drugs? Is it possible to disentangle the determination of what is publicly funded (medically necessary) from questions of physician reimbursement?

Another important set of questions that arise once we contemplate increasingly shifting physician services in and out of the publicly funded sector involve what we do about conflicts of interest if we expand the range of services that should be publicly funded. For example, if we acknowledge that sometimes a magnetic resonance imaging (MRI) scan is medically necessary and sometimes it is not, and if the physician has the discretion to make that determination, then how do we make sure that the physician will not have a conflict of interest in sending a patient for a private MRI?

Our review of the existing local processes in Ontario suggests that the path for reform is to explore whether new accommodations can be reached with physicians so that it is possible to unbuckle determinations of remuneration for physicians from decisions about what is in and out of Medicare. Further exploration of the prospects for sorting services across the spectrum of public and private financing and measures to cut through the sectoral boundaries that have historically characterized Canada's health care system (full public funding for hospital and physician services and mixed funding for prescriptions and home care) is also required, particularly given the conflicts of interest that physicians face when discretion is accorded to them to determine what falls in or out of the publicly funded health basket.

Public Values and Public Participation in Decision-Making

Although evidence is important, so are values.[50] Indeed, there may not be good evidence for the kinds of care that citizens value. For example, caring services and palliative care are difficult to measure in terms of health outcomes, as are traditional healing practices and treatments. Also difficult to measure is the extent to which patients are treated with respect and dignity and in accordance with their culture. The importance of values is increasingly recognized, as is the idea that citizens need a voice in governance structures and are no longer content to assume that governments or physicians sufficiently represent the public interest in these matters.[51] However, public participation is at present given little weight in the decision-making regarding what to fund publicly. While communication and participation are considered 'essential' in determining access to services at the clinical level, between doctors and their patients,[52] they are virtually non-existent between the state and its citizens in determining the same issues at the policy level.[53] As one participant in the consultation process told the Romanow Commission, '[O]ur system lacks communication, lacks clear accountability.'[54]

Questions that need to be addressed include the following: Given the historical and political complexities inherent in Medicare, could (and should) the public be involved? What role could public values have in determining which health care services are publicly funded and which are left to the private sector? What, in particular, is the role of legal institutions (for example, national legislation enshrining rights to health care) in shaping and reinforcing values? Also, as we try to move beyond care that we have been conditioned to accept in the past and the predominance of physicians and hospitals in our health care system, how do we address the fact that we value this kind of care even though there may be no evidence that much of it is effective? There are already entrenched expectations and public values; we do not have a clean slate on which to work. Values are not developed in a vacuum, but are shaped by existing institutions.

The Role of Law and Legal Institutions

Law and legal institutions can be both barriers and facilitators to an equitable and efficient health care system. For example, in Canada, the *Canada Health Act* gives primacy to hospital and physician services. Although the CHA has protected Canadians well through the years, it has skewed public resources towards hospital and physician services rather than community care, home care, public health, preventive care, drugs, and new technologies. Thus, while law can be a powerful force, entrenching values and protecting entitlements, it can also result in inflexibility and present barriers to reform if it fails to keep pace with changing technology, expectations, and health care needs.[55]

Again our research to date leaves us with some questions that need to be addressed and some prescriptions for reform. With regard to the former, specifically, can legal rights be framed to ensure that they are meaningful through changing circumstances? In other words, is it possible to create robust rights that ensure equitable access to care and that keep pace with changing technology, expectations, and resources? As for prescriptions for reform, the existing legal framework is inappropriate, inaccessible, and ineffective, and changes need to be made to facilitate redress and challenge on the part of patients and citizens unsatisfied with decisions about the scope of Medicare. This is not simply because of concerns vis-à-vis fairness for individual claimants but as a check to keep the process of decision-making both rigorous and principled. Appeal mechanisms such as exist in Ontario through the Health Services Appeal and Review Board should be available in all provinces, so that patients and citizens do not have to rely on access to the general courts alone to provide a check on decision-making. Also, review should be done on a principled basis, and such principles should be articulated in provincial legislation, including analysis of relative cost-effectiveness, a commitment to funding new and relatively beneficial treatments, delisting older and less beneficial treatments, and consideration of fundamental Canadian values, such as the equality provisions of the *Charter*.

Conclusion

In this chapter we have explored in depth the processes for determining entitlements to publicly funded Medicare in Ontario. To some such a survey may be too particular to be of use in that it fails to describe in some overarching way the 'Canadian' system. We don't agree. It is necessary to both understand the national framework and local processes for decision-making as any reforms will be layered on top of existing and deep-seated dynamics. Consequently, we don't advocate any form of broad, sweeping, overarching, grand, normative prescription for change. Instead, we have made some very specific recommendations for reform, relating to improving the appeal process, making more transparent the principles on which determinations are made to list and delist, and seeking solutions to unbuckling physician remuneration from questions of entitlement. Setting entitlements and determining priorities will always be messy and difficult, and the whole process is complicated by the expectations and interests of the various players and interest groups that cumulatively comprise Medicare. Policymakers must work through, incrementally, every stage in the decision-making process and where possible improve the legitimacy and fairness of that process.

NOTES

This is a revised version of Working Paper No. 5 of the CHSRF-OMHLTC Research Project 'Defining the Medicare Basket' (RC2-0861-06) available online at http://www.law.utoronto.ca/healthlaw/basket/index.html. We would like to thank our research associates Mona Awad, Caroline Pitfield, and the CHSRF project director, Greig Hinds, for their research and administrative assistance. Special thanks to the CHSRF and the Ontario Ministry of Health and Long-Term Care for funding our research. All errors and omissions remain our own.

1 The Fyke Commission established by Saskatchewan's NDP government; the Clair Commission established by the Parti Québécois government of Quebec; the Mazankowski Council commissioned by Alberta's Conservative government; the Standing Senate Committee on Social Affairs Science, and Technology (the Kirby Committee); and, finally, the Royal Commission on the Future of Health Care in Canada chaired by Roy Romanow, who was appointed by Jean Chrétien, then Liberal prime minister.

2 Canada, Commission on the Future of Health Care in Canada, *Building on Values: The Future of Health Care in Canada – Final Report* (Chair: Roy Romanow) (Saskatoon: Commission on the Future of Health Care in Canada, 2002) at 24–6. at 45 online: http://www.hc-sc.gc.ca/english/pdf/

romanow/pdfs/HCC_Final_Report.pdf (accessed 20 August 2005) [*Romanow Report*].

3 The International Convention on Economic, Social and Cultural Rights (ICESCR) Committee considerably developed the normative content of the right to health in Article 12 of the Convention as well as the nature of state obligations. For a discussion, see Audrey Chapman, ed., *Health Care Reform: A Human Rights Approach* (Washington: Georgetown University Press, 1994) and Brigit Toebes, *The Right to Health as a Human Right in International Law* (Antwerp: Intersentia, 1999).

4 Part I of the *Constitution Act, 1982,* being Schedule B to the *Canada Act 1982* (U.K.), 1982, c. 11.

5 For an excellent discussion see Tim Tenbensel, 'Interpreting Public Input into Priority-Setting: The Role of Mediating Institutions' (2002) 62:2 Health Policy 173–94 at 193.

6 See generally Chris Ham and Glenn Robert (eds), *Reasonable Rationing: International Experience of Priority Setting in Health Care* (Maidenhead: Open University Press, 2003). Also see Office of Medical Assistance Programs, Oregon Department of Human Services. *The Oregon Health Plan: It May Be for You* (Oregan: Oregon Department of Human Services, 2001), http://www.omap.hr.state.or.us/ohp/3256_0401.html (accessed 28 January 2002); Oregon Health Services Commission, *Oregon Health Services Commission Report: Prioritized List of Packages for OHP Standard* (Salem: Office of Oregon Health Policy and Research, 2001); Wendy Edgar, 'Rationing Health Care in New Zealand: How the Public Has a Say,' in Angela Coulter and Chris Ham, eds., *The Global Challenge of Health Care Rationing* (Buckingham and Philadelphia: Open University Press, 2000) at 175–91; Ministry of Health, Welfare and Sport, *Health Care, Health Policies and Health Care Reforms in the Netherlands,* review paper by Kieke Okma (The Hague: Ministry of Health Welfare and Sport, 2001); and Raisa Deber, 'Discussion Paper 17: Delivering Health Care Services: Public, Not-for-profit, or Private?' submission to Canada, Commission on the Future of Health Care in Canada.

7 R.S.C. 1985, c. C-6.

8 For a discussion of the specific features of the Canadian system relative to other health care systems, see Carolyn Tuohy, Colleen M. Flood, and Mark Stabile, 'How Does Private Finance Affect Public Health Care Systems? Marshalling the Evidence from OECD Nations' (2004) 29:3 J. of Health Politics, Policy and Law 359.

9 Carolyn H. Tuohy, *Accidental Logics: The Dynamics of Change in the Health Care Arena in the United States, Britain, and Canada* (New York: Oxford University Press, 1999).

10 Pursuant to section 3 of the *Health Care Accessibility Act*, R.S.O. 1990, c. H.3, the MOHLTC may enter into agreements with the OMA 'to provide for methods of negotiating and determining the amounts payable under the [Ontario Health Insurance] Plan in respect of the rendering of insured services to insured persons.'

11 See Cathy Charles *et al.*, 'Medical Necessity in Canadian Heath Policy: Four Meanings and ... a Funeral?' (1997) 75:3 Milbank Quarterly 365, and Colleen Flood and Sujit Choudhry, 'Strengthening the Foundations: Modernizing the Canada Health Act,' in Tom McIntosh, Pierre-Gerlier Forest, and Gregory Marchildon, eds, *The Governance of Health Care in Canada, vol. 3 of Selected Papers from the Commission on the Future of Health Care in Canada* (Toronto: University of Toronto Press, 2004) 346.

12 OMA-MOHLTC Comprehensive Agreement 1997–2000 (December 1996), http://www.oma.org/member/negotiat/agreemnt/agree.htm (accessed 2 March 2004) [1997 Agreement].

13 OMA-MOHLTC 2000–4 Agreement, online at http://www.srpc.ca/librarydocs/ omaagrmt.htm (accessed 2 March 2004) [2000 Agreement].

14 Pursuant to the 1997 agreement the MOHLTC and the OMA agreed to various initiatives designed to lessen the impact of utilization growth including an annual cap of 1.5% on increases in funding for medical services. The revised 2000 Agreement provided for a 1.95% increase in all fees listed in the schedule of benefits effective April 2000. For each of the remaining three years of the agreement, the PSC could recommend either an across-the-board increase of 2% in all fees, or it could target certain services for larger increases (and maintain the status quo or even decrease fees for other services) within a general cap of 2% for total funding of the listed services on the Schedule of Benefits (with increases being effective on April 1 of each year). 1997 Agreement, *supra* n. 12; 2000 Agreement, *supra* n. 13.

15 Rudolph Klein, 'Puzzling Out Priorities' (1998) 317 Brit. Med. J. 959–60 (10 October).

16 These were 12.39 million people in Ontario as at July 2004 – http://www.gov.on.ca/FIN/english/demographics/demog04e.pdf (accessed 2 March 2004).

17 For more detail on the PSC see Colleen M. Flood and Joanna Erdman, 'The Boundaries of Medicare: The Role of Ontario's Physician Services Review Committee' CHSRF-OMHLTC Research Project 'Defining the Medicare Basket' (RC2-0861-06), Working Paper No. 2, and Tom Archibald and Colleen M. Flood, 'The Physician Services Committee: The Relationship between the Ontario Medical Association and the Ontario Ministry of

Health and Long-Term Care,' CHSRF-OMHLTC Research Project 'Defining the Medicare Basket' (RC2-0861-06), Working Paper No. 3, http://
www.law.utoronto.ca/healthlaw/basket/index.html.

18 There is, however, some evidence that even in the arena of drug assess-
ment that cost-effectiveness analysis is not consistently used. Rather
evidence of clinical efficacy is what primarily drives decision-making.
See A.M. PaussJensen, Peter A. Singer, and Alan S. Detsky, 'How
Ontario's Formulary Committee Makes Recommendations' (2003) 21:4
Pharmacoeconomics 285–94.

19 *Shulman v. College of Audiologists and Speech-Language Pathologists of Ontario,*
[2001] O.J. No. 5057

20 R.S.O. 1990, c. F.31.

21 Its predecessor was the Federal–Provincial/Territorial Coordinating
Committee on Reciprocal Billing.

22 The Director of Access to Information at Health Canada has advised that
although there are relevant documents, they will likely not be released to
us as they fall within the exemption of information obtained 'in confidence' from other governments, the disclosure of which could be 'injuri-
ous to federal-provincial consultations' (ss. 13 and 14).

23 For an in-depth discussion, see Mona Awad, Julia Abelson, and Colleen
Flood, 'The Boundaries of Canadian Medicare: The Role of Medical Direc-
tors and Public Participation in Decision Making,' CHSRF-OMHLTC
Research Project 'Defining the Medicare Basket' (RC2-0861-06), Working
Paper No. 4, http://www.law.utoronto.ca/healthlaw/basket/index.html.

24 Vanessa Lu, 'More Cuts Coming to Medical Procedures,' *Toronto Star,*
2 February 2002, at H4.

25 For discussion about how setting substantial limits on Medicare's benefit
package could actually increase costs because legislators and health
ministers are placed in the position of confronting public pressures, see
Jonathon Oberlander, Theodore Marmor, and Lawrence Jacobs, 'Rationing
Medical Care: Rhetoric and Reality in the Oregon Health Plan' (2001)
164:11 Can. Med. Assoc. J. 1583.

26 Norman Daniels and James Sabin, 'The Ethics of Accountability in Managed Care Reform' (1998) 17:5 Health Affairs 50–64 at 57.

27 *Ibid.* at 57.

28 *Ombudsman Act*, R.S.O. 1990, c. O.6 defines the role of the Ombudsman,
who investigates complaints about any governmental organization's
decisions, recommendations, acts, or omissions. The ombudsman's
website specifically mentions jurisdiction over complaints on health
insurance (OHIP) issues and patient care in psychiatric hospitals.

29 See section 'What Does the Ombudsman Do?' on the Ombudsman's
    website, http://www.ombudsman.on.ca/examples.asp#cantdo (accessed
    2 March 2004).
30 *An Act Respecting the Health and Social Services Ombudsman* R.S.Q.,
    ch. P-31.1.
31 *Loi sur la justice administrative*, L.R.Q. c. J-3, s. 14 and the following.
32 *Ministry of Health Appeal and Review Boards Act*, 1998 S.O. 1998, c. 18,
    Sched. H.
33 *Ibid.*, s. 7(1).
34 R.S.O. 1990, c. H.6.
35 R.R.O. 1990, Reg. 552.
36 *Ibid.*, s. 28.4(2).
37 *Ibid.*, s. 28.4(5).
38 *Ibid.*, ss. 28.4(2), (5); emphasis added.
39 Donna Greschner, 'How Will the Charter of Rights and Freedoms and
    Evolving Jurisprudence Affect Health Care Costs?' in Tom McIntosh *et al.*,
    eds., *Romanow Papers, supra* note 11 at 25.
40 [1999] Q.J. No. 2724 (QL).
41 [2001] O.J. No. 5057 (Sup. Ct.) (QL).
42 One exception involves a lower-court decision around the right of women
    to access abortion services. In *Doe et al. v. The Government of Manitoba*,
    [2004] MBQB 285, the Court of Queen's Bench found that there had been a
    s. 7 breach as a result of the government's failure to publicly fund abortion
    services at a private clinic, forcing women to wait for much longer periods
    for treatment in a publicly funded hospital. Justice Oliphant notes (at 78)
    'In my view, legislation that forces women to have to stand in line in an
    overburdened publicly-funded health care system and to have to wait for
    a therapeutic abortion, a procedure that provably must be performed in a
    timely manner, is a gross violation of the right of women to both liberty
    and security of the person as guaranteed by s. 7 of the Charter.'
43 *Chaoulli v. Québec (Attorney General)*, [2005] S.C.C. 35. A copy of the judg-
    ment of the trial judge, the Court of Appeal, and the Supreme Court and
    copies of the briefs and related materials are available at http://www
    .utoronto.ca/healthlaw (accessed 20 August 2005). See also Collen M.
    Flood, Kent Roach, and Lorne Sossin, *Access to Care, Access to Justice : The
    Legal Debate over Private Health Insurance in Canada* (Toronto: University of
    Toronto Press, 2005).
44 Cases have included challenges to restrictions on funding for translation
    services for the deaf, anti-retroviral drugs, funding for in vitro fertilization
    services, and funding for autistic treatments.

45 Greschner, *supra* note 39.

46 [1997] 3 S.C.R. 624.

47 *Auton (Guardian ad litem of) v. British Columbia (Attorney General)*, [2004] 3 S.C.R. 657.

48 See Greg Stoddart *et al., Why Not User Charges? The Real Issues: A Discussion Paper* (Toronto: Premier's Council on Health, Well-being and Social Justice, 1993) at 7

49 David Cutler, *Your Money or Your Life* (New York: Oxford University Press, 2004).

50 For a discussion, see John M. Eisenberg, 'Globalize the Evidence, Localize the Decision: Evidence-based Medicine and International Diversity' (2002) 21:3 Health Affairs 166.

51 *Romanow Report* note 2.

52 As LaForest J. commented in *Eldridge v. British Columbia (A.G.)*, the fact that 'adequate communication is essential to proper medical care is surely so incontrovertible that the Court could, if necessary, take judicial notice of it' ([1997] 3 S.C.R 624 at para. 70).

53 We are grateful to Caroline Pitfield for making this point.

54 *Romanow Report, supra* note 2 at 63.

55 Flood and Choudhry, *supra* note 11.

2 *Charter* Challenges and Evidence-Based Decision-Making in the Health Care System: Towards a Symbiotic Relationship

DONNA GRESCHNER

The health care system has become increasingly subject to judicial scrutiny, as patients and providers bring court challenges under the *Canadian Charter of Rights and Freedoms*.[1] At the same time, health care providers and policy-makers have devoted increasing attention to developing and implementing evidence-based decision-making (EBDM).[2] However, legal actions have given little, if any, explicit consideration to the objectives and methods of EBDM. This chapter hopes to bridge that gap. With a view to improving the health care system overall, it seeks to encourage cross-disciplinary discussions about EBDM and the *Charter* among lawyers, judges, doctors, and health policy experts. Turning first to law, the second part of the chapter briefly summarizes *Charter* challenges to health care policies and notes several difficulties with judicial review. Turning next to health care, the third part briefly describes EBDM, both with respect to clinical decisions and broader policy questions. The last section then begins the cross-disciplinary discussion by arguing that when courts adjudicate *Charter*-based claims about health care policies, they ought to adopt approaches that will encourage EBDM throughout the health care system. Since EBDM promotes sound health care practices, judicial encouragement of EBDM would improve the system overall, as well as strengthen patients' *Charter* rights.

The *Charter* and Health Care Policies

The *Charter of Rights and Freedoms* requires all governmental decisions to comply with its constitutional standards. The health care system, which is described in chapter 1 and elsewhere in this volume, is no exception. The *Charter* covers diverse health care matters from the involuntary treatment of persons with mental illnesses to employment relationships between governments and health care workers.[3] During its first twenty years, from 1982 to 2002, there were approximately fifty constitutional challenges to governmental health care policies. In about one-third of the actions, plaintiffs were successful, with courts ordering governments to change health care policies in conformity with *Charter* rights or preventing them from implementing reform proposals.[4] With respect to the Medicare system, challenges have fallen into two broad and related categories: (1) structure of payment and delivery of health care and (2) scope of coverage with respect to insured services.[5]

The first category involves challenges to Medicare's framework, delivery system, and fundamental principles. The cases range from successful litigation initiated by physicians to prevent provincial governments from changing their remuneration to unsuccessful attempts by community groups to stop hospital closures. In aid of their claims, plaintiffs have called upon numerous *Charter* rights, including mobility rights in section 6, equality rights in section 15, and most frequently perhaps, section 7's rights of liberty and security of the person.[6]

The second category seeks to add services to the list of those that are publicly insured through the Medicare program. In these actions, plaintiffs do not usually question one of Medicare's basic planks. Rather, they want Medicare's umbrella expanded to cover more services. The actions always engage section 15's equality rights because patients argue, in essence, that they are not receiving a benefit (that is, public funding of a desired medical service) that they say the government gives to other people.[7]

In 2004 the Supreme Court of Canada heard appeals in two cases about health care policies. *Chaoulli* v *Quebec*[8] falls squarely within the first category because the plaintiffs argue that the Quebec ban on private insurance for Medicare services – a fundamental feature of the provincial insurance scheme – violates their section 7 rights to liberty and security of the person. To put the issue in terms of the public/ private division in health care financing, the plaintiffs want the publicly financed side of Medicare to lose its state-mandated monopoly status, thereby permitting private financing for the same service (see Martha Jackman's contribution in this volume for an analysis of the critical issues in the *Chaoulli* appeal). The second case, *Auton v. British Columbia*,[9] is from the second category, 'scope of funding,' because it sought expansion of the Medicare umbrella. Parents of children with autism argued that the British Columbian government violated their children's right to equal benefit of the law by denying Medicare funding for a specific behavioural therapy. They wanted the therapy to be declared a health care service, which would have moved the service from the privately financed side of health care to the publicly financed side.[10] The claimants were successful in the lower courts,[11] but not in the Supreme Court of Canada. In November 2004 the Court released a unanimous judgment that the government's failure to fund behavioural therapy did not violate section 15.[12]

Both types of challenges are difficult, and judicial review poses both positive and negative risks for the health care system's efficiency and fairness. The health care system is fiendishly complex. Court actions will involve medical, scientific, and economic evidence, and judges are not usually doctors, scientists, or economists. Health care policy decisions are polycentric: changing one aspect in one corner of the system sends ripples in all directions. Moreover, many plaintiffs will evoke instant sympathy because of their illnesses and need for treatments; sometimes they are children, whose situations will seem especially tragic. To complicate matters further, courts have telescopic vision. Of necessity they focus on the case before them, but that focus magnifies the case's features and blocks out almost everything else, which is a troublesome perspective for scrutinizing a system with interlocking parts.[13] These factors and others present the danger that judicial review will tilt the health care system even more towards persons with resources, in this instance those patients with the economic and social resources to initiate legal action.[14] In Professor Jackman's apt phrase, courts may misdiagnose rather than cure.

Until the decision of the Supreme Court in *Chaoulli v. Quebec*,[15] one could happily report that the courts had been generally sensitive to the polycentrism of health care policies, and had given governments a wide margin of appreciation in health policies.[16] Courts had recognized that Medicare's principles already exemplified *Charter* values, as the Quebec courts did in *Chaoulli* litigation.[17] The *Auton* judgments in the British Columbia courts, which dispensed a highly interventionist order without cogent evidence or consideration of its impact on the system, were more of an exception than a rule.[18] The trend of cautious engagement with health care policies seemed to receive the Supreme Court's seal of approval in its *Auton* judgment. Then into the mix came the Court's ruling in *Chaoulli*. Time and space preclude dissection of the majority opinion's deployment of evidence; suffice it to say that the majority opinion has made judicial appreciation of evidence-based decision-making more urgent.

Evidence-Based Decision-Making and the Health Care System

EBDM began with evidence-based medicine, which has been influentially defined as follows: '[T]he conscientious, explicit, and judicious use of current best evidence in making decisions about the care of individual patients. [It] means integrating individual clinical expertise with the best available external clinical evidence from systematic research.'[19] It now encompasses evidence-based health care, which aspires to extend the principles of evidence-based medicine to every corner of the health care system, including management, purchasing, and professional regulation.[20] EBDM, with origins that are significantly Canadian,[21] is altering fundamentally the practice and delivery of health care. In Canada and around the world, EBDM now has its own journals, research centres, educational curricula, and other indicia and levers of influence. For instance, in the past ten years, its literature has grown exponentially, 'from 1 MEDLINE citation in 1992 to more than 13000 in 2004.'[22] Obviously, one short chapter cannot do justice to the shifts occasioned by EBDM. Here is a sketch.

Within every branch of EBDM, decision-makers find, appraise, and incorporate evidence about relevant issues into their decision-making processes. In the context of treating an individual patient, EBDM requires a health care provider to locate evidence about different treatments for the patient's condition and apply the one supported by the best evidence about effectiveness. With health policy, the process is similar. A decision-maker examines the research (the evidence) about different strategies for achieving a particular policy goal.[23] In large part EBDM relies upon computerized databases and online publication of research that put the latest and best research on everyone's computer screens. In practising EBDM, decision-makers need skills in designing search techniques and in retrieving appropriate information from the enormous amount of data that are increasingly inexpensively and readily available. To describe the process pithily, EBDM sees medical problems as research questions.

What counts as evidence is the critical question, of course. Health care knowledge is socially constructed in the same multifarious way that all scientific information is, and it is subject to the same well-known critiques and concerns. Accordingly, in searching for the best evidence, EBDM uses levels of evidence.[24] With respect to clinical decisions, at the top of the evidence hierarchy is systematic reviews with homogeneity,[25] in which a large number of high quality,[26] randomized controlled trials (RCTs) are analysed for their findings about the effects of particular treatments. These studies, according to the Oxford Centre for Evidence-Based Medicine, give the least-biased estimate of the effects of an intervention, and thus have the greatest reliability. If this evidence is not available, decision-makers turn to the next most reliable type, which is systemic reviews with heterogeneity. As decision-makers move down the evidence hierarchy, they find evidence with decreasing reliability, that is, increasing distortions of results: individual, high quality RCTs; individual lower quality RCTs; cohort studies;[27] case-series;[28] and, at the bottom, expert opinion by itself. The bottom rung is defined, in the words of the Oxford Centre, as 'expert opinion, without explicit critical appraisal, or based on physiology, bench research, or "first principles."'[29]

The placing of unadorned expert opinion at the bottom of the EBDM hierarchy illustrates rather neatly how evidence-based medicine portends a shift in clinical practice. Seniority and authority are no longer, by themselves, superior hallmarks of good judgment. The most reliable sources of advice about the best treatment are results of well-designed clinical studies, rather than the expert's personal experiences with patients. Or, to put the matter another way, if the expert authority's opinion differs from the findings of well-designed research studies, the latter trumps the former.[30] The shift in philosophy and practice is pointedly asserted in the title of a recent, related article: 'Statistics, Not Experts.'[31]

EBDM has many benefits for both health care providers[32] and patients. From the patients' perspective, perhaps the most important benefit is improving outcomes, which is, indeed, the overriding objective of health care generally. Patients are more likely to receive treatments that ameliorate or cure their conditions and avoid interventions that cause harm. Physicians practising EBMD are advising patients on the best treatments currently known to medical science. As one consequence, they give patients more accurate and up-to-date information about treatment options. Because EBDM improves the quality and accuracy of information, which is the basis of informed consent, it also enhances patient autonomy.[33]

Implementing EBDM, however, is not without its problems and detractors.[34] Unfortunately, but not unexpectedly, reliable evidence is not always available for clinical decisions. Doctors who want to practise EBDM exclusively will be unable to do so, especially since many treatments have not received empirical study, let alone been the subject of RCTs. EBDM also takes time and money to practise, although computerized databases are becoming increasingly inexpensive or even free, and the time invested is shortened by practice and the availability of evidence-based clinical guidelines. In the medical literature these criticisms and other concerns have received considerable attention.[35]

EBDM meets even greater challenges when it moves outside the realm of clinical practices that focus on individual treatment. In many areas of population health policies, for instance, evidence is highly complex, uncertain, and variable.[36] Evidence gathered for clinical practice guidelines, which focus on the benefits of interventions aimed at *individuals*, may not assist in designing policies to improve the health of *populations* or reduce health inequalities among *communities*.[37] Little good evidence may be available about the validity of assumptions that guide specific public health policies.[38] Different sorts of evidence, such as socioeconomic data, may assume critical relevance. While socioeconomic data are not foreign to clinical practice guidelines, and indeed often must be incorporated into guidelines for particular medical conditions,[39] in public health policy decisions they are usually essential. Moreover, such evidence may reasonably generate diverse and hotly contested interpretations. One consequence of these factors is that the hierarchy of evidence may look different when assessing population health strategies. Thus, it is not surprising that in many corners of governmental policies EBDM has a spotty record of influence. Too often, policy decisions remain opaque, ad hoc, or apparently without scientific foundation,[40] leading a former Minister of Health to wonder if Canada has a health care 'system' at all.[41]

The good news is that several recent reports on health care reform have stressed the importance of EBDM throughout the health care system. In line with the Romanow Report's recommendations, governments have established the Health Council of Canada with a mandate to facilitate systemic changes in the health care system. The Canadian Institutes for Health Research actively promote sound research on a comprehensive range of health care issues. Provinces have created agencies to promote EBDM, such as the Saskatchewan Health Quality Council. Undeniably, a major impetus for these initiatives is the prospect of cost-efficiencies. The health care budget, although very generous, is not unlimited. Decision-making processes must consider not only the effectiveness of a particular policy (that is, does it produce its intended consequences?) but also the resources required to achieve the desired outcomes. Cost-benefit analysis is often politically charged, rendering its incorporation within EBDM additionally problematic.[42] Nevertheless, agencies and governments hope that EBDM will cull outdated or dubious therapies, and manage service delivery and public health programs more efficiently.[43]

Many areas of health policy are good candidates for applying the techniques of EBDM, and progress is apparent. In this category are health policies that focus on treatments for individual patients, since these policies are generalizations about individualized treatment decisions. One such area in which governments already widely practice EBDM is drug formularies. In deciding which drugs to include in their formularies, provincial pharmacare programs use scientific review committees that assess and compare drugs. EBDM helps draw the line between the drug prescriptions that receive public funding and those that will remain privately financed by patients. As well, EBDM has taken hold with cancer therapy protocols, which are often strongly science-based and subject to continuous evaluation and revision in light of current research. Moreover, EBDM is helpful in other areas, such as management practices with respect to administering hospital and provider services. For instance, Ontario developed the world's first evidence-based queuing guidelines and registry for patients waiting for open-heart surgery. Variations of its model have been adopted nationally and internationally.[44]

Within governmental decision-making, an obvious candidate for EBDM is the topic of this book and the conference that gave rise to it, namely, the question of which health care services should be within the Medicare basket. Here, just as in its pharmacare programs, the government is deciding which health care treatments it will fund and which ones it will leave to private resources. In these determinations, clinical practice guidelines developed by evidence-based medicine should play a significant role. For instance, if systematic reviews of treatments for diabetes conclude that a particular treatment has little effectiveness, the government would have a compelling argument for not funding that treatment. To date, decisions about the scope of insured services are mostly a matter of negotiation between provincial governments and doctors' professional associations, a process ripe for political trade-offs and other non-medical influences.[45] The initiatives mentioned in the preceding paragraph, such as the Canadian Institutes for Health Research, may assist in encouraging EBDM. So, too, would the recommendation of Flood, Stabile, and Tuohy in Chapter 1 of in this volume to unbuckle physician remuneration from questions of entitlement.

Charter Adjudication and Promoting EBDM

From a health care policy perspective, implementing EBDM broadly should be an uncontroversial goal because of its superiority to other methods of decision-making. For, when governments make health care decisions, what are the alternatives to using the best available evidence? Consider this book's topic, namely, decisions about what services to insure in the Medicare program. Instead of scientific evidence, should funding decisions be made on the basis of political power? This method of allocating resources may quickly become the 'squeaky wheel,' the 'big stick,' or the 'secret trade-off' method, with the obvious negative effects that these labels imply. What about prejudice, that is, making decisions based on stereotypes about groups or animosity towards them? Using that ground is clearly inconsistent with both sound medical judgment and constitutional values, as Lisa Forman's chapter in this volume clearly illustrates in her discussion about access to essential HIV/AIDS medicine in South Africa. Another criterion for decisions is tradition ('that's the way we've always done it') but it does not promote innovation, to say the least, and only haphazardly promotes the goal of equality in health care; indeed, this justification is more likely to entrench inequitable practices more deeply. Another ground is expertise, but as noted above, expertise by itself, without testing, is subject to similar flaws as other methods. In sum, the alternatives do not seem particularly attractive.

When we turn to the courts and *Charter* challenges to health care policies, the goal of encouraging EBDM continues to appear meritorious. EBDM is a structured method of decision-making and for that reason alone may be more likely to foster the *Charter* values of equality and non-discrimination than other decision-making methods. To bolster this claim, one can rely on lessons from other human rights areas. Human rights experience has taught that developing and following fair and general rules for decision-making are important safeguards against unacceptable discrimination. For instance, when an organization develops non-discriminatory employment policies, it increases the likelihood that its workforce will represent the labour market with respect to gender, ethnic origin, age, and other traits. If an organization does not establish objective employment policies, it will contain many more avenues for irrationality and bias; for instance, managers will have an easier time hiring their family members (nepotism) or acting on old-fashioned stereotypes about gender roles (sexism), or using other questionable factors. In the health care system, EBDM serves a similar function. It requires decision-makers to examine the best evidence available before making a decision, in much the same way as human rights laws tell employers to consider demographic, sociological, and testing evidence before deciding employment practices. Just as EBDM can show that an old saw of medical practice lacks scientific foundation,[46] it can reveal biases built into previously unquestioned assumptions and unexamined policies, and also correct and contextualize popular beliefs about health care treatments. Generally, EBDM can act as a bulwark against decisions that are unduly influenced by extraneous factors (such as political pressures, including interest group lobbying), which detract from the fairness and equity of a health care system. Fairness and equity are of especial importance for a health care system that delivers its services to people with illness and disability, a protected group under section 15 of the *Charter*.

Of course, EBDM does not guarantee *Charter* values such as equality. As noted earlier, EBDM is not impervious to the tilts and skews embedded in any social practice. The 'evidence' in evidence-based decision-making can be collected or interpreted in unfair or biased ways. And if the evidence is biased, so, too, will be the policy or guideline. But implementing EBDM does increase the likelihood of fair results. For one thing, because the hierarchy of evidence places systematic reviews, which combine the results of many high-quality studies, at its apex, the influence of inequitable or biased results is diminished. EBDM's methods will expose superstitions that masquerade as science, such as the AIDS denialist theories described in Lisa Forman's chapter.

In its *Auton* judgment, the Supreme Court of Canada applied its standard section 15 analysis and, in doing so, furthered the methods and values of EBDM. As noted above, parents claimed that the British Columbia government violated their children's rights to equal benefit of the law by denying Medicare funding for Lovas treatment, a form of intensive behavioural therapy for children with autism. The Court's decision has two major components. First, it held that the benefit sought by the claimants did not come within section 15's ambit. In examining the federal and provincial statutes that establish Medicare, the Court emphasized that the laws distinguish between core services (medically necessary services provided in hospitals or by physicians) and non-core services. The benefit at issue in the litigation – funding for intensive behavioural therapy – was not a core service. Rather, it was a non-core service that provinces could fund at their discretion by designating its providers as health care professionals. Since the government had exercised its discretion not to designate intensive behavioural therapists as health care professionals, the treatment offered by these therapists was not a benefit provided *by law*.[47] Accordingly, the claim did not fall within section 15. The Court did not need to say more, as this ruling disposed of the legal action. However, because the case was the first one of this kind to reach it, the Court went on to consider whether the claimants would have succeeded if they had established that behavioural therapy was a benefit provided by law.

In the second major part of its analysis, the Court pointed out that claimants in section 15 actions always have to show that they are denied a benefit that an appropriate comparator group is receiving. Selecting the appropriate comparator group is invariably the critical question, and a legal question that the Court decides. In this case, the claimants were seeking funding for a non-core therapy that was emergent and only just becoming recognized as medically necessary. In the Court's view, it would be inapt to compare funding for an experimental non-core therapy to funding for well-established non-core therapies. Rather, the appropriate comparator group would be a group receiving benefits of the same type, in this case, emerging non-core therapies. Since the claimants had not adduced any evidence that another group was receiving emergent, non-core therapies as part of Medicare's funding scheme, a finding of discrimination could not be sustained.[48]

The Court can be applauded for its careful and adept handling of the issues. In the first part, it grappled expertly with the interlocking federal and provincial laws that together comprise the Canada's Medicare system.[49] In the second part, its analysis of comparator groups showed sensitivity to the dynamic nature of health treatments and the role of evidence in evaluating and implementing them. The Court recognized that until sufficient evidence is available about emergent treatments, governments can be cautious about funding them. In the Court's words, '[F]unding may be legitimately denied or delayed because of uncertainty about a program and administrative difficulties related to its recognition and implementation.'[50] While plaintiffs may be disappointed in not receiving funding for emergent treatment, this cautious approach has considerable merit, and not only because continued testing and experimentation may uncover dangers with experimental therapies. Every patient has an interest in a safe and sustainable health care system, and few policies are more likely to bankrupt a system than quick funding of every new treatment.

In future cases when claimants can adduce evidence of how a province has responded to requests for therapies or treatments by other patients in the appropriate comparator group, what will the claimants need to show? To begin, EBDM tells us that governments can refuse to fund treatments for which there is no good evidence of effectiveness. An obvious example is laetrile treatment for cancer patients, which has no proven effectiveness at all, no matter what its fans have loudly proclaimed. Accordingly, claimants must first adduce evidence that the treatment in question treats their condition effectively. EBDM tells us that a claimant's subjective assessment of benefit is insufficient.[51] Rather, the claim will require sound scientific evidence that the non-funded treatment meets a minimum standard. Second, claimants will need to show that the appropriate comparator group has been receiving treatments with lower effectiveness rates. This step is necessary because section 15 claims involve *disparate* treatment. If patient A wants funding for treatment X, which has a 10 per cent effectiveness rate, then for the purposes of a section 15 claim she will need to show that patients B and C in the appropriate comparator group are receiving funded treatments that have 10 per cent effectiveness or less, for example, 1 per cent. If all other patients are receiving treatments with at least 20 per cent effectiveness, patient A is not prima facie suffering discrimination. EBDM provides the evidence of effectiveness. This is not a novel injection into section 15 claims; rather, it usefully contributes the means by which to refine and analyse claims of discriminatory health care funding.

The last stage in a *Charter* challenge is section 1, in which the government can attempt to justify section 15 violations as reasonable limits. EBDM may have an important role in section 1 justifications. If the government has engaged in EBDM in formulating its funding policies, it will have the evidence to demonstrate reasonable limits. At this stage, court decisions could encourage EBDM by requiring justifications for reasonable limits to be evidence that governmental funding decisions are the outcomes of a decision-making process for health care treatments that is relatively divorced from political pressure, stereotypes about particular conditions, and other factors that provide a breeding ground for inequities.[52] In *Auton*, the Supreme Court did not need to deal with any section 1 issues, and an explication of incorporating EBDM into section 1 analysis awaits another day.

Conclusion

This chapter described EBDM and suggested that courts should promote EBDM when they hear *Charter* challenges. Deciding where to draw the line between public and private funding for health treatments often involves tragic choices, and in making those choices the *Charter* rights of patients must be respected. EBDM has the potential of creating a health care system that delivers not only excellent health care, but also greater patient equality and autonomy. Accordingly, judicial review of health care decisions should use standards that promote EBDM. Clearly, much more needs to be said about the relationship between court actions and the health care system, but these comments may assist in the conversation among lawyers and health care providers. From the foregoing, it is fair to conclude that detractors of EBDM bear the burden of showing that another method of making health care decisions will better promote *Charter* values.

NOTES

1 *Canadian Charter of Rights and Freedoms*, Part I of the *Constitution Act, 1982*, being Schedule B to the *Canada Act, 1982* (U.K.), 1982, c.11 [*Charter*].
2 For a description of EBDM, see Part 3 in this volume.
3 For a description of various *Charter* actions, see Donna Greschner, 'How Will the Charter of Rights and Freedoms and Evolving Jurisprudence Affect Health Care Costs?' in Tom McIntosh *et al.*, eds., *Romanow Papers*, Vol. 3, *The Governance of Health Care in Canada* (Toronto: University of Toronto Press, 2004) at 84–7.
4 *Ibid.* at 87–90
5 Barbara von Tigerstrom, 'Human Rights and Health Care Reform: A Canadian Perspective,' in Timothy Caulfield and Barbara von Tigerstrom, eds., *Health Care Reform and the Law in Canada: Meeting the Challenge* (Edmonton: University of Alberta Press, 2002) 157.
6 For an overview of these actions from 1982 to 2002, see Greschner, *supra* note 3 at 111–21.
7 *Ibid.* at 90–3.
8 [2002] C.S.C.R. No. 280 (QL), on appeal from [2002] R.J.Q. 1205 (C.A.) (QL).

9 *Auton (Guardian ad litem of) v. British Columbia (Attorney General)*, [2004] 3 S.C.R. 657.

10 The claim in *Auton* shows also that the distinction between the two categories is not stark. *Auton* was a scope-of-funding case because the plaintiffs wanted public funding of behavioural therapy as part of Medicare funding. At the same time, the lawsuit challenged a basic plank of Medicare, namely, the restriction of core services (those funded under the *Canada Health Act*) to hospital and physician services. Since the requested treatment is offered by behavioural therapists outside of hospitals, a court order requiring governments to fund it would have altered significantly Medicare's boundaries.

11 [2000] BCCA 538, affirming [2000] BCSC 1142, with supplementary reasons [2001] BCSC 220. For an extended critique of the lower court judgments in *Auton*, see Donna Greschner and Steven Lewis, 'Auton and Evidence-Based Decision-Making: Medicare in the Courts' (2003) 82 Can. Bar Rev. 501.

12 *Supra* note 9.

13 See generally, Christopher Manfredi and Antonia Maioni, 'Courts and Health Policy: Judicial Policy Making and Publicly Funded Health Care in Canada' (2002) 27 J. of Health Pol. 213; Greschner and Lewis, *supra* note 11.

14 Consider, e.g., the plight of many children with fetal alcohol syndrome, who do not have parents arguing on their behalf for treatment, or initiating legal action to obtain it.

15 *Chaoulli v. Quebec (Attorney General)*, [2005] S.C.C. 35 (Q.L.).

16 For an overview of the cases from 1982 to 2002, see Greschner, *supra* note 3 at 98–101.

17 *Chaoulli c. Québec*, [2000] J.Q. No. 479 (C.Q) (QL); aff'd. [2002] R. J.Q. 1205 (C.A.) (QL). Reversed *Chaoulli v. Quebec (Attorney General)*, [2005] S.C.C. 35 (Q.L.).

18 See Greschner and Lewis, *supra* note 11.

19 David Sackett *et al.*, 'Evidence-Based Medicine: What It Is and what It Isn't' (1996) 312 Brit. Med. J. 71. See also the influential work of the Health Information Research Unit at McMaster University, which defines evidence-based medicine as 'an approach to health care that promotes the collection, interpretation, and integration of valid, important and applicable patient-reported, clinician-observed, and research-derived evidence. The best available evidence, moderated by patient circumstances and preferences, is applied to improve the quality of clinical judgments.' K. Ann McKibbon *et al.*, *The Medical Literature as a Resource for Evidence Based*

Care, working paper from the Health Information Research Unit, McMaster University, Hamilton, Ontario, 1995, http://hiru.mcmaster.ca/hiru/ medline/asis-pap.htm (accessed 20 March 2004).

20 See the definition of evidence-based health care in Oxford Centre for Evidence-Based Medicine, 'Evidence-Based Medicine Glossary,' http:// www.cebm.net/glossary.asp (accessed 20 March 2004). See also Mark Dobrow, Vivek Goel, and R.E.G. Upshur, 'Evidence-based Health Policy: Context and Utilisation' (2004) 58 Social Science and Medicine 207–217; J.A. Muir Gray, *Evidence-Based Healthcare,* 2nd ed. (City: Churchill Livingstone, 2001).

21 The coining of the phrase has been attributed to McMaster University Medical School, which created the label for its clinical learning strategy. See William Rosenberg and Anna Donald, 'Evidence-Based Medicine: an Approach to Clinical Problem-solving' (1995) 310 Brit. Med. J. 1122.

22 Sharon Straus, 'What's the E for EBM?' (2004) 328 Brit. Med. J. 535.

23 See David Naylor, 'Evidence-Based Health Care: A Reality Check,' the Second Annual Amyot Lecture at Health Canada, 2000, http://www .hc-sc.gc.ca/english/for_you/hpo/amyot/amyot2000.htm (accessed 15 January 2005).

24 See Oxford Centre for Evidence-Based Medicine, 'Levels of Evidence and Grades of Recommendation,' http://www.cebm.net/levels_of_evidence .asp (accessed 15 January 2005) ['Levels of Evidence']; and 'Frequently Asked Questions on Levels of Evidence,' http://www .cebm.net/levels_ faq.asp (accessed 15 January 2005).

25 'Levels of Evidence': 'By homogeneity we mean a systematic review that is free of worrisome variations (heterogeneity) in the directions and degrees of results between individual studies.'

26 RCTs with the following characteristics are high quality: randomized with concealment, double-blinded, complete follow-up, and intention-to-treat analysis.

27 Cohort studies identify two groups (cohorts) of patients, one of which receives the specified treatment and the other which does not, and records the outcomes for both groups.

28 A case series reports on a number of patients with a particular condition or outcome, without any involvement of a control group. Even less reliability is assigned to single case reports, but while they are the weakest clinical evidence of causation, they are not ignored because they may alert clinicians to previously unrecognized associations.

29 'Frequently Asked Questions on Levels of Evidence,' *supra* note 24: 'We mean the pathophysiological principles used to determine clinical prac-

tice.' First principles that are not proven by clinical trials may be disastrously wrong. For examples, see Naylor, *supra* note 23.

30 Rosenberg and Donald, *supra* note 21, comment on how EBDM may shift fundamentally the dynamics of a medical team, removing hierarchical distinctions based on seniority.

31 William Meadow and Cass Sunstein, 'Statistics, Not Experts' (2001) 51 Duke L. J. 629 (in medical malpractice litigation, courts should rely on statistical data about doctors' performance, rather than expert opinion, in assessing the customary practice of doctors).

32 For a discussion of EBDM's benefits for physicians, see Rosenberg and Donald, *supra* note 21.

33 A. Schattner and R.H. Fletcher, 'Research Evidence and the Individual Patient' (2003) 96 Q. J. Med. 1.

34 Sharon Straus and Finlay McAlister, 'Evidence-Based Medicine: A Commentary on Common Criticisms' (2000) 163 Can. Med. Assoc. J. 837.

35 From this voluminous material, several topics will resonate with *Charter* lawyers because they raise issues of values. For instance, critics argue that EBDM is 'cook-book' medicine, ignoring the unique needs and problems of the individual patient. The supporters respond that EBDM is an essential component of patient-centered medicine. See Straus and McAlister, *ibid.*

36 Dobrow, Goel, and Upshur, *supra* note 20.

37 George Davey Smith, Shah Ebrahim, and Stephen Franket, 'How Policy Informs the Evidence' (2001) 322 Brit. Med. J. 184.

38 Sally Macintyre *et al.*, 'Using Evidence to Inform Health Policy: Case Study' (2001) 322 Brit. Med. J. 222; Steven Cummins and Sally Macintyre, '"Food Deserts" – Evidence and Assumption in Health Policy Making' (2002) 325 Brit. Med. J. 436.

39 Rosemary Aldrich *et al.*, 'Using Socioeconomic Evidence in Clinical Practice Guidelines' (2003) 327 Brit. Med. J. 1283.

40 For a more extensive description, see Greschner and Lewis, *supra* note 11 at 505–7, 527–33.

41 Alan Rock, as quoted in Naylor, *supra* note 23.

42 See the Australian study by the National Health and Medical Research Council (NHMRC), 'How to Compare the Costs and Benefits: Evaluation of the Economic Evidence' (Canberra: NHMRC, 2001), http://www.nhmrc.gov.au/publications/pdf/cp73.pdf (accessed 19 March 2004).

43 EBDM does not necessarily lead to fewer services. Naylor describes an example of EBDM where the studies led to creating more hip and knee replacement services in metropolitan Toronto.

44 See Naylor, *supra* note 23.

45 For analysis of the process and a recommendation to create a more
evidence-based process, see Colleen M. Flood and Sujit Choudhry,
'Strengthening the Foundations: Modernizing the Canada Health Act,' in
McIntosh, *supra* note 3 at 355–60.

46 See, e.g., Michelle Guppy, Sharon Mickan, and Chris Del Mar, '"Drink
Plenty of Fluids": A Systematic Review of Evidence for This Recommendation in Acute Respiratory Infections' (2004) 328 Brit. Med. J. 499.

47 *Supra* note 9 at paras. 27–47.

48 *Ibid.*, paras. 48–62.

49 The judgment also contains an appendix that succinctly describes
Medicare's funding scheme.

50 *Supra* note 9 at para. 55.

51 The basic tenet of EBDM is that subjective opinions be subject to testing
and proof. To accept subjective assessment of benefits with respect to
health treatments, without more, violates this tenet.

52 For an extended discussion, see Greschner and Lewis, *supra* note 11.

3 Misdiagnosis or Cure? *Charter* Review of the Health Care System

MARTHA JACKMAN

Following the Supreme Court of Canada's decision in *Eldridge v. British Columbia (Attorney General)*,[1] the potential application of the *Canadian Charter of Rights and Freedoms*[2] in the health context, and the role for the courts in determining the boundaries of the Canadian Medicare system have expanded significantly.[3] As Donna Greschner points out in chapter 2, the *Charter* has been invoked to challenge both the underlying principles of Medicare and the type of services that are publicly funded.[4] In the following paper I will discuss a recent case that challenges not government limits on public funding but rather the fundamental concept of one-tier Medicare: the case of *Chaoulli v. Quebec*,[5] now before the Supreme Court of Canada.[6] The appellants in the *Chaoulli* case are not arguing for higher levels of Medicare spending or for funding for particular services. Instead they allege that legislative limits on the provision of private health and hospital insurance coupled with a lack of timely access to provincially funded health care services in Quebec, violate their rights under section 7 of the *Charter*. In her decision, upheld by the Quebec Court of Appeal,[7] Quebec Superior Court Justice Ginette Piché found that section 7 of the *Charter* guarantees the right to health care, but statutory restrictions on private health insurance accord with the 'principles of fundamental justice.'[8]

Recent health care system reviews have underscored the importance that Canadians attach to Medicare as a defining social program and as a symbol of Canadian values.[9] In the Final Report of the Commission on the Future of Health Care in Canada, Commissioner Roy Romanow observed that 'Canadians consider equal and timely access to medically necessary services on the basis of need as a right of citizenship, not as a privilege of status or wealth.'[10] Notwithstanding increasing pressures placed upon it, Canadians have remained constant in their view that equality of access to health care must be preserved as a core and defining feature of the publicly funded Medicare system: 'The Canadian approach to the provision of health care services continues to receive strong and passionate support. The public does not want to see any significant changes which would alter the fundamental principles of our health care system. They have an abiding sense of the values of fairness and equality and do not want to see a health care system in which the rich are treated differently from the poor.'[11]

At the same time, Canadians are increasingly concerned about problems within the publicly funded system, especially lengthening waiting times for some acute care services.[12] These concerns have, in turn, resulted in heightened attention, including from government-appointed review bodies such as the Clair and Mazankowski commissions,[13] to proposals for greater privatization of health care funding and services as a means of increasing individual patient choice and of relieving pressure on the public system.

Against this backdrop, I will consider the potential implications of section 7 of the *Charter* for current debates over health care funding and reform, including the potential role of the Courts in determining what services are covered by Medicare. To that end, I will first examine the facts and lower-court rulings in the *Chaoulli* case, as a concrete illustration of the application of section 7 in the health care context. I will go on to assess the broader social implications of a section 7–based review of the health care system and conclude by considering the choices facing the Supreme Court of Canada in *Chaoulli*.

The Facts and Evidence in *Chaoulli*

At issue in *Chaoulli* is the constitutional validity of section 15 of Quebec's *Health Insurance Act*[14] and section 11 of the province's *Hospital Insurance Act*.[15] These provisions, the equivalent to which exist in most other provinces,[16] prohibit private insurance contracts for publicly insured health and hospital services and, thus, effectively ensure a publicly funded single-payer system in Canada. In the context of resource constraints and delays within the public system, the appellants in *Chaoulli* claim that, by making delivery of private care uneconomical and thereby effectively depriving them of access to it, these legislative provisions violate their right to health under section 7 of the *Charter*.

In her judgment at trial, Justice Piché began by describing the obstacles that the appellants themselves faced in attempting to obtain, or to provide, health care services in Quebec. Mr Gregory Zéliotis, who was sixty-seven years old at the time of trial and suffering from various health problems, complained of having to wait from June 1994 until May 1995 for a left hip replacement and from February until September 1997 for a right hip replacement.[17] Dr Jacques Chaoulli, who completed his medical training in France prior to immigrating to Quebec in the late 1970s, reported several unsuccessful attempts to obtain government approval and funding for a twenty-four-hour ambulance service, a twenty-four-hour physician house-call service, and a private not-for-profit hospital.[18]

After outlining the appellants' interactions with the publicly funded system, Justice Piché reviewed the expert evidence adduced by the appellants in support of their claim, including evidence from a number of medical specialists in the fields of orthopaedic surgery, ophthalmology, oncology, and cardiology. These experts pointed to lengthy waiting lists; shortage of operating room time; shortage of nursing staff; shortage of, and outdated, equipment; erratic decision-making; 'politicking'; and lack of planning within the publicly funded system.[19] The appellants also called Barry Stein, a Montreal lawyer who, faced with treatment delays in Quebec, successfully challenged the provincial health insurance plan's refusal to reimburse him for the costs of obtaining cancer care in New York State.[20] Based on this evidence, Justice Piché agreed with the appellants' claim that waiting lists were too long. In her view 'même si ce n'est pas toujours une question de vie ou de mort, tous les citoyens ont droit à recevoir les soins dont ils ont besoin, et ce, dans les meilleurs délais.'[21]

Justice Piché went on to consider the evidence put forward by the federal and Quebec governments in response to the appellants' claim.[22] Yale School of Management Professor Ted Marmor, whom Justice Piché quoted at length, identified a number of recurring concerns in the expert evidence called by the federal government and the province. Marmor argued that allowing the development of a parallel private health insurance system in Quebec and Canada generally would have a number of negative consequences. In particular, Marmor argued that introducing private insurance funding would lead to decreased public support for Medicare and, in particular, to a loss of support from more affluent and thus politically influential groups most likely to exit the system.[23] As Marmor put it, 'it is axiomatic that those who exit a public system no longer have a strong stake in its effective operation. This, in turn, can and frequently does lead to an erosion of public support.'[24]

Marmor also cited unfair subsidies to the private system and private providers resulting from past and future public investment in hospitals, capital improvements, and research; diversion of financial and human resources away from, and lengthening of waiting lists in, the public system; increased government administrative costs required to regulate the private health insurance market; advantaging of those able to afford and to secure private coverage; and increased overall health spending with no clear improvement in health outcomes.[25] As Marmor concluded, 'the grounds used to bolster arguments for parallel insurance are uniformly weak empirically.'[26]

Other experts called by the respondent governments pointed to the efficiency of the Canadian health insurance system relative to that in the United States, where administrative costs are almost four times higher;[27] the fact that rationing occurs in all health care systems – in the United States based on price, resulting in 39 per cent of the U.S. population having no health insurance coverage at all;[28] the problem of 'cream skimming' within the private system, where providers 'siphon off high revenue patients and vigorously try to avoid providing care to patient populations who are at financial risk';[29] and the overall contribution of the public health care system to social cohesion in Canada.[30]

Lastly, Justice Piché summarized the evidence of Dr Edwin Coffey, a specialist in obstetrics and gynaecology and the Director of the Montreal District Executive of the Quebec Medical Association, called by the appellants. Coffey argued, based on his own experience and a comparative review of the situation in other member-states of the Organization for Economic Cooperation and Development (OECD), that prohibitions on private health insurance create a 'unique and outstanding disadvantage that handicaps the health system in Québec and Canada' and 'have contributed to the dysfunctional state of our present health system.'[31] Having earlier noted the failure by the appellants' other experts to endorse the view that allowing parallel private care would necessarily address waiting times and other access issues,[32] Justice Piché concluded that Coffey's opinion on the advantages of allowing private funding was inconsistent with the weight of expert evidence in the case: 'le Dr Coffey fait cavalier seul avec son expertise et les conclusions auxquelles il arrive.'[33]

The *Charter* Analysis in *Chaoulli*

Justice Piché began her legal analysis of the appellants' section 7 *Charter* claim[34] by reviewing existing Supreme Court of Canada jurisprudence on the scope of the right to life, liberty, and security of the person under section 7, including in *Singh* v *Canada*,[35] *R.* v *Morgentaler*,[36] *Irwin Toy* v *Québec (Attorney General)*,[37] and *Rodriguez* v *British Columbia (Attorney General)*.[38] Based on her review of the case law, Justice Piché concluded that the Supreme Court had left the door open to recognizing economic rights intimately connected to life, liberty, or personal security.[39] In answer to the question whether access to health care services was such a right, she concluded in the affirmative. In her view, 'S'il n'y a pas d'accès possible au système de santé, c'est illusoire de croire que les droits à la vie et à la sécurité sont respectés.'[40]

On the specific question of whether the right to contract for private health and hospital insurance, restricted under the legislative provisions at issue, was also protected under section 7, Justice Piché also found the answer to be yes. To the extent that the legislative restrictions on private insurance created economic barriers rendering access to private health care illusory, Justice Piché held that the appellants' rights to life, liberty, and security were affected. As she explained, 'ces dispositions sont une entrave à l'accès à des services de santé et sont donc susceptibles de porter atteinte à la vie, à la liberté et à la sécurité de la personne.'[41] In Justice Piché's view however, limits on access to private health services would violate section 7 only where the public system was unable to effectively guarantee access to similar care. As Justice Piché put it, '[L]e tribunal ne croit pas par contre qu'il puisse exister un droit constitutionnel de choisir la provenance de soins médicalement requis.'[42] Justice Piché acknowledged that the appellants were not in actual need of health care, nor of services that they had been unable to obtain within the publicly funded system. Rather, she accepted their claim that resource constraints within the public system, reflected in waiting lists and other access-related problems, combined with the impugned prohibitions on private insurance, meant that the appellants' future health care needs might not be met. Justice Piché agreed that this constituted a sufficient threat to the appellants' life, liberty, and security of the person: 'nous devons conclure, vu l'imprevisibilité de l'état de santé d'une personne, qu'il y a une menace d'atteinte imminente en l'espèce.'[43]

In light of her finding that the appellants' section 7 rights had been threatened, Justice Piché went on to consider whether the prohibition on private health insurance was 'in accordance with the principles of fundamental justice.' In doing so, she first reviewed the Supreme Court's decisions in *Rodriguez*[44] and other cases establishing that, in order to determine whether a violation of the right to life, liberty, or security of the person is in accordance with the principles of fundamental justice, the interests of the individual must be balanced against those of the state and society as a whole.[45] Applying this balancing test, Justice Piché pointed out that Quebec's health insurance legislation was designed to create and maintain a public health care system, universally accessible to all residents of the province, without barriers related to individual economic circumstances.[46] Restrictions on the development of a parallel private system, she found, were put in place by the province to prevent a transfer of resources out of the public system, to the detriment of all members of society.[47] She explained:

> La preuve a montré que le droit d'avoir recours à un système parallèle privé de soins, invoqué par les requérants, aurait des répercussions sur les droits de l'ensemble de la population … L'établissement d'un système de santé parallèle privé aurait pour effet de menacer l'intégrité, le bon fonctionnement ainsi que la viabilité du système public. Les articles [contestés] empêchent cette éventualité et garantissent l'existence d'un système de santé public de qualité au Québec.[48]

This balancing of interests in favour of the collective benefit to all residents of Quebec of preserving a viable and effective public health care system, Justice Piché found, was motivated by equality and dignity concerns, and was consistent with Canadian and Quebec constitutional and human rights norms.[49] Such a legislative choice was therefore clearly in conformity with the principles of fundamental justice. Thus, Justice Piché concluded, restrictions on access to private insurance and private health care under provincial health and hospital insurance legislation did not violate section 7 of the *Charter*.[50] While a section 1 justification was therefore not required, Justice Piché expressed the view that such an analysis would demonstrate that the provisions at issue constituted a reasonable limit in a free and democratic society.[51]

The Court of Appeal decision in *Chaoulli*

Justice Piché's decision was upheld by the Quebec Court of Appeal in three concurring judgments.[52] Justice Delisle found that access to a publicly funded health care system was a fundamental right protected under section 7. In contrast to Justice Piché, he held that the right to contract for private health insurance being claimed by the appellants was a purely economic interest that was not essential to human life and that it was therefore excluded from section 7 of the *Charter*.[53] Justice Delisle warned:

> Il ne faut pas inverser les principes en jeu pour, ainsi, rendre essentiel un droit économique accessoire auquel, par ailleurs, les gens financièrement défavorisés n'auraient pas accès. Le droit fondamental en cause est celui de fournir à tous un régime public de protection de santé, que les défenses édictées par les articles précités ont pour but de sauvegarder.[54]

Justice Forget agreed with Justice Piché that, while the appellants' section 7 health rights were affected by the statutory limits on private health insurance, the province's decision to favour the collective interest in maintaining the public health care system was in accordance with section 7 principles of fundamental justice.[55] For his part, Justice Brossard agreed with Justice Delisle that the contractual rights restricted under the health and hospital insurance provisions at issue were economic rights that were not fundamental to human life. To the extent that the evidence failed to show that the statutory restrictions on private insurance had, in fact, imperilled the appellants' rights to life or health, Justice Brossard concluded that no violation of section 7 had been shown.[56]

The Broader Social Implications of Section 7 Review of the Health Care System

As noted at the outset of this chapter, publicly funded Medicare occupies a pre-eminent place in Canadian society. It therefore stands to reason that fundamental health-related interests should be constitutionally recognized and that health care decision-making should respect basic constitutional norms. As Justice Piché affirmed, the right to life, liberty, and security of the person has little meaning for someone who lacks access to medically necessary care in the event of sickness. To the extent that section 7 gives clear constitutional expression to the idea that 'all are entitled – as a matter of citizenship – to equal access to quality care,'[57] and that compliance with section 7 norms is likely to generate more open, accountable, and inclusive health care decision-making,[58] a section 7 review can be characterized as a possible 'cure' for some of the problems facing the current health care system.

From a broader, determinants of health perspective, however, the risks of a section 7 'misdiagnosis' of the health care system are also apparent. In recent years, health care has become the dominant social policy concern in Canada, for governments and the public alike.[59] While the 1995 federal budget repealed the national standards for social welfare programs and services that existed until that point under the *Canada Assistance Plan*,[60] national conditions under the *Canada Health Act*[61] have been maintained and continue to be vigorously defended, if not necessarily enforced,[62] by successive federal governments. The result is that in many parts of Canada, for those forced to rely on social assistance, almost the only certainty of food, clothing, and shelter is to fall so ill as to require hospitalization.[63]

Notwithstanding overwhelming evidence that poverty and related social and economic factors such as education and unemployment are the most significant determinants of health, Canadians remain wedded to the idea that access to biomedical services is the best guarantee of individual and public health.[64] At the same time, powerful stakeholder interests, drawing significant media attention, reinforce the view that the publicly funded system is broken and that more acute care spending, both by government and through increased privatization of health funding and services, is required to fix it.[65] As the Mazankowski Advisory Council on Health framed the issue, '[i]f we continue to depend only on provincial and federal revenues to support health care services, we have few options other than rationing health care services. On the other hand, if we are able to diversify the revenue sources used to support health care, we have the opportunity of improving access, expanding health care services, and realizing the potential of new techniques and treatments to improve health.'[66]

In the current neo-liberal policy climate, both the demand for more public funding for acute health care services and the call for increased health care privatization have serious negative implications for low-income Canadians. Public and stakeholder demands for more public spending on acute health care, coupled with governments' own deficit- and tax-cutting agendas, have provided a major impetus for significant reductions in social welfare spending. Over the past decade, as health care spending has gone up, social assistance programs and benefits have been cut across the country by governments of all political stripes. Ironically, these social welfare cuts have occurred without consideration of their impact on the health of the individuals affected or the broader economic and social costs in terms of public health and health care spending.[67]

Demands for increased private health care funding have equally significant negative implications for the poor, inasmuch as they represent a profound threat to the access of low-income Canadians to the health care services that are currently provided within the framework of the *Canada Health Act*. As the evidence accepted by Justice Piché in the *Chaoulli* case demonstrates, allowing the development of a parallel private insurance system will have serious adverse consequences for the health care rights of low-income Canadians, both by advantaging those who are able to purchase private health insurance and care and by drawing resources away from and eroding public support for the publicly funded system upon which people living in poverty disproportionately rely.[68]

As the *Chaoulli* case illustrates, not only the argument for more public spending, but also the demand for increased private funding and privatization of services, can find support under section 7 of the *Charter*. In their intervention before the Supreme Court of Canada in the *Chaoulli* case, for example, the Canadian Medical Association and the Canadian Orthopaedic Association,[69] along with a group composed of a number of private surgery and diagnostic clinics in British Columbia,[70] are supporting the appellants' claim, based on the argument that if governments are unwilling to devote the necessary resources to eliminate waiting periods for acute care, the system must be opened up to private funding as a matter of section 7 right. The B.C. Clinics argue:

> To the extent that individuals are given a reasonable opportunity to secure, in a timely manner, such medically necessary treatment as is not provided by the state, the failure of the state to provide such treatment does not result in a deprivation of s. 7 rights. Personal autonomy in that case would be protected ...
>
> Likewise, the current public health care provisions aimed at preventing the development of a parallel private health care system, including the bar on private health insurance, would arguably not violate the liberty and security of individuals provided that unlimited, or at least adequate, health care resources were available from the state.[71]

For their part, Committee Chair Michael Kirby and other members of the Senate Standing Committee on Social Affairs, Science and Technology, are advancing similar arguments in their intervention in *Chaoulli*. While professing support for the publicly funded system, the Kirby Committee argues that 'Health Care Guarantees' would be sufficient to preserve its main features and that Quebec's private health insurance prohibitions should be struck down.[72] The inference is that governments can bring themselves into compliance with section 7, either by increasing public funding to reduce waiting times to a level the Committee deems acceptable, or by allowing the introduction of private funding to achieve the same results. As the Committee repeatedly asserts, 'governments can no longer have it both ways – they cannot fail to provide access to medically necessary care in the publicly funded health care system and, at the same time, prevent Canadians from acquiring those services through private means.'[73]

Quite apart from the fact that the Kirby Committee's benign assessment of the effects of striking down the impugned provisions is contradicted by the evidence, neither the choice of more public spending on acute care services, nor the prospect of increased private funding, reflect the interests of low-income Canadians. Canadians living in poverty continue to suffer the consequences of governments' overemphasis on acute health care and their corresponding underinvestment in social welfare programs, social services, and other positive measures to address social determinants of health. People living in poverty also have the most to lose from a move to private funding and a two-tiered health care system.[74]

The Choices Facing the Supreme Court in *Chaoulli*

To her credit, Justice Piché did not limit her analysis in *Chaoulli* to the narrow issue of individual autonomy and choice that the rhetoric of health care privatization relies on, and that a narrow reading of section 7 of the *Charter* permits. Rather, she considered the broader social policy issues raised in the case. In examining the scope of section 7 and the meaning of fundamental justice within the health care context, Justice Piché considered the life, liberty, and security of the person interests of those Canadians for whom access to health care is contingent on rationing that is unrelated to ability to pay.[75] To put it more starkly, Justice Piché's judgment recognizes that, from the perspective of people living in poverty, a system that imposes some waiting period for all is infinitely preferable to a system in which poor people may wait forever for care.

In deciding the *Chaoulli* case, the Supreme Court of Canada can either uphold or reverse Justice Piché's decision and the judgment of the Quebec Court of Appeal. Whether or not the Court adopts Justice's

Piché's interpretation of section 7, in light of its decision in *Gosselin* v *Québec (Attorney General)*,[76] the Court should be expected to defer to her conclusions of fact as to the impact of striking down the current restrictions on private health and hospital insurance funding. As Dr Marmor pointed out in his testimony at trial, opponents of the single-tier system portray the introduction of parallel private insurance funding as being a reform option with no downside: 'The case for changing the present Canadian prohibition against parallel private health insurance for core medical services rests upon an appealing, but unrealistic theory. It is the view that parallel insurance can be introduced and operated so that no one in Canada would be worse off ... This "win-win" theory has a surface plausibility ... however, a closer examination reveals its theoretical and empirical flaws.'[77]

Justice Piché accepted the evidence presented at trial that striking down the prohibition on private health and hospital insurance would have serious negative consequences for the public system.[78] Nevertheless, the appellants and supporting interveners have continued to argue before the Supreme Court that the harm of striking down the impugned provisions has not been proven. For example, the B.C. Clinics contend that 'the evidence simply does not support the proposition that the public health care system in Canada will suffer significantly if private payment for insured services is permitted.'[79] The Kirby Committee makes a similar assertion that '[a] declaration that the impugned legislation is unconstitutional will not sound the death knell for the Canadian system of publicly funded health care for medically necessary services.'[80] The Supreme Court's decision whether to accept the appellants' arguments on this point over Justice Piche's findings of fact will undoubtedly have a major impact on the outcome of the case.

Beyond the weight of expert evidence, the Supreme Court has been clear that private contractual rights of the type being claimed by the appellants in *Chaoulli* are not included under section 7 of the *Charter*.[81] In essence, the appellants and supporting interveners are arguing, not only that they have a right to purchase private insurance, but that governments cannot legislate in such a way that it becomes economically unattractive for the market to provide it. The idea that section 7 includes private corporate-commercial rights of this nature was firmly rejected by the Court in *Irwin Toy*.[82] The argument that physicians, and by analogy other private health care providers, have a section 7 right to provide health care services has also been dismissed.[83]

However, as the appellants and supporting interveners in *Chaoulli* argue effectively, the idea that an individual should be able to choose private care, and that such a choice is fundamental to personal autonomy and dignity, finds significant support in Supreme Court case law. The Court has recently reiterated that the right to liberty under section 7 'grants the individual a degree of autonomy in making decisions of fundamental importance, without interference from the state.'[84] The appellants and supporting interveners invoke this jurisprudence in support of a purely negative conception of section 7 as a guarantee against measures that 'prevent individuals from utilizing their own resources' to obtain private care.[85] As the B.C. Clinics assert, 'there is no right to have one's health care ... paid for by the government. However ... the individual has a right to be protected from government interference with his or her ability to take care of his or her own health.'[86] Or, as the members of the Kirby Committee state their position, '[t]hese interveners are not asserting a free-standing constitutional right to health care. Rather, these interveners assert a constitutional right not to be prevented from obtaining 'timely access to medically necessary care' in Canada that is not currently available through the publicly-funded system.'[87]

In this regard the appellants and supporting interveners are proposing an underinclusive and discriminatory interpretation of the section 7 right to health: one that recognizes and protects the health care rights of the economically advantaged while denying those of the poor, whose access to health care depends on the existence of the public system. This approach to the right to health care is incompatible both with domestic equality rights principles,[88] and with health and equality guarantees under international treaties ratified by Canada, which the Court has identified as an important guide for Section 7 principles of fundamental justice,[89] and for *Charter* interpretation generally.[90] In particular, an interpretation of section 7 that entrenches the right to buy private care free from state interference, but not the right to health care per se, is inconsistent with Canada's international treaty obligations under the *International Covenant on Economic, Social and Cultural Rights* to guarantee 'medical service and medical attention in the event of sickness' without discrimination based on 'social origin, property, birth or other status.'[91]

The appellants' and supporting interveners' definition of the right to health is considerably narrower than the one adopted by Justice Piché, who held that section 7 protects the right to access health care services and the health care system generally.[92] On appeal, Justice Delisle also found that that the right guaranteed under section 7 is to publicly funded care and rejected the appellants' argument precisely because it amounted to a claim to a right that would be inaccessible to low-income people. [93] The Supreme Court's choice of either the narrow and de-contextualized reading of section 7 put forward by the appellants, or an interpretation of the right to health informed by equality and interna-tional human rights principles, will be a determining factor, not only for the outcome of the *Chaoulli* case, but for the future application of section 7 in the health care context.

In addition to defining the right to health care more narrowly, the interveners supporting the appellants point out that the balancing ap-proach to fundamental justice adopted by Justice Piché at trial was thrown into doubt by the Supreme Court's recent decision in *R. v. Malmo-Levine; R. v. Caine*, where the Court cautioned: 'The balancing of individual and societal interests within section 7 is only relevant when elucidating a particular principle of fundamental justice ... Once the principle of fundamental justice has been elucidated; however, it is not within the ambit of s. 7 to bring into account such "societal inter-ests" as health care costs. Those considerations will be looked at, if at all, under s. 1.'[94]

While section 7 may no longer allow for the balancing approach to fundamental justice applied by Justice Piché at trial, the evidence does make it clear that, aside from promoting broader collective interests in a viable publicly funded health care system, Quebec's decision to pro-hibit private health and hospital insurance is neither arbitrary, irratio-nal, nor inconsistent with fundamental social values – the principal requirements of fundamental justice identified by the Court in *Malmo-Levine*.[95] As Justice Piché found, the prohibitions accord with funda-mental justice by ensuring that both individual treatment and broader health policy and resource allocation decisions are based on need, rather than dictated by market pressures shown to generate not only inequi-table, but inefficient and irrational health care choices.[96] By ensuring that access to health care is not conditional upon ability to pay, the impugned provisions also reflect and promote the fundamental *Charter* value of respect for human life, recognized as a matter of societal consensus by the Court in *Rodriguez*,[97] as well as the widely shared Canadian value that access to health care should be determined by need, not wealth.[98]

As Justice Piché's judgment recognizes, and as Justice Delisle reiterates on appeal, a failure by governments to ensure access to health care services without barriers based on ability to pay would have a discriminatory impact on the life, liberty, and security of the person of people living in poverty and on others for whom access to publicly funded health care is crucial. In his decision in *Eldridge v British Columbia (Attorney General)* outlining the positive obligations imposed by the *Charter* in the context of health care services for the deaf, Justice LaForest argued: 'If we accept the concept of adverse effect discrimination, it seems inevitable, at least at the s. 15(1) stage of analysis, that the government will be required to take special measures to ensure that disadvantaged groups are able to benefit equally from government services.'[99] On that basis, it is not the impugned prohibitions on private health and hospital insurance, as the appellants allege, but rather the absence of legislative measures to ensure equal access to health care that should give rise to constitutional question under the *Charter*.

Conclusion

A recent CBC national broadcast declared that, while health care dominates political debate in Canada, 'the most important decision about the future of health care is actually taking place inside the halls of the Supreme Court of Canada' in *Chaoulli*.[100] As suggested at the outset of this chapter, lower courts in Canada have generally been unwilling to consider the scope of the publicly funded system as justiciable under section 7 of the *Charter*.[101] As the B.C. Court of Appeal summarily concluded in a recent case, '[w]hen the *Charter* was first presented considerable debate ensued as to whether it could apply to provide a positive entitlement to health care. In my view … it does not.'[102] In this regard, Justice Piché's decision represents a clear change in direction and, as the CBC media clip highlights, the *Chaoulli* hearing before the Supreme Court of Canada signifies a major turning point both for the *Charter* and for the Canadian health care system.

As the comparative South African experience (described by Lisa Forman in this volume) illustrates, 'rights and law [have the capacity] to function as powerful gate openers to health care access unreasonably denied by government.' From a health policy perspective, a section 7–based review of health care decision-making represents a potential cure for some of the problems within the current Canadian health care system. Compliance with section 7 principles of fundamental justice may generate more open, accountable, and participatory decision-making, including in relation to decisions about what services are publicly funded. However, as Greschner and as Flood, Stabile, and Tuohy argue elsewhere in this volume, *Charter* review of health care decision-making also presents risks. In particular, as suggested earlier, a section 7 review of the health care system runs the very real danger of focusing not on the systemic inadequacies and inequities within the public health care system, but rather on a narrow conception of individual autonomy and choice that fails to acknowledge the positive and collective dimensions of health care entitlements. As outlined above, this danger is clearly illustrated in the *Chaoulli* case. To the extent that *Charter* review contributes to or exacerbates the current disconnect between acute health care and broader social welfare and determinants of health as a focus of government concern and spending, a section 7 review risks producing a serious misdiagnosis of the system. In particular, acceptance of the appellants' and supporting interveners' claim in *Chaoulli* that restrictions on private insurance funding are unconstitutional and must be struck down would represent a serious perversion of the right to health – one from which the patient, be it the publicly funded health care system or section 7 of the *Charter*, would not easily recover.

In the early *Charter* case of *R. v. Edwards Books and Art Ltd.*,[103] former Chief Justice Brian Dickson warned: 'In interpreting and applying the *Charter* … the courts must be cautious to ensure that it does not simply become an instrument of better situated individuals to roll back legislation which has as its object the improvement of the conditions of less advantaged persons.' More recently, in a discussion paper for the Romanow Commission examining the distributional implications of various health funding options currently under consideration in Canada, health economist Robert Evans explained support for increased privatization of health care services and funding as follows: 'The real motive underlying proposals for more private financing is very simple. The more private funding we have, the more those with high incomes can assure themselves of first class care without having to pay taxes to help support a similar standard of care for everyone else.'[104] Consistent with its recent judgment in *Harper v. Canada (Attorney General)*,[105] it is to be hoped that in deciding the *Chaoulli* case the Supreme Court will prove as sensitive as Justice Piché was at trial to the life, liberty, and security-related health interests of all Canadians, and not simply of the most advantaged.

NOTES

1 [1997] 3 S.C.R. 624.
2 *Canadian Charter of Rights and Freedoms*, Part I of the *Constitution Act, 1982*, being Schedule B to the *Canada Act, 1982* (U.K.), 1982, c. 11 [*Charter*].
3 Martha Jackman, 'The Application of the *Canadian Charter* in the Health Care Context' (2000) 9 Health Law Review 22.
4 See, generally, Donna Greschner, *How Will the Charter of Rights and Freedoms and Evolving Jurisprudence Affect Health Care Costs? Discussion Paper No. 20* (submission to the Commission on the Future of Health Care in Canada) (Saskatoon: Commission on the Future of Health Care in Canada, 2002); Martha Jackman, *The Implications of Section 7 of the Charter for Health Care Spending in Canada, Discussion Paper No. 31, ibid.*
5 *Chaoulli c. Québec (Procureure générale)*, [2000] J.Q. no. 479 (Cour supérieure du Québec – Chambre civil) [*Chaoulli* (C.S.)].
6 This chapter was completed before the Supreme Court of Canada rendered its 9 June 2005 decision in the *Chaoulli* case, now reported at [2005] S.C.C. 35. The author represented the Charter Committee on Poverty Issues and the Canadian Health Coalition in their intervention in the case. For commentary on the Supreme Court's decision see: Colleen M. Flood, Kent Roach, and Lorne Sossis, eds., *Access to Care, Access to Justice: The Legal Debate over Private Health Insurance* (Toronto: University of Toronto Press, 2005); Martha Jackman, 'Health and Equality: Is There a Cure?' in Sheila McIntyre and Sanda Rodgers, eds., *Diminishing Returns: Inequality and the Canadian Charter of Rights and Freedoms* (Toronto: Irwin Law, in press).
7 *Chaoulli c. Québec (Procureur général)*, [2002] J.Q. No. 759 (Cour d'appel du Québec) [*Chaoulli* (C.A.)].
8 Section 7 provides: 'Everyone has the right to life, liberty and security of the person and the right not to be deprived thereof except in accordance with the principles of fundamental justice.'
9 Canada, Commission on the Future of Health Care in Canada, *Building on Values: The Future of Health Care in Canada – Final Report* (Saskatoon: Commission on the Future of Health Care in Canada, 2002) (Chair: Roy Romanow) at xvi [Romanow Commission]; Standing Senate Committee on Social Affairs, Science and Technology, *The Health of Canadians: The Federal Role, Interim Report on the State of the Health Care System in Canada*, vol. 1, *The Story So Far* (Ottawa: Standing Senate Committee on Social Affairs, Science and Technology, 2002) (Chair: Michael Kirby) chap. 3 [Kirby Committee, *Interim Report*]; Commission d'étude sur les services de santé et les

services sociaux, *Emerging Solutions: Report and Recommendations* (Quebec: Ministry of Health and Social Services, 2001) (Chair: Michel Clair) at 7 [Clair Commission]; Commission on Medicare, *Caring for Medicare: Sustaining a Quality System* (Regina: Saskatchewan Health, 2001) (Chair: Ken J. Fyke) at 5; Institute for Research on Public Policy Task Force on Health Care Reform, *Recommendations to First Ministers* (Montreal: Institute for Research on Public Policy, 2000) at 5.

10 Romanow Commission, at xvi.

11 National Forum on Health, 'Values Working Group Synthesis Report' in *Canada Health Action: Building on the Legacy,* vol. 2 (Ottawa: Minister of Public Works and Government Services, 1997) at 11 [National Forum on Health, 'Values Working Group Synthesis Report'].

12 Romanow Commission, *supra* note 9 at 138–9; Kirby Committee, *Interim Report, supra* note 9 at 45; Premier's Advisory Council on Health, *A Framework for Reform: Report of the Premier's Advisory Council on Health* (Edmonton: Premier's Advisory Council on Health, 2001) (Chair: Donald Mazankowski) at 19 [*Mazankowski Report*].

13 Clair Commission, *supra* note 9; Mazankowski Report.

14 R.S.Q., c. A-29 [*Health IA*].

15 R.S.Q., c. A-28 [*Hospital IA*].

16 Colleen M. Flood and Tom Archibald, 'The Illegality of Private Health Care in Canada' (2001) 164:6 Canadian Medical Association Journal 825.

17 *Chaoulli* (C.S.), *supra* note 5 at paras. 19–23.

18 *Ibid.* at paras. 24–39.

19 *Ibid.* at paras. 44–51.

20 *Ibid.* at paras. 52–4; for a discussion of the *Stein* case, see Stanley Hartt and Patrick Monahan, 'The *Charter* and Health Care: Guaranteeing Timely Access to Health Care for Canadians' (2002) 164 C.D. Howe Institute Commentary 1–28.

21 Translation: 'even if it isn't always a question of life or death, all citizens have the right to receive the care they need, and within the shortest possible delay.' *Chaoulli* (C.S.), *supra* note 5 at para. 50.

22 *Ibid.* at paras. 71–115.

23 *Ibid.* at paras. 109–12.

24 *Ibid.* at para. 109.

25 *Ibid.* at paras. 102–15.

26 *Ibid.* at para. 115.

27 *Ibid.* at para. 75, per Dr Fernand Turcotte.

28 *Ibid.* at para. 89, per Dr Howard Bergman; at para. 95, per Dr Jean-Louis Denis.

29 *Ibid.* at para. 91, per Dr Charles Wright.

30 *Ibid.* at para. 101, per Dr Jean-Louis Denis.

31 *Ibid.* at para. 119.

32 *Ibid.* at para. 51.

33 Translation: 'Dr Coffey is a lone horseman in his expertise and the conclusions to which he arrives.' *Ibid.* at para. 120.

34 The appellants also argued, unsuccessfully, that the prohibitions on private insurance were matters of federal criminal law and thereby exceeded provincial jurisdiction over health under ss. 92(7), (13), (15) and (16) of the *Constitution Act, 1867*; that the provisions violated the guarantee against 'cruel and unusual treatment or punishment' under s. 12 of the *Charter*; and that they discriminated between Quebec residents and non-residents, contrary to s. 15(1) of the *Charter*.

35 [1985] 1 S.C.R. 177 [*Singh*].

36 [1988] 1 S.C.R. 30 [*Morgentaler*].

37 [1989] 1 S.C.R. 927 [*Irwin Toy*].

38 [1993] 3 S.C.R. 519 [*Rodriguez*].

39 *Chaoulli* (C.S.), *supra* note 5 at para. 221.

40 Translation: 'If there is no access to the health care system, it is illusory to think that rights to life and security are respected.' *Ibid.* at para. 223.

41 Translation: 'these provisions are an obstacle to access to health services and may therefore infringe life, liberty and security of the person.' *Ibid.* at para. 225.

42 Translation: 'The Court does not think, however, that there is a constitutional right to choose where medically required health care will come from.' *Ibid.* at para. 227.

43 Translation: 'we must conclude, given the unpredictability of a person's state of health, that there is an imminent threat of deprivation in the present case.' *Ibid* at para. 242.

44 *Supra* note 38. As Justice Sopinka expressed it, at 594, 'where the deprivation of the right in question does little or nothing to enhance the state's interest ... a breach of fundamental justice will be made out.'

45 *Chaoulli* (C.S.), *supra* note 5 at para. 256.

46 *Ibid.* at para. 258.

47 *Ibid.* at para. 259.

48 Translation: 'The evidence shows that the right, claimed by the plaintiffs, to have recourse to a parallel private health care system would have repercussions for the rights of the entire population ... The creation of a parallel, private health care system would threaten the integrity, the effective operation and the viability of the public system. The [challenged]

provisions prevent such an occurrence and guarantee the existence of a quality, public health care system in Québec.' *Ibid.* at para. 263.

49 *Ibid.* at para. 260.

50 *Ibid.* at para. 267.

51 *Ibid.* at para. 268. Section 1 of the *Charter* provides: 'The *Canadian Charter of Rights and Freedoms* guarantees the rights and freedoms set out in it subject only to such reasonable limits prescribed by law as can be demonstrably justified in a free and democratic society.'

52 *Chaoulli* (C.A.), *supra* note 7.

53 *Ibid.* at para. 25.

54 Translation: 'The principles at issue must not be inverted so as to make an ancillary economic right essential, and further, one to which economically disadvantaged people would not have access. The fundamental right at issue is that of providing a public health protection system to all, a right which the prohibitions set out under the abovementioned provisions are designed to safeguard.' *Ibid.* at para. 25.

55 *Ibid.* at para. 63.

56 *Ibid.* at para. 66.

57 National Forum on Health, 'Values Working Group Synthesis Report' *supra* note 11 at 11.

58 See Martha Jackman, 'The Right to Participate in Health Care and Health Resource Allocation Decisions Under Section 7 of the *Canadian Charter*' (1995) vol. 4:2 Health Law Review 3–11.

59 Romanow Commission, *supra* note 9 at xvi; Kirby Committee, *Interim Report*, *supra* note 9 chap. 5; Ted R. Marmor, Kieke G.H. Okma, and Stephen R. Latham, *National Values, Institutions and Health Policies: What Do They Imply for Medicare Reform? Discussion Paper No. 5* (submission to the Commission on the Future of Health Care in Canada) (Saskatoon: Commission on the Future of Health Care in Canada, 2002) at 15–16 [Marmor et al., *National Values*]; National Forum on Health, 'Values Working Group Synthesis Report,' *supra* note 11 at 5.

60 R.S.C. 1985, c. C-1; Martha Jackman, 'Women and the Canadian Health and Social Transfer: Ensuring Gender Equality in Federal Welfare Reform' (1995) 8 Canadian Journal of Women and the Law 371.

61 R.S.C. 1985, c. C–6.

62 Office of the Auditor General of Canada, 'Federal Support for Health Care Delivery,' in *1999 Report of the Auditor General of Canada* (Ottawa: Office of the Auditor General of Canada, 1999) chap. 19; Sujit Choudhry, 'The Enforcement of the Canada Health Act' (1996) 41 McGill Law Journal 461.

63 For an account of the impact of social welfare changes over the past decade, see Bruce Porter, 'Rewriting the Charter or Reading It Right: The Challenge of Poverty and Homelessness in Canada,' in W. Cragg and C. Koggel, eds., *Contemporary Moral Issues* (Toronto: McGraw-Hill Ryerson, 2004) 373; Jean Swanson, *Poor-Bashing: The Politics of Exclusion* (Toronto: Between the Lines, 2001); National Council of Welfare, *Another Look at Welfare Reform* (Ottawa: Minister of Public Works and Government Services Canada, 1997).

64 Kirby Committee, *Interim Report, supra* note 9 chap. 5; Dennis Raphael, 'From Increasing Poverty to Social Disintegration: The Effects of Economic Inequality on the Health of Individuals and Communities,' in Hugh. Armstrong, Pat Armstrong, and David Coburn, eds., *Unhealthy Times: The Political Economy of Health Care in Canada* (Toronto: Oxford University Press, 2001) 223; Monica Townson, *Health and Wealth: How Social and Economic Factors Affect Our Well-Being* (Ottawa: Canadian Centre for Policy Alternatives, 1999); National Forum on Health, 'Determinants of Health Working Group Synthesis Report,' in National Forum on Health, *Canada Health Action: Building on the Legacy,* vol. 2 (Ottawa: Minister of Public Works and Government Services, 1997) at 5–6.

65 Robert G. Evans, *Raising the Money: Options, Consequences and Objectives for Financing Health Care in Canada, Discussion Paper No. 27* (submission to the Commission on the Future of Health Care in Canada) (Saskatoon: Commission on the Future of Health Care in Canada, 2002); Donna Greschner and Steven Lewis, '*Auton* and Evidence-Based Decision-Making: Medicare in the Courts' (2003) 82 Can. Bar Rev. 501; Marie-Clare Prémont, *The Canada Health Act and the Future of Health Care Systems in Canada, Discussion Paper No. 4* (submission to the Commission on the Future of Health Care in Canada) (Saskatoon: Commission on the Future of Health Care in Canada, 2002); Raisa B. Deber, 'Getting What We Pay For: Myths and Realities about Financing Canada's Health Care System' (2000) 21:2 Health Law in Canada 9–40.

66 *Mazankowski Report, supra* note 12 at 52.

67 National Council of Welfare, *The Cost of Poverty* (Ottawa: Minister of Public Works and Government Services Canada, 2001) at 7–8; Raphael, 'From Increasing Poverty to Social Disintegration,' *supra* note 64; National Anti-Poverty Organization, *Government Expenditure Cuts and Other Changes to Health and Post-Secondary Education: Impacts on Low-Income Canadians* (Ottawa: National Anti-Poverty Organization, 1998), c. 3.

68 Evans, *supra* note 65 at 37; National Anti-Poverty Organization, *ibid.*

69 *Factum of the Interveners Canadian Medical Association and the Canadian Orthopaedic Association in Chaoulli v. Québec (Attorney General)* [*Factum of the Interveners CMA and COA*].

70 *Factum of the Interveners Cambie Surgeries Corporation, False Creek Surgical Centre Inc. and Others in Chaoulli v. Québec (Attorney General)* [*Factum of the Interveners Cambie Surgeries Corporation et al.*].

71 *Ibid.* at paras. 26–7; *Factum of the Interveners CMA and COA*, *supra* note 69 at para. 19.

72 *Factum of the Interveners Senator Michael Kirby, Senator Marjory Lebreton, Senator Catherine Callbeck, Senator Joan Cook, Senator Jane Cordy, Senator Joyce Fairbarin, Senator Wilbert Keon, Senator Lucie Pepin, Senator Brenda Robertson, and Senator Douglas Roche in Chaoulli v. Québec* at paras. 24 and 62 [*Factum of the Interveners Senator Michael Kirby et al.*]

73 *Ibid.* at paras. 7 and 16; Standing Senate Committee on Social Affairs, Science and Technology, *The Health of Canadians: The Federal Role, Final Report, Vol. 6, Recommendations for Reform* (Ottawa: Standing Senate Committee on Social Affairs, Science and Technology, 2002) (Chair: Michael Kirby) at 120.

74 NAPO, 'Government Expenditure Cuts,' *supra* note 67; see also National Coordinating Group on Health Care Reform and Women, *Reading Romanow: The Implications of the Final Report of the Commission on the Future of Health Care in Canada for Women* at 7–11 (at ch. 7, p. 11).

75 *Chaoulli (C.S.) supra* note 5 at para. 262.

76 [2002] 4 S.C.R. 429.

77 *Chaoulli (C.S.) supra* note 5 at para. 104.

78 *Ibid.* at paras. 91–3; 103–5.

79 *Factum of the Interveners Cambie Surgeries Corporation et al.*, supra note 70 at para. 56.

80 *Factum of the Interveners Senator Michael Kirby et al.*, *supra* note 72 at para. 62.

81 *Irwin Toy*, *supra* note 37 at 1004.

82 *Ibid.*

83 Jackman, 'The Implications of Section 7 of the Charter,' *supra* note 4 at 9–10.

84 *R. v. Malmo-Levine; R. v. Caine*, [2003] 3 S.C.R. 571 at para. 85 citing *Morgentaler*, *supra* note 35 at 166; *Godbout v. Longueuil (City)*, [1997] 3 S.C.R. 844 at para. 66; *R.B. v. Children's Aid Society of Metropolitan Toronto*, [1995] 1 S.C.R. 315 at para. 80.

85 *Factum of the Interveners Cambie Surgeries Corporation et al.*, *supra* note 70 at para. 9; *Factum of the Interveners CMA and COA*, *supra* note 69 at para. 22.

86 *Factum of the Interveners Cambie Surgeries Corporation et al., ibid.* at para. 26.
87 *Factum of the Interveners Senator Michael Kirby et al., supra* note 72 at para. 32.
88 Greschner, *supra* note 4 at 21; *Factum of the Charter Committee on Poverty Issues and the Canadian Health Coalition in Chaoulli v. Quebec.*
89 *Re B.C. Motor Vehicle Act,* [1985] 2 S.C.R. 487 at 503; *United States* v. *Burns,* [2001] 1 S.C.R. 283 at paras. 79–81; *Malmo-Levine, supra* note 84 at para. 270.
90 *Baker v. Canada (Minister of Citizenship and Immigration),* [1999] 2 S.C.R. 817 at para. 70.
91 993 U.N. s. 3 (1966); Can. T.S. 1976 No. 47, Articles 2(2), 12(2)(d). For a discussion of the right to health under international law see Barbara von Tigerstrom, 'Human Rights and Health Care Reform: A Canadian Per- spective,' in Tim A. Caulfield and Barbara von Tigerstrom, eds., *Health Care Reform and the Law in Canada: Meeting the Challenge* (Edmonton: University of Alberta Press, 2002) 157–85; B.C.A. Toebes, *The Right to Health as a Human Right in International Law* (Oxford: Intersentia – Hart, 1999).
92 *Chaoulli* (C.S.), *supra* note 5 at para. 223.
93 *Chaoulli* (C.A.), *supra* note 7 at para. 25.
94 *Malmo-Levine, supra* note 84 at para. 98.
95 *Ibid.* at paras. 113, 135.
96 *Chaoulli* (C.S.), *supra* note 5 at paras. 66, 76; Evans, *supra* note 65.
97 *Rodriguez, supra* note 37 at 608.
98 Romanow Commission, *supra* note 9 at xvi; National Forum on Health, 'Values Working Group Synthesis Report,' *supra* note 11 at 11; Marmor et al., *National Values, supra* note 59 at v.
99 [1997] 3 S.C.R. 624 at para. 77.
100 CBC Radio One, *The Current,* Medical Special, 26 May 2004 http://www .cbc.ca/thecurrent/2004/200405/20040526.html.
101 Jackman, *supra* note 3.
102 *Auton (Guardian ad Litem of) v. British Columbia (Minister of Health),* [2002] B.C.J. 2258 at para. 73.
103 [1986] 2 S.C.R. 713 at 779.
104 Evans, *supra* note 65 at 42.
105 [2004] S.C.C. 33.

4 Claiming Equity and Justice in Health: The Role of the South African Right to Health in Ensuring Access to HIV/AIDS Treatment

LISA FORMAN

Ensuring access to health care for poor and vulnerable populations is a challenge regardless of a country's level of development. But it is obviously far greater in a country like South Africa, where almost half the population lives in poverty and people are serviced by a public health care system not originally constructed with the intention of providing universal and equitable health services. This challenge is exponentially greater in light of the emergence of a massive and explosive HIV/AIDS epidemic, the largest in the world. In South Africa progress towards the goal of universal and equitable health care access has been marked by the convergence of two relatively contemporaneous legal and political developments. While the post-apartheid Constitution entrenches an explicit right to access to health care services, under President Mbeki, the government has been both neglectful and intransigent in providing access to essential HIV/AIDS medicines.

The interaction of these factors tells an illuminating story about how a constitutional right to health care can ensure access on the part of poor and vulnerable populations unfairly excluded from public health care benefits, and ensure reasonable and accountable governance of health care. Flood, Stabile, and Tuohy point out in their chapter that '[w]ith respect to the question of what services to fund, it is impossible to generalize across nations given their different resource constraints and values.' Although South Africa's development levels and resources are of a different order from Canada's, what is illuminating for the Canadian context is the way that law, particularly a constitutional right to health care, has played an instrumental role in shaping government health care policies in relation to HIV/AIDS treatment. Martha Jackman, in this volume, persuasively argued for section 7 of the *Canadian Charter of Rights and Freedoms* to be read to encapsulate a right to publicly funded health care. The South African experience clearly illustrates the potential for such a right to provide better for the most vulnerable in society.

To draw out the nuances and implications of the South African story, this chapter is structured in three sections. The first sketches the challenge posed by the national AIDS epidemic and the South African government's policy responses in providing treatment for HIV/AIDS. The second describes constitutional obligations regarding the right of access to health care services, as interpreted by the courts. The final section assesses the contribution made by judicial enforcement of the constitutional right to health care and its relationship to changes in the government's stand on HIV and AIDS treatments.

The HIV/AIDS Epidemic in South Africa

South Africa hosts the largest number of people with HIV and/or AIDS in the world, and what was until recently the world's fastest growing epidemic. This is an unfortunate achievement in a region that is the epicentre of the global HIV/AIDS pandemic, and where an estimated 25 to 28.2 million people have HIV and/or AIDS.[1] Official national estimates are of 5.3 million people with HIV/AIDS,[2] although independent studies indicate that around 6.5 million could be infected.[3] In a country of approximately 43 million people, this amounts to infections in between 12 to 15 per cent of the total population. AIDS has become the single biggest cause of death in the country, with over 300,000 people dying per year.[4] If the epidemic's course is not interrupted by effective prevention and treatment, by 2015 more than 7 million people will die, leaving 2 million orphaned children.[5]

People in all age groups are testing positive for HIV, but the predominant demographic of infection is in the 20–29 age group, with lower but still significant rates of infection in the group 30–35 years old. While infections are found in all races and at all economic levels, they predominate among populations already experiencing social and economic vulnerabilities, especially poverty and other structural inequalities, such as those in relation to gender. Poverty intensifies susceptibility to infection, as well as magnifying the suffering experienced as a result of infection: '[I]t is the poorest South Africans who are most vulnerable to HIV/AIDS and for whom the consequences are inevitably most severe. The average age of the AIDS-sick person in the households surveyed was 35 years – in most cases these were breadwinners and the parents of young children ... [I]n already poor households HIV/AIDS is the tipping point from poverty into destitution.'[6]

The epidemic is also associated with significant levels of stigma and marginalization, manifested in pervasive discrimination in employment, health care, education, and violations of privacy rights. This deadly combination of social and economic vulnerabilities has resulted in the judicial recognition of people living with HIV and AIDS as one of the most vulnerable groups in South African society, such that 'any discrimination against them can ... be interpreted as a fresh instance of stigmatization and ... an assault on their dignity.'[7]

Impact on the Health Care Sector

Illness and death on this scale among reproductively and economically active people has vast concentric social and economic consequences, beyond the obvious devastating impact on individuals and families. Experts estimate that the longer term impact of the epidemic will be to deepen household poverty, reverse gains in human development, worsen gender inequality, erode the ability of governments to maintain essential services, and reduce labour productivity.[8] In addition there is international consensus, reflected in the 2001 U.N. Declaration of Commitment on HIV/AIDS, that AIDS is threatening social cohesion, political stability, and food security.[9]

The health sector in particular is deeply affected. A recent report commissioned by the South African Department of Health from the Human Sciences Research Council (HSRC) showed that 46.2 per cent of patients served in public medical and pediatric wards tested positive for HIV,[10] while another study found infections in 60 per cent of pediatric admissions in an urban public hospital.[11] At the same time there have been significant HIV/AIDS–related losses of health care staff, because of illness, absenteeism, and death, as well as low staff morale from the high AIDS-related patient burden.[12] The study indicates that in the absence of life-prolonging drugs such as antiretroviral therapy (ARV), South Africa can expect to lose at least 16 per cent of its health workers to AIDS in the future – a heavy burden given the current shortages of skilled personnel in public health care.[13]

Antiretroviral Drugs

While there is currently no cure for HIV infection, antiretroviral drugs can effectively halt the fatal progression of the virus and restore good health. Wherever they are used, AIDS-related illness and death rates have been slashed, shifting the definition of AIDS from a progressive fatal illness to a chronic manageable disease. The problem, however, is that until recently the drugs cost $15,000 per year for each patient, making universal access in developing countries all but impossible.[14] The average cost of ARV therapies has dropped considerably in recent years, to around $250, and in October 2003 the Clinton Foundation negotiated prices of $140 a year with generic manufacturers in South Africa and India for use in sub-Saharan African countries.[15] There are also significant new international and bilateral sources for this purpose, primarily the Global Fund for HIV/AIDS, Tuberculosis and Malaria, the World Bank Multi-Country AIDS Program for Africa and the Caribbean, and the U.S. President's Emergency Plans for AIDS. These institutions are becoming important sources of funding for countries seeking to introduce ARV; for example, Botswana's national antiretroviral program, which is currently being implemented, relies on Merck and the Gates Foundation for resources and drugs. At the same time, the World Health Organization (WHO) is championing a major advocacy drive to place three million people in developing countries on ARV by 2005, and will provide technical support to countries to do so. These measures are enabling many African countries to initiate antiretroviral drug programs, including Namibia, Zambia, Botswana, Ghana, Malawi, and Senegal.[16]

Health Care in South Africa and National Treatment Policies

While many of its poorer neighbours were starting to provide treatment, South Africa, which is one of the wealthiest countries on the African continent, continued to delay doing so. Although it is classified as a middle-income developing country, South Africa has a gross domestic product comparable to that of far more developed countries.[17] However, while South Africa has a relatively well-resourced government, its wealth is less equally distributed than in almost any country in the world,[18] with more than 50 per cent of households living in conditions of poverty,[19] and unemployment levels at over 40 per cent[20] and rising. It has a two-tier health care system that largely echoes this economic divide. The inequality has its historical roots in apartheid, which created a separate health care system for black South Africans. At the advent of democracy in 1994 the system was 'highly fragmented, biased towards curative care and the private sector, inefficient and inequitable.'[21] While one goal of the newly elected ANC government was 'a complete transformation of the national health care delivery system and all relevant institutions,'[22] access to health care in South Africa is still severely unequal. Public health care is responsible for meeting the needs of 80 per cent of the population,[23] yet it receives only 40 per cent of total funding and employs a minority of health care personnel.[24] Meanwhile, the private sector, which is accessible to less than 20 per cent of the population, consumes more than 60 per cent of the health care budget and employs more than 70 per cent of health care personnel, including psychologists, pharmacists, dentists, general practitioners, and specialists.[25] The inequities between public and private health care in South Africa are matched by interprovincial inequities in public health per capita expenditure and the distribution of health care personnel.[26]

No one can deny that the large-scale provision of AIDS drugs, which are costly and demand trained health care workers and monitoring, would place significant demands on a highly unequal health care system, and require increased public funding. However, in South Africa, the real obstacles to treatment have been more ideological than logistical.

President Mbeki and AIDS Dissidents

Shortly after he assumed the presidency, President Thabo Mbeki began to champion publicly AIDS denialist theories, which refute a causal link between HIV and AIDS, and in some cases deny the existence of an AIDS epidemic. These theories argue that immune failure from AIDS is caused by a drug-oriented and promiscuous gay lifestyle or, in the case of Africa, from malnutrition and illness associated with poverty. The demonization of antiretroviral drugs is central to this ideology: they are viewed as fatally toxic and themselves the cause of a significant number of deaths wrongly attributed to AIDS.

President Mbeki's subscription to AIDS denialist theories first became evident in 1999, at a time when there was extensive civil society lobbying for the government to provide AZT to pregnant mothers to prevent pediatric transmission of HIV. This public clamour intensified, particularly after the government's withdrawal in late 1998 of its sponsorship of a range of pilot projects around the country that would have provided short courses of AZT to pregnant women. Maternal transmission is a significant source of pediatric infections, with between 80,000 and 90,000 children infected in this way each year. In October 1999

President Mbeki addressed the National Council of Provinces, where he argued that there 'exists a large volume of scientific literature alleging that, among other things, the toxicity of [AZT] is such that it is in fact a danger to health,' and announced that he had asked the Minister of Health as a matter of urgency to research these issues to be 'certain of where the truth lies.'[27] Mbeki's support of these theories attracted international attention in 2000, when he addressed a widely publicized letter to U.S. President Clinton and other Western leaders. In the letter Mbeki argued that the particular features of the African AIDS epidemic indicated that 'a simple superimposition of Western experience on African reality would be absurd and illogical [and] would constitute a criminal betrayal of our responsibility to our own people.'[28] Rather, what Mbeki saw as necessary was a 'search for specific and targeted responses to the specifically African incidence of HIV-AIDS.'[29]

Accordingly, in 2000 Mbeki convened a Presidential AIDS Advisory Panel to advise the government on an appropriate response to the epidemic. The panel, which comprised both denialist and orthodox scientists and health professionals, was asked to answer a number of questions drawing from the central themes of denialism, including the 'viral aetiology of AIDS and related concerns about pathogenesis and diagnosis,' as well as the more generally relevant question of the 'role of therapeutic interventions in the context of developing countries.'[30] The final report reflects the unbridgeable divide between the two groups, with separate recommendations on all issues from 'panellists who do not subscribe to the causal linkage between HIV and AIDS' and those who did.[31]

To the extent that Mbeki clearly favours the dissident perspective on HIV and AIDS,[32] the report's conclusions on treatment and the use of ARV drugs are of particular interest. The denialist group 'felt strongly that anti-retroviral drugs were toxic to the point of producing disease conditions in otherwise healthy people'[33] and that 'anti-retroviral drugs and any other immune suppressive drugs should *under no circumstances* be used to treat AIDS patients or any other patients that are immune-compromised.'[34]

Despite public avowals to the contrary, South Africa's government policy has hewed closely to the recommendations made by the denialists on the Presidential Advisory Panel Report. The South African government has refused, delayed, and even actively opposed the use of ARV drugs in the public sector. Opposition is justified on the grounds of cost and the toxicity of the drugs, despite extensive scientific evidence supporting their efficacy and safety. Moreover, cost considerations clearly did not apply to the use of nevirapine, the antiretroviral drug used to interrupt mother-to-child transmission of HIV, as it was offered free by its manufacturer to the government for five years. This drug held the potential to prevent infections in 30 to 40 per cent of children infected each year. Nonetheless, the government both refused to provide the medicine and stymied others' attempts to provide access to it.

The South African Constitution

This failure to act rationally and urgently when millions of lives hang in the balance[35] seems to demand the invocation of protections at the heart of South Africa's constitutional – protections erected to guard against irrational and unaccountable governance. The South African Constitution, which is very much a product of that country's history, seeks to create an open and democratic state based on equality, dignity, and freedom – the antithesis of the apartheid state.[36] This emphasis on the creation of an open and democratic country is the primary constitutional commitment, reflected throughout the Bill of Rights.[37] The entrenchment of socioeconomic rights like health truly animate these commitments by ensuring the basic necessities of a free, equal, and dignified life and holding the state explicitly accountable for doing so. Rights to health are included as part of a bundle of socioeconomic rights to food, water, social security, housing, and education.[38]

From a North American perspective the entrenchment of justiciable social and economic rights is somewhat unorthodox. Yet, given the history and consequences of apartheid, the imperative to include these rights was strong. While apartheid was ideologically grounded in systematic racial oppression, its practical outcome was to amass wealth and develop infrastructures for the exclusive benefit of the country's white minority. This left the majority of black South Africans living in poverty, with many areas lacking adequate social services.[39] In this context, to protect only civil and political freedoms would have ignored the unjust social conditions created by apartheid, creating a paradox powerfully identified at the time by Nelson Mandela: 'The right to vote, without food, shelter and health care will create the appearance of equality and justice, while actual inequality is entrenched. We do not want freedom without bread, nor do we want bread without freedom ... A denial of such claims would be to accept the dehumanising effects of deprivation and mass poverty as the lot of the majority of our people.'[40]

Rights to Health in the Constitution

The Constitution entrenches a universal right to health care as well as health rights for specific populations, including children's rights to basic nutrition and to basic health and social services, and the rights of prisoners to adequate medical treatment.[41] The primary health right is contained in section 27, which also entrenches rights to food, water, and social security. Section 27 requires the state to provide everyone with access to health care services, including reproductive health care. It also provides that no one may be refused emergency medical treatment. Subsection 2 requires the state to take reasonable legislative and other measures, within available resources, to achieve the progressive realization of this right.

Constitutional Court Jurisprudence

The formulation of section 27 reveals little about the nature of health care services that must be provided or about the state's flexibility to refuse health care services under the limitations clause. Greater clarity with respect to the state's obligations given these limitations has emerged from the Constitutional Court's first two socioeconomic rights cases, *Soobramoney,*[42] which dealt with the right to health, and the *Grootboom*[43] case, which dealt with housing. A third case, the *Treatment Action Campaign (TAC)* decision,[44] dealing with the right to health, is discussed in the last section of this chapter.

Thiagraj Soobramoney v. Minister of Health (Kwa-Zulu Natal)
At first blush, the Court's decision in *Soobramoney* might seem to support the government's refusal to support access to expensive drugs like antiretrovirals. Mr Soobramoney approached the Constitutional Court after being refused life-prolonging renal dialysis by a state hospital. Although the hospital treated people with acute renal failure, it rationed treatment for patients suffering from chronic renal failure, who could only receive dialysis if they were also eligible for a kidney transplant. Mr Soobramoney was forty years old and suffering from various physical ailments, including diabetes, ischemic heart disease, and cerebrovascular disease which left him ineligible for a kidney transplant – and therefore for renal dialysis. His condition was irreversible and he approached the Court in the final stages of chronic renal failure.

In a judgment rendered by Justice Chaskalson, the Constitutional

Court dismissed Soobramoney's claim, finding that it had not been shown that the state's failure to provide renal dialysis facilities for all people suffering from chronic renal failure was a breach of its obligations under section 27. The Court considered that the provincial department had significantly and persistently overspent its budget in three successive years preceding the case, and that the resource limitations faced at this renal unit were shared in renal clinics throughout the country. In these circumstances, the Court found that the guidelines were a rational response to scarce resources and necessary to assist people working in clinics to 'make the agonising choices which have to be made in deciding who should receive treatment and who not.'[45] As a practical response to scarce resources, the guidelines also served to maximize the number of people who could access dialysis.[46]

While the Court denied Soobramoney's claim, its deference to the hospital's and state's rationing of health care in this case came with an important caveat. In its most significant dictum, Justice Chaskalson held that 'a court would be slow to interfere with rational decisions taken in good faith by the political organs and medical authorities whose responsibility it is to deal with such matters.'[47]

This emphasis on rational and principled decision-making is reflected in the *Grootboom* case which followed, where the Constitutional Court chose a standard of reasonableness to measure the state's compliance with its obligations with respect to socioeconomic rights.

Government of the Republic of South Africa and Others v. Irene Grootboom and Others[48]

The state's obligations vis-à-vis housing in section 26(2) of South Africa's *Constitution* are articulated in the same terms as its obligation to provide health care services – namely, to take reasonable legislative and other measures within available resources to achieve the progressive realization of the right. Thus, the *Grootboom* decision, albeit about housing rights, has important ramifications for the provision of publicly funded health care generally.

In a judgment delivered by Justice Yacoob, the Court indicated that reasonableness is determined on a case-by-case basis, looking at the social and historical context of problems and the context afforded by the Constitution.[49] Given great poverty and the constitutional commitment to equality, dignity, and freedom, the Court indicated that the state's primary obligation was to act reasonably to provide the basic necessities of life to those who lacked them.[50] The Court stressed that socioeconomic rights were entrenched because 'we value human beings and want to ensure that they are afforded their basic human needs' and that 'the poor are particularly vulnerable and their needs require special attention.'[51] These were precisely the interests at stake in the *Grootboom* case, which dealt with the rights to shelter of poor and homeless people who had been forcibly evicted by the state from the land they occupied as they waited for low-cost housing. They had been left without any shelter or sanitation, and state policy on housing, although extensive, made no provision for people deprived of housing in situations of crisis.

The Court's judgment extensively interprets the limitations clause common to sections 26 and 27, providing a road map for state compliance with the constitutional standard of reasonableness.

'Reasonable Legislative and Other Measures.' The Court indicated that at a minimum, reasonable measures require the state to devise a comprehensive and workable plan to meet its obligations, providing for all needs, including short-, medium-, and long-term needs, as well as crises.[52] Thus, legislation, policies and programs that exclude 'a significant segment of society' will be unreasonable.[53] A particular emphasis was placed on meeting the needs of the most vulnerable, especially the poor, as well as people experiencing particularly urgent and desperate needs.[54] The Court stressed that to be reasonable 'measures cannot leave out of account the degree and extent of the denial of the right they endeavour to realize. Those whose needs are the most urgent and whose ability to enjoy all rights therefore is most in peril, must not be ignored by the measures aimed at achieving realization of the right.'[55] In this light, health care policies solely grounded in utilitarianism would not be constitutionally sufficient: 'if the measures, though statistically successful, fail to respond to the needs of those most desperate, they may not pass the test.'[56]

The Court emphasized that the requirement of reasonableness applies to all elements of governance, not only the content of legislation, programs, and policies, but also their manner of implementation.[57] So, for instance, programs should be balanced and flexible, with the national government bearing the responsibility of ensuring sufficient laws and polices to fulfil their obligations.[58]

Progressive Realization. While progressive realization recognizes that full and immediate realization of everyone's rights is not always possible, it nonetheless does place time-bound and explicit obligations on the state. These include 'taking steps' to ensure that basic needs can be met and progressively facilitating access, with legal, administrative, operational, and financial hurdles examined and where possible lowered over time.[59] In addition, the state must move expeditiously and effectively in doing so, and it may not take any deliberately retrogressive measures.[60]

Resources. The Court recognized that resources are an important determinant of reasonableness, and the state is not required to do more than its available resources permit.[61] Resources, therefore, govern 'the content of the obligation in relation to the rate at which it is achieved as well as the reasonableness of the measures employed to achieve the result.'[62]

The Court's order declared that in terms of section 26, a comprehensive program to realize the right of access to adequate housing would have to include reasonable measures to provide relief to those with no access to land and no roof over their heads, living in intolerable conditions or in crisis. State housing fell short of compliance for its failure to do so.

Implications for AIDS Drugs

These decisions are a telling guide to the state's obligations on health care, and AIDS medicines in particular. *Grootboom* suggests that failing to address the health care needs of a significant segment of society is prima facie unreasonable, especially if the population affected is predominantly poor and experiencing urgent and desperate needs. By implication, and in the absence of persuasive justification, the state's failure to respond appropriately and in a timely fashion to the great need for AIDS treatments is constitutionally unreasonable, since these are the essential medicines necessary to treat a pandemic experienced by predominantly poor and often exceedingly vulnerable people.

Further persuasive support for this interpretation comes from international law, which holds that providing essential medicines as defined by the WHO is a 'minimum core' obligation under the right to health, with obligations to treat and control epidemic disease comparably important.[63] The minimum core is the minimum essential level of health that states have priority obligations to provide; a state cannot justify its failure to comply with its core obligations, which are non-derogable.[64] In April 2002 the WHO placed several ARV medicines onto its essential medicines list, thus bringing these drugs within the minimum core of the international right to health.[65] Indeed that access to medicines is a fundamental element of the right to health, is emphasized in three successive resolutions of the U.N.'s Commission on Human Rights.[66]

Although South Africa's Constitutional Court has chosen not to directly import the minimum core concept into domestic constitutional law, it has nonetheless indicated that the notion may be relevant to a determination of the reasonableness of state policy.[67]

The inclusion of ARV within the minimum core in international law confirms at a general level what is abundantly clear in a sub-Saharan African context: that the provision of essential AIDS drugs engages priority obligations under the right to health and requires urgent action. This observation holds important interpretive value independent of whether the minimum core concept is domestically applicable. At a minimum, international law suggests that state policy in this area should be held to a stringent standard of accountability and that, in denying such services, a state would have to mount a highly persuasive justification for its inability to do so within its resources.

The Cost of Treatment

There is no scientific evidence to support the government's contention that the toxicity of antiretrovirals justifies its failure to act.[68] Nor is there is any reason to believe that the government lacked the resources to initiate a national program, even though it would have required significant expenditures. South Africa has far more resources than other African countries that have nonetheless made treatment a possibility. Moreover, the South African government has legislative authority under both the *Patents Act*[69] and the *Medicines and Related Substances Control Amendment Act*[70] to significantly reduce the cost of essential medicines for public health care, using price controls, generic substitution, parallel importing, and compulsory licensing. Brazil provides an excellent example and through similar measures and negotiated discounts has reduced antiretroviral costs for use in its national antiretroviral program. Any shortfalls in funding could be supplemented with international and bilateral funding.

The cost argument has another key weakness. While comprehensive treatment for all HIV-infected people would be costly, over time, not treating them will be far costlier, since the state will have to bear the direct health care costs of the ill and dying and the costs of caring for orphans, as well as the broader social and economic impacts. The cost-saving benefit of ARV is confirmed in Brazil's national antiretroviral program, which literally paid for itself in averted costs of hospitalization.[71]

The up-front cost of antiretroviral medicines therefore suggests only that universal access may not be immediately realizable and must be realized progressively. In South Africa there was no legitimate justification for failing to work towards this goal, by taking steps to lower drug costs and initiating treatment where possible. Moreover, it was quite impossible to justify not providing treatment to prevent mother-to-child transmission, where the drugs had been offered free of charge to the government.

Resolution of AIDS Policies on Treatment

State policy on mother-to-child transmission became one of the most contentious issues in South Africa, attracting extensive civil society protest and media criticism, with the state's refusal seen as irrational and even genocidal. As a result in 2000 the government announced its intentions to provide nevirapine to pregnant women through a two-year pilot program of eighteen sites, at which point the government would assess whether to provide the intervention more comprehensively.

Minister of Health and Others v. Treatment Action Campaign and others

Despite this undertaking, after a year not all sites were operational and the government had actively blocked the availability of the drug in the public sector pending the completion of its pilot program. As a result, in 2001, civil society groups instituted legal action, and in Minister of Health and Others v. Treatment Action Campaign and Others[72] (the TAC case) argued that these actions breached a range of rights, including those provided for in section 27 of the Constitution. The government argued that its approach was reasonable given concerns about the safety and efficacy of the drug, resistance to the drug, and the cost of the comprehensive program required. The High Court ruled against the government, and the government appealed to the Constitutional Court, which handed down its decision in July 2002.

The Constitutional Court indirectly acknowledged President Mbeki's support of AIDS-denialist theories. According to the Court, 'in our country the issue of HIV/AIDS has for some time been fraught with an unusual degree of political, ideological and emotional contention.'[73]

The issue is not raised directly anywhere else in the judgment, but the implication that the government has based its policy on something other than its stated reasons is a strong subtext throughout the TAC decision.

Two aspects of the judgment support this sub-textual reading. The first is the way in which the Court swiftly brushed aside the government's central arguments against the comprehensive use of the medicines on the basis of safety, efficacy, and resistance to nevirapine, and the cost of a comprehensive national program. In the Court's estimation, '[m]ost if not all of [this] disputation is beside the point [and] the essential facts, *as we see them*, are not seriously in dispute.'[74] Indeed, the Court dismisses these arguments in a mere ten paragraphs, emphasizing the abundant scientific evidence supporting the intervention and the insufficiency of the concerns raised in relation to the overwhelming life interests of affected children at stake.[75] As Donna Greschner points out in her chapter in this volume, governments can legitimately refuse to fund treatments for which there is no good evidence of effectiveness. But in this case the efficacy of nevirapine was well supported by scientific evidence, albeit evidence disputed by the government. The second element of the Court's decision, implicitly hinting at the government's underlying ideological motivations, is its finding that state policy was unreasonable because of its excessive rigidity and inflexibility particularly in light of the interests at stake.[76]

The Court found that the government's policy of confining nevirapine to research and training sites failed 'to address the needs of mothers and their newborn children who do not have access to these sites. It fails to distinguish between the evaluation of programmes for reducing mother-to-child transmission and the need to provide access to health care services required by those who do not have access to the sites.'[77] The Court stressed that the case was concerned with newborn babies whose lives might be saved by the administration of a simple and cheap intervention, whose safety and efficacy had been established and which the government itself was providing in pilot sites in every province.[78]

The children's rights at stake in this case are provided in sections 28(1)(b) and (c) of the Constitution, which hold that 'every child has the right ... (b) to family care or parental care, or to appropriate alternative care when removed from the family environment; and (c) to basic ... health care services.'[79] The Court reiterated the holding in *Grootboom*, which found that 'a child has the right to parental or family care in the first place, and the right to alternative appropriate care only where that is lacking.'[80] In this case, 'the provision of a single dose of nevirapine to mother to child for the purpose of protecting the child against the transmission of HIV is, as far as the children are concerned, essential. Their needs are "most urgent" and their inability to have access to nevirapine profoundly affects their ability to enjoy all rights to which they are entitled. Their rights are "most in peril" as a result of the policy that has been adopted and are most affected by a rigid and inflexible policy that excludes them from having access to nevirapine.'[81]

The state was therefore 'obliged to ensure that children are accorded the protection contemplated by section 28 that arises when the implementation of the right to parental or family care is lacking.' This was particularly so in this case which concerned 'children born in public hospitals and clinics to mothers who are for the most part indigent and unable to gain access to private medical treatment which is beyond their means. They and their children are in the main part dependent upon the state to make health care services available to them.'[82]

The Court found that government policy failed to meet constitutional standards because it excluded those who could reasonably be included where such treatment was medically indicated.[83] It acknowledged the nature and extent of the problems facing government in its fight to combat HIV/AIDS and in particular to reduce the transmission of HIV from mother to child. However, the Court stressed that 'the nature of the problem is such that it demands urgent attention.'[84] While the Court recognized that there is a need to assess operational challenges and monitor issues relevant to the safety, efficacy, and resistance of nevirapine, it stressed that there is however also 'a pressing need to ensure that where possible loss of life is prevented in the meantime.'[85]

The Court accordingly declared that sections 27(1) and 27(2) require the government to devise and implement within its available resources a comprehensive and coordinated program to realize progressively the rights of pregnant women and their newborn children to have access to health services to combat mother-to-child transmission of HIV, with reasonable measures for counselling and testing. Present government policy fell short of compliance in two respects. First, doctors at public hospitals and clinics other than the research and training sites were not enabled to prescribe nevirapine to reduce the risk of mother-to-child transmission, *even* where it was medically indicated and adequate facilities existed for the testing and counselling of the pregnant women concerned. Second, the policy failed to make provision for counsellors at hospitals and clinics other than at research and training sites to be trained in counselling for the use of nevirapine as a means of reducing the risk of mother-to-child transmission of HIV.

The Court ordered that the government, without delay, remove the restrictions on nevirapine outside research and training sites; permit and facilitate the use of the drug and make it available at hospitals and clinics when medically indicated; make provision for the training of counsellors at public hospitals and clinics outside the research and training sites; and take reasonable measures to extend the testing and counselling facilities at hospitals and clinics throughout the public health sector.

National Treatment Plan

The *TAC* decision illustrates the tremendous potential of constitutional rights to health to hold the state to account for the provision of equitable health care and to challenge what was clearly irrational decision-making.

This decision has undoubtedly had significant influence on the outcome of the battle for a national AIDS treatment plan. On this issue, too, the state hemmed and hawed and obfuscated, attracting tremendous public protest and international condemnation, with media criticism reflecting it as a grave failure of governance. Joint efforts by labour, business, and civil society to get the government to sign onto a national treatment plan came to naught. However, in July 2002, the government established a Joint Health and Treasury Task Team to investigate issues relating to the financing of an enhanced response to HIV/AIDS, focusing on treatment. The Task Team's report was only submitted to cabinet a year later, in August 2003, and that same month the government announced plans to introduce a national treatment program.

An operational plan for a comprehensive national plan was released in November 2003.[86] The intention is to provide one HIV/AIDS service point in every health district by the end of the first year of implementation and one service point in every local municipality within five years. By 2009 the government intends to be treating 1.47 million people, the projected number of people who will have developed AIDS-related illnesses by that time. The cost of the program will grow from an initial $44.7 million to $680 million by 2008.[87] It is to be funded with entirely new public money and supplemented, where appropriate, using donor resources.[88]

Interestingly, a fundamental principle and goal of the plan is to strengthen the national health system as a whole through significant staffing and facility upgrades, including improved drug procurement and distribution, enhanced management systems, and consolidating the National Health Laboratory Service. More than half of the total expenditures will be directed towards these purposes. In deference to its constitutional obligations, the plan indicates that implementation will be equitable, with greater human and financial resources placed at the disposal of historically underserved districts.

Why Did the Government Change Its Mind?

A number of factors converged to bring about a reversal in the South African government's stance, including social pressure and persistently negative media coverage. However, enforcement of the constitutional right to health care, and in particular the *TAC* decision, arguably played a critical role. The decision showed civil society's capacity to effectively litigate this issue, and the Constitutional Court's willingness to subject health care policy to vigorous judicial review, including, where necessary, ordering constitutionally compliant programs. It made the prospect of litigation over national treatment inevitable and arguably, inevitably successful. This provided a tremendous incentive for the government to become responsive to the urgent calls for action that came from civil society as well as the media.

TAC threatened to be politically damaging for the African National Congress (the ruling party), as it approached an election year in 2003. The policy change was probably intended in large part to shore up the government's political support by addressing growing perceptions of it as irrational and uncaring. That the failure to treat AIDS had become a political liability for the state is itself a tremendous achievement, since in most countries violating the rights of people with HIV/AIDS has not traditionally attracted broad public condemnation. Clearly, in South Africa the scale of the epidemic contributed to this outcome. However, it also speaks to the efficacy of AIDS advocates in communicating the violation of rights committed by not treating, which focused media attention on the issue and mobilized broader popular support.

This brings to mind Amartya Sen's famous observation that there has never been a famine in a democratic country: because of the political incentives generated by elections, multi-party politics and investigative journalism.[89] The South African government's change in policy illustrates how effective use of the civil and political freedoms of expression, association, and media can enable better democratic responsiveness on health care. But these are imperfect guarantees of equity or justice in health care, especially for health care violations on a smaller scale, or those affecting minority populations. It is arguable that it would have been the case here, too, if not for the *TAC* decision, although clearly AIDS in South Africa had reached the magnitude of a famine to the extent that tens of millions of lives stood to be lost as a result of government inaction. In this light, the government's change in policy may have been inevitable, although at far greater cost in terms of lives lost through further delayed action. If the impact of the right to health care and the *TAC* case was only to hurry along the inevitable, in an epidemic where hundreds of people are dying every day, the contribution remains significant.

Conclusion

The South African constitutional right to access health care services makes equitable access to health care a binding obligation on the government. To some extent it ensures that decisions regarding fair access to health care are removed from the vagaries of political good will or historical contingencies. Where a state is bound by such a constitutional commitment, the courts may hold the state accountable for fulfilling it, thus preventing it from hiding behind the blind spots afforded by an overly broad judicial deference on health care policy. This gives some power to poor and vulnerable people who lack the economic, social, and political clout to influence decision-making through ordinary democratic avenues. This was certainly the case for the poor and for pregnant women and for infants, on whose behalf the *TAC* order secured a critical health service, effectively overturning irrational policies where extensive protest and advocacy had failed. As the decision in *Soobramoney* illustrates, section 27 of South Africa's Constitution will not support all claims for health care services. However, *TAC* illustrates that it does provide a substantive entitlement to more basic forms of health care, particularly where poor and vulnerable people are concerned.

Martha Jackman argues elsewhere in this book, that governmental compliance with constitutional values in Canada's *Charter of Rights and Freedoms* 'may generate more open, accountable and participatory decision-making' in health care. This insight applies equally to the South African context and to the role of judicial review of constitutional health rights. The decision in *TAC* suggests that in addition to being a substantive entitlement, section 27 demands fair, rational, and transparent decision-making with regard to health care services. In this way it becomes a critical element of the responsive, reasonable, and transparent government that constitutional democracy aspires to create, adding strength to the constitutional culture of justification. As Etienne Mureinik argues: 'leadership ... depends on the cogency of the case offered in defence of its decisions.'[90] The South African experience shows that rights of any nature hold the capacity to transform particular manifestations of inequality and poverty, as well as unresponsive and irrational governance, and that this transformative power is not simply a function of the way that rights are constitutionally entrenched, but depends quite fundamentally on the willingness of a vibrant civil society to use its rights creatively and effectively and of an independent judiciary to give these rights force and meaning. The South African experience therefore illustrates the capacity for rights and law to function as powerful gate openers to health care unreasonably denied by government.

NOTES

1 UNAIDS, *AIDS Epidemic Update 2003* (Geneva: UNAIDS, 2003).

2 South African Department of Health, *National HIV and Syphilis Sero-Prevalence Survey of Women Attending Public Antenatal Clinics in South Africa 2002,* http://www.doh.gov.za/docs/reports/2002/hiv-syphilis.pdf (accessed 29 August 2005).

3 Rob E. Dorrington, Debbie Bradshaw, and Debbie Budlender, *HIV/AIDS Profile in the Provinces of South Africa: Indicators for 2002* (Cape Town: Center for Actuarial Research, Medical Research Council and the Actuarial Society of South Africa, 2002) at 2, http://www.mrc.ac.za/bod/AIDSindicators2002.pdf (accessed 29 August 2005).

4 Rob Dorrington, David Bourne, Debbie Bradshaw, Ria Laubscher, and Ian M. Timaeus, *The Impact of HIV/AIDS on Adult Mortality in South Africa,* Technical Report, Burden of Disease Research Unit (Medical Research Council, 2001), http://www.mrc.org.za (accessed 29 August 2005).

5 Alan Whiteside and Clem Sunter, *AIDS: The Challenge for South Africa* (Cape Town: Human and Rousseau (Pty) Ltd, 2000) at 69.

6 Malcolm Steinberg *et al.,* 'Hitting Home: How Households Cope with the Impact of the HIV/AIDS Epidemic – A Survey of Households Affected by HIV/AIDS in South Africa,' October 2002, Henry J. Kaiser Family Founda-

tion, http://www.health-e.org.za/resources/household.pdf. See also Human Sciences Research Council, *Nelson Mandela/HSRC Study of HIV/ AIDS South African National HIV Prevalence, Behavioural Risks and Mass Media Household Survey 2002* (Cape Town: Human Sciences Research Council Publishers, 2002), http://www.hsrcpublishers.co.za/user_uploads/ tb1PDF/2009_00_Nelson_Mandela_HIV_Full_Report.pdf (accessed 29 August 2005) indicating that infections are highest among black South Africans, women, and in informal urban settlements.

7 *Hoffman v. South African Airways*, [2001] 1 S.Afr.L.R. 1 (S.Afr.Const.Ct) at para. 28.

8 Rene Loewenson and Alan Whiteside, 'HIV/AIDS Implications for Poverty Reduction,' United Nations Development Program Policy Paper, 2001, at 1–27, http://www.undp.org/dpa/frontpagearchive/2001/june/ 22june01/hiv-aids.pdf (accessed 29 August 2005). *See also* UNAIDS, *Report on the Global HIV/AIDS Epidemic 2002* (Geneva: UNAIDS, 2002).

9 United Nations General Assembly, 'Declaration of Commitment on HIV/ AIDS,' A/RES/S-26/2, 2 August 2001, at para. 8.

10 *Ibid*. at xiv.

11 P.M. Jeena, P. Pillay, T. Pillay, and H.M. Coovadia, 'Impact of HIV-1 Co-infection on presentation and hospital-related mortality in children with culture proven pulmonary tuberculosis in Durban, South Africa,' (2002) 6:8 Int. J. of Tuberculosis and Lung Disease, at 672–8.

12 Olive Shisana *et al.*, *The Impact of HIV/AIDS on the Health Sector: National Survey of Health Personnel, Ambulatory and Hospitalised Patients and Health Facilities, 2002* (Cape Town: Human Sciences Research Council, Medical University of South Africa and Medical Research Council, 2003), at xii, http://www.hsrcpress.co.za/user_uploads/tb1PDF/1986_pre_Impact_ HIV/ AIDS_Health_sector.pdf

13 *Ibid*.

14 All dollar figures used in this chapter refer to U.S. dollars.

15 United Nations Foundation, 'Clinton Foundation Helps Cut Cost of AIDS Drugs for Poor States,' *United Nations Wire* (24 October 2003), http:// www.unwire.org/UNWire/20031024/449_9756.asp (accessed 29 August 2005). Under the terms of the settlement of a recent court case at the South African Competition Commission between the South African Treatment Action Campaign and GlaxoSmithKline South Africa (Pty) Ltd (GSK) and Boehringer Ingelheim, companies would voluntarily license various ARV to generic manufacturers to manufacture for domestic and export use within all Sub-Saharan African countries medicines at this cost of $140 per annum. *See* Treatment Action Campaign, 'Competition Commission

Settlement Agreements Secure Access to Affordable Life-Saving Anti-retroviral Medicines,' *Newsletter* (10 December 2003), http://www.tac
.org.za/newsletter/2003/ns10_12_2003.htm (accessed 29 August 2005).

16 World Health Organization, 'The 3 by 5 Initiative,' http://www.who.int/
3by5/en/ (accessed 29 August 2005).

17 The latest UNDP human development report indicates that although
ranked 111th, South Africa's GDP is $11,290. By comparison, Chile
ranked at 43rd, has a GDP of $9,190, and Argentina, ranked at 34th, has a
GDP of $11,320. See United Nations Development Programme (UNDP),
*Human Development Report 2003: Millennium Development Goals – A Compact
Among Nations to End Human Poverty* (New York: Oxford University Press,
2003).

18 Debbie Bradshaw and Krisela Steyn (eds.), *Poverty and Chronic Diseases in
South Africa: Technical Report 2001* (Cape Town: Medical Research Council,
2001), available at www.mrc.ac.za/bod/povertyfinal.pdf (accessed
29 August 2005). South Africa has a gini co-efficient of 0.58, second globally only to Brazil.

19 Statistics South Africa, *Comparison of October Household Surveys* (Pretoria:
Statistics South Africa, 2000).

20 Statistics South Africa, *Census 2001: Census in Brief* (Pretoria: Statistics
South Africa, 2001).

21 African National Congress (ANC), 'A National Health Plan for South
Africa,' May 1994, www.anc.org.za/ancdocs/policy/health.htm, at 1
(accessed 29 August 2005).

22 See ANC, *Reconstruction and Development Programme: A Policy Framework*
(Policy Outline) (1994) at para. 2.12.5.2; see also ANC, 'National Health
Plan,' at 1.

23 Public health care spending in South Africa is $364 per capita, approx.
3.7% of the GDP. When private care is included, total health care spending
jumps to 10.3% of the GDP, with $770 per capita. Philip Musgrove, Riadh
Zeramdini, and Guy Carrin, 'Basic Patterns in National Health Expenditure,' (2002) 80:2 Bulletin of the World Health Organization 134 at 145.

24 Antoinette Ntuli, Delrida Ijumba, David McCoy, Ashnie Padarata, Lee
Berthiaume, 'HIV/AIDS and Health Sector Responses in South Africa –
Treatment Access and Equity: Balancing the Act,' Equinet Discussion
Paper No. 7, September 2003, www.equinetafrica.org/bibl/docs/
DIS7aids.pdf (accessed 29 August 2005).

25 *Ibid*.

26 *Ibid*. at chap. 3.3.

27 President Thabo Mbeki, 'Address to the National Council of Provinces' (Public Address, Cape Town, 28 Oct. 1999), www.anc.org.39/ancdocs/history/mbeki/1999/tm1028.html (accessed 29 August 2005).

28 President Mbeki, open letter to world leaders on AIDS in Africa (3 Apr. 2000). See Treatment Action Campaign (TAC), 'Statements by South African President Thabo Mbeki on the Subject of HIV/AIDS October 1999–October 2003,' www.tac.org.za/Documents/Mbeki-on-HIVAids-October2003.doc (accessed 29 August 2005).

29 *Ibid.*

30 Government of South Africa, *Presidential AIDS Advisory Panel Report: A Synthesis Report of the Deliberations by the Panel of Experts Invited by the President of the Republic of South Africa, the Honourable Mr Thabo Mbeki* (Presidential Advisory Report) (South Africa, March 2001), www.info.gov.za/otherdocs/2001/aidspanelpdf.pdf (accessed 29 August 2005).

31 The impossibility of reaching consensus is unsurprising given the chasm between accepted science on AIDS and that of the dissidents. See, e.g., the Panel Report's description of the denialist panelists' approach to HIV/AIDS, *ibid.* at 15.

32 In 2000 President Mbeki publicly withdrew from the 'public debate over HIV/AIDS.' See Carol Paton, 'AIDS: Mbeki Backs Off' Sunday Times, 15 October 2000, available at www.aegis.com/news/suntimes/2000/ST001003.html (accessed 29 August 2005). However, many of the government's statements on HIV/AIDS continue to hint at a lack of conviction of the causal link between HIV and AIDS, with policies stated to be based on the 'assumption' and the 'premise' that HIV causes AIDS. See Edwin Cameron, 'AIDS Denial and Holocaust Denial: AIDS, Justice and the Courts in South Africa' (2003) 120:3 S. Afr. L. J. 525, at 533.

33 Presidential Report, *supra* note 30 at 56.

34 *Ibid.* at 59, emphasis added.

35 The government has persistently disputed statistics on the prevalence and mortality of HIV/AIDS. When the Medical Research Council study (*supra* note 4) illustrating the extent of AIDS deaths in South Africa was released, the government refuted the accuracy of its findings, arguing that it had inflated the figures by failing to account for the general population increase as a result of the inclusion of the previously independent homelands into the country.

36 *Constitution of the Republic of South Africa*, Act 108 of 1996.

37 *Ibid.*, sections 1(a), 7(1), 36(1), and 39(1)(a).

38 *Ibid.*, sections 27 (food, water, and social security), 26 (housing), and 29

(education). Specific social and economic rights for children are entrenched in section 28.

39 Despite some progress since then, these disparities in wealth and infrastructure largely persist. In the context of rising unemployment, and despite economic growth since 1994, poverty and inequality may if anything have deepened. See Siegmar Schmidt, 'South Africa: The New Divide' (2003) 4 International Politics and Society 148.

40 Nelson Mandela, address at his investiture as Doctor of Laws, Soochow University, Taiwan, 1 August 1993, http://www.anc.org.za/ancdocs/history/mandela/1993/sp930801.html (accessed 29 August 2005).

41 *Supra,* note 36. Children's rights to basic health care services are contained in section 28(1)(c), and prisoner's rights to adequate medical treatment are contained in section 35(2)(e).

42 *Thiagraj Soobramoney v. Minister of Health (Kwa-Zulu Natal),* [1998] 1 S. Afr. L. R. 765 (CS. Afr. Const. Ct.) [*Soobramoney*].

43 *Government of the Republic of South Africa and Others v. Irene Grootboom and Others,* [2000] 11 B.Const. L.R. 1169 (S. Afr. Const. Ct.) [*Grootbroom*]

44 *Minister of Health and Others v. Treatment Action Campaign and Others,* [2002] 5 S. Afr. L.R. 721 (S. Afr. Const. Ct.) [*TAC*]

45 Soobramoney, *supra* note 42 at para. 24.

46 *Ibid.* at paras 24–5.

47 *Ibid.* at para. 29.

48 *Ibid.* note 41

49 Grootboom, *supra* note 43 at paras. 20 and 22.

50 *Ibid.* at paras. 24 and 44.

51 *Ibid.* at paras. 36 and 44, respectively.

52 *Ibid.* at paras. 38, 40, 42 and 43.

53 *Ibid.* at para.44.

54 *Ibid.* at paras. 35 and 43.

55 *Ibid.* at para. 44.

56 *Ibid.*

57 *Ibid.* at para. 42.

58 *Ibid.* at paras. 40 and 43.

59 *Ibid.*

60 U.N. Committee on Economic, Social and Cultural Rights, *General Comment 3: The Nature of State Party Obligations,* U.N. Doc. HRI\GEN\1\Rev.1 at 45 (1994), at para. 9, cited with approval in *Grootboom.*

61 *Grootboom, supra* note 43 at para. 46.

62 *Ibid.*

63 UN Committee on Economic, Social and Cultural Rights, *General Comment*

14: The Right to the Highest Attainable Standard of Health, UN Doc. E/C.12/ 2000/4 (2000) at paras. 43 and 44 [*General Comment 14*].

64 *Ibid.* at para. 47.

65 WHO, 'WHO Takes Major Steps to Make HIV Treatment Accessible: Treatment Guidelines and AIDS Medicines List Announced by WHO,' *Press Release WHO/28* (22 April 2002).

66 Commission on Human Rights resolutions 2001/33, 2002/32, and 2003/29, 'Access to Medication in the Context of Pandemics such as HIV/AIDS,' E/ CN.4/2002/2000; E/CN.4/RES/2001/33, and E/CN.4/2003/L33, respectively. The resolutions hold that 'access to medications in the context of pandemics like HIV/AIDS is one fundamental element for achieving progressively the full realization of the right of everyone to the enjoyment of the highest attainable standard of health.'

67 *Grootboom, supra* note 43 at para. 33; TAC, *supra* note 44 at para. 34.

68 While the drugs do have a high toxicity, this does not mean that they are not safe, since as the U.S. Food and Drug Administration indicate 'a safe drug is not risk free, but has reasonable risks given the magnitude of the benefit expected and the alternatives available.' However, Carr indicates that given the high morbidity associated with HIV disease, a higher degree of toxicity is considered reasonable for HAART than for other drugs. This makes patient monitoring for adherence, side effects, and toxicity a critical part of treatment regimes. See Andrew Carr, 'Improvement of the Study, Analysis, and Reporting of Adverse Events Associated with Antiretroviral Therapy' (2002) 360 Lancet 81–5, at 81, quoting from U.S. Food and Drug Administration, 'Managing the Risk from Medical Product Use: Creating a Risk Management Framework,' www.fda.gov/ oc/tfrm/riskmanagement.html (accessed 29 August 2005).

69 No. 57 of 1978 as revised.

70 No. 59 of 2002.

71 Paulo R. Teixeira, Paulo R. Teixeira, Marco Antônia Vitória, Jhoney Barcarolo, 'The Brazilian Experience in Providing Universal Access to Antiretroviral Therapy,' in Agence Nationale de Recherches sur le Sida, *Economics of AIDs and Access to HIV/AIDS Care in Developing Countries: Issues & Challenges* 2003, www.igen.org/papers.anm.php/ (accessed 29 August 2005). http://www.unaids.org/acc_access/acc_care_support/ DiscursoDrPauloARVContactGroup.doc.

72 *Supra* note 44.

73 *Ibid.* at para. 20.

74 *Ibid.* at para. 21, emphasis added.

75 All four elements of the government's defence are addressed by the Court

in *ibid.* at paras. 57–66. On efficacy, the Court indicates at para. 57 that 'the wealth of scientific material produced by both sides makes plain that … nevirapine … remains to some extent efficacious in combating mother-to-child transmission even if the mother breastfeeds her baby.' On safety, at para. 60: 'the evidence shows that safety is no more than a hypothetical issue.' On resistance, at para. 59: '[t]he prospects of the child surviving if infected are so slim and the nature of the suffering so grave that the risk of some resistance manifesting at some time in the future is well worth running.'

76 *Ibid.* at para. 78: '[Children's] rights are 'most in peril' as a result of the policy that has been adopted and are most affected by a rigid and inflexible policy that excludes them from having access to nevirapine.' At para. 95: 'The rigidity of government's approach when these proceedings commenced affected its policy as a whole.' At para. 118: 'During the course of these proceedings the state's policy has evolved and is no longer as rigid as it was when the proceedings commenced.'

77 *Ibid.* at para. 67.

78 *Ibid.* at paras. 71 and 72.

79 *Ibid.* at para. 74.

80 *Grootboom, supra* note 43 at paras. 76–7.

81 *Supra* note 44 at para. 78.

82 *Ibid.* at para. 79.

83 *Ibid.* at para. 125.

84 *Ibid.* at para. 131.

85 *Ibid.*

86 Department of Health, *Operational Plan for Comprehensive HIV and AIDS Care, Management and Treatment for South Africa 19 November 2003* (Care Plan), http://www.info.gov.za/otherdocs/2003/aidsplan.pdf (accessed 29 August 2005).

87 The costs in South African rands for 2003/4 are R296 million, growing to nearly R4.5 billion in 2007/8.

88 Operational Plan, *supra* note 86, executive summary, at para. 9.6.4.

89 Amartya Sen, *Development as Freedom* (New York: Anchor Books, 1999) at 178–84.

90 Etienne Mureinik, 'A Bridge to Where? Introducing the Interim Bill of Rights' (1994) 10 south African J. of Human Rights 31 at 32.

PART TWO

Access to Abortion and
Reproductive Health Services

5 Abortion Denied: Bearing the Limits of Law

SANDA RODGERS

The roots of these social disparities go well beyond the Abortion Law itself. They reflect how much Canadian society has dealt with a socially sensitive issue involving much stigma and fear. These disparities cannot be easily or effectively resolved by any law until there is a more widespread openness about the issue coupled with a deepened sense of social responsibility about a procedure which has involved several hundred thousand Canadian women in recent years, a number increased several fold when their partners and families who are involved are also included.[1]

Badgley Report

The study of abortion is the study of law's limitations and of the women who bear them. In 1988, the Supreme Court of Canada struck down section 251 of the *Criminal Code*,[2] thus decriminalizing abortion. Yet despite this decision in *Morgentaler*,[3] there has been little improvement for Canadian women in the availability of abortion services. Prior to 1988, Canadian women had limited access to therapeutic abortion services and could be prosecuted for obtaining an abortion outside of the parameters of the *Criminal Code*.[4] Sixteen years later, Canadian women still have limited access to these services, although the provisions of the criminal law are silent. In contrast to the power of a constitutional right to health care in the South African context, described in the preceding chapter by Lisa Forman, the constitutional decriminalization of abortion in Canada has created the illusion rather than the reality of access to abortion.

Decriminalizing Abortion in Canada

The 1969 reforms to the Canadian *Criminal Code* provide a starting point for a brief history of abortion.[5] In that year reforms introduced section

251, providing limited legalization of abortion.[6] Section 251 provided that a woman could have an abortion if she obtained the permission of a committee of three physicians. The committee could approve an abortion at any time during pregnancy, so long as the pregnancy would or likely would 'endanger her life or health.' Without permission, both the woman and her physician were subject to incarceration, the physician for life and the woman for a maximum of two years.

The 1969 amendments proved a disappointment to women. In 1975 the federal government commissioned a report on whether section 251 operated equitably across Canada.[7] The 1977 *Badgley Report* provided the first comprehensive study of abortion and concluded: 'It is not the law that has led to the inequities in its operation or the sharp disparities in how therapeutic abortions are obtained by women within cities, regions, or provinces. It is the Canadian people, their health institutions and the medical profession, who are responsible for this situation. The social cost has been the tolerance of widespread and entrenched social inequality ...'[8]

The *Badgley Report* found that although deaths from illegal abortions had dropped after section 251 was enacted[9] complications could be reduced if abortions were performed earlier and in specialized units. It found that the criterion of 'danger to life or health' was being applied unevenly. Additional criteria were imposed, including spousal consent,[10] gestational limitations, residency restrictions, and hospital quotas. Many hospitals had no committee, while others had a committee which never met.[11] Some hospitals were too small. Only 20.1 per cent of hospitals[12] had established committees. Obtaining permission usually took eight weeks. Abortions generally occurred at sixteen weeks, increasing risks.[13] One in five women was extra-billed[14] – that is, charged an additional out-of-pocket fee by the physician, who also received the government tariff. Among the women who were extra-billed many were 'socially vulnerable – the young, less well educated and newcomers to Canada.'[15] Data on abortion were sometimes not collected, and where collected were neither analysed nor published. In 1975, 9,627 Canadian women had an abortion in the United States.[16]

The *Badgley Report* demonstrated that abortion services were deeply compromised. Access was inadequate, in fact deceptive. Barriers were multiple and serious, jeopardized women's health and had their most serious impact on the most vulnerable. Not one government in Canada responded to the *Badgley Report*'s indictment or to the craven betrayal of Canadian women and the manipulation of the *Criminal Code* provisions.[17]

Ten years later, little had changed. In 1987 an Ontario report revealed no significant improvement in access.[18] The *Powell Report* found three to seven contacts were required to access an abortion, physician availability was limited, there was an absence of committees and, committees applied additional restrictive criteria. Of Ontario hospitals, 46 per cent had no committee, and of those with committees twelve performed no abortions. Others imposed quotas and gestational limits. Committees required as many as three letters of referral. Some required reports from a social worker or psychiatrist.[19] Administrative fees from $20 to $500 were imposed, which women were required to pay out of pocket. To obtain access to an abortion many women had to pay their own travel and accommodation expenses. Marriage or repeat abortions were grounds for refusal. Operating room time influenced the number of procedures a hospital would perform.[20] Some hospitals failed to use techniques known to reduce complications.[21] Powell noted that committee permission was an anomaly in health care. She noted that women were subjected to unprofessional and negligent conduct, to unsupportive behavior and outright hostility by staff, to treatment that was based on stereotypes of women as irresponsible and promiscuous, to punitive care including minimal anaesthetic, breaches of confidentiality, and forced sterilization before a repeat abortion would be authorized.[22] In 1984, legislation had been introduced in Ontario banning extra-billing. Powell noted that some of the reduction in abortion services was a result of physician protest towards that ban.[23]

In the years following the *Badgley Report*, Dr Henry Morgentaler ignored section 251. He performed abortions in private clinics without committee permission and did not limit them to women whose 'life or health' was in danger. Remarkably, in Quebec and Ontario, Canadian juries refused to convict him of unlawfully performing abortions.[24]

In 1981 Canada repatriated its constitution, adding the *Canadian Charter of Rights and Freedoms*.[25] The *Charter* contained a list of the fundamental rights from which federal and provincial governments may not derogate easily. When Dr Morgentaler was charged with performing an abortion in a private clinic, he argued that section 251 violated his constitutional rights under the *Charter*. The Supreme Court of Canada agreed, striking down section 251. Abortion was no longer a crime.

The *Badgley* and the *Powell* reports formed the factual and contextual basis for the decision of the Supreme Court in *Morgentaler*.[26] Dickson, C.J., began by noting that 'as is so often the case in matters of interpretation ... the straightforward reading of this statutory scheme is not fully revealing. In order to understand the true nature and scope of s. 251, it is necessary to investigate the practical operation of the provisions.'[27] He referred to the reports on issues of delay,[28] complication and mortality rates,[29] psychological injury,[30] the low number of hospitals with functioning committees,[31] the arbitrary definition of 'danger to life or health,'[32] and the need for women to travel or leave Canada to obtain an abortion.[33] There are nine references to the *Badgley Report* and nine to the *Powell Report* in his reasons. Beetz, J. (Estey, J., concurring) referred to *Badgley* sixteen times and to *Powell* thirteen times.[34] Without these studies, it is questionable whether the appellants could have marshaled a sufficient evidentiary basis to support their claim that section 251 violated women's *Charter* rights.

Chief Justice Dickson (Lamer, J., concurring) was of the view that section 251 infringes a woman's right to security of the person as well as her section 7 right to control her body.[35] Justice Wilson took an even broader approach holding that section 251 violated both section 2 freedom of conscience and section 7 rights to liberty and security.[36] Justice Beetz (Estey, J., concurring) found a breach of section 7 of the *Charter*. In his view access to a committee was often unavailable.[37] Delays increased the physical and psychological risk to the woman, creating constitutionally impermissible increased risk and delay. Justice McIntyre (LaForest, J., concurring), in dissent, found section 251 to be constitutional. In his view, any delay was caused by women who requested an abortion but failed to meet the requirements of the section 251 defence.[38] These requests caused queues and delays that impacted on women who were entitled to an abortion.[39] The decision of McIntyre, J., is a classic example of blaming the victim.

The Federal and Provincial Governments Respond

The Supreme Court's decision in *Morgentaler* spotlighted the importance of provincial governments in the provision of abortion services. Provision of health care is within provincial jurisdiction, and federal authority is limited at best. However, the federal government may criminalize behavior which is appropriately the subject of criminal law. It also makes significant funding available to the provinces to finance provincial health plans. Once section 251 was struck down, provincial regulation of doctors, hospitals, and access to health care services applied to abortion as to any other procedure.

The federal government's response was to introduce legislation to replace section 251. In November 1989 Justice Minister Lewis introduced Bill C-43,[40] recriminalizing abortion. The Bill was approved 140 to 131 in the House of Commons; however, on 31 January 1991 it was defeated in the Senate by a vote of 44 to 43. By that time Justice Minister Kim Campbell announced that no further legislation would be introduced.

Following the defeat of *Bill C-43* provincial responses differed dramatically. Ontario funded abortion in hospitals and in clinics. Other provinces reinstituted limits to abortion that the Supreme Court of Canada had found unconstitutional. British Columbia, Manitoba, New Brunswick, Nova Scotia, and Prince Edward Island passed legislation or regulations designed to recreate section 251. British Columbia implemented regulations providing that abortion would not be insured unless performed in a hospital, where a 'significant threat exists to that person's life.' These regulations were struck down.[41] Manitoba regulations refusing coverage for abortions performed outside of a hospital also were struck down.[42] A New Brunswick amendment which provided that abortions outside a hospital constituted professional misconduct was found unconstitutional.[43] Nova Scotia legislation, which prohibited the privatization of health care services outside of hospitals, was struck down.[44] Provisions in Prince Edward Island, providing coverage only for abortions performed in hospital and authorized as medically necessary by a committee of five doctors, were upheld. Arguably, this case was wrongly decided.[45]

Following the *Morgentaler* decision, anti-abortion activists increased their protests. They picketed clinics, engaged in sidewalk counselling and organized prayer vigils. They displayed graphic protest signs. They blocked staff and clients who were entering clinics. They damaged property. The Morgentaler Clinic in Toronto was fire-bombed and a guard was killed. In 1994, Dr Garson Romalis was shot in his home in British Columbia. In 2000 he was stabbed. The following year Dr Hugh Short of Ontario was shot. Two years later, Dr Fainman was shot in Winnipeg.

Ontario and British Columbia responded to increased picketing and increasing violence by establishing a 'bubble zone' within which protest was prohibited. In 1994 Justice Adams allowed an application by the Ontario government for an interlocutory injunction restricting abortion protest activity.[46] Similarly, in 1995, the British Columbia legislature passed the *Access to Abortion Services Act*[47] creating a protected access zone around clinics. This legislation also was upheld.

Accessing Legal Abortion after 1988

Following the invalidation of section 251 and the decriminalization of abortion, only three governments commissioned studies of access. All three found no real improvement in the availability of abortion. Instead, they described the continuing barriers women faced.

The first, commissioned by Ontario in 1992, used a broader definition of accessibility than that used by *Badgley* and *Powell*. The intention was to document social as well as medical barriers to access including 'first language, how much money she has, her race or origin, or where she lives.'[48] The authors considered accessibility for young women, poor women, women living with disabilities, aboriginal women, women of colour, and immigrant and refugee women, as well as for women in rural, remote, and northern communities. The *Report on Access* concluded that abortion services remained inequitable and inaccessible. It noted that training opportunities for providers needed expansion and asserted that no public facility should be allowed to refuse to provide abortions. It exposed cases where anti-abortion physicians and others were purposely delaying or refusing to refer women to providers. It noted that providers were subject to increasing harassment and that protesters targeted the most vulnerable, including women alone, immigrant women, and women of colour, subjecting them to more extreme harassment than they did white women or those accompanied by a man. It confirmed that breaches of confidentiality, mistreatment, and insensitivity remained frequent and that the young, disabled, aboriginal, and refugee women and women of colour were particularly mistreated.

A second report was commissioned the same year by the Northwest Territories,[49] where the Stanton Yellowknife Hospital was the only facility performing abortions. The Status of Women Council had reported a flood of complaints of excessively painful procedures and uncaring attitudes from staff. The *NWT Report* described a lack of communication and the refusal to provide appropriate anaesthetic and pain relief to women.[50] Doctors opposed to abortion were refusing to provide referrals.[51] Delays were serious and increased risk. Women travelled long distances. The barriers of travel and cost were significant. Many women were members of the First Nations community. Three women received an intrauterine device (IUD) immediately following the abortion procedure, which is contraindicated and increases the risk of infection. The *NWT Report* noted numerous instances of failure to communicate; raising the question of the legitimacy of consent obtained for abortion procedures or for the insertion of an IUD. It seems highly unlikely that a woman fully apprised of the risks of inserting an IUD immediately following an abortion would agree to the procedure. The *NWT Report* documented barriers to filing a complaint and complaints that had been ignored.

A 1994 British Columbia report provided further evidence of racist delivery of services and the imposition of contraception on Aboriginal women and on women with disabilities.[52] Poor women, women with disabilities, and Aboriginal women all experienced coercive contraception, pressure to terminate a pregnancy or to use permanent or long-term forms of contraception such as sterilization or Depo-Provera.[53]

Despite these barriers, issues of access have fallen from both federal and provincial agendas, leaving the non-governmental, privately financed Canadian Abortion Rights Action League (CARAL)[54] to provide us with a current picture of access to services. CARAL has issued two outstanding reports, the first marking the tenth anniversary of the *Morgentaler* (1988) decision, the second the fifteenth anniversary.[55] The *CARAL 1998 Report* found that access to abortion had decreased since 1988. The 2003 study documented a further erosion of abortion services.[56] The 2003 study was designed to measure the accessibility of services offered by those hospitals which do provide abortion services.

The *CARAL 2003 Report* identified the myriad difficulties that women face. The most serious barriers identified included travel, followed by anti-choice doctors, lack of information, long waiting periods, gestational limits, and unsolicited anti-choice counselling. Other barriers included increased violence by anti-choice activists, fewer service providers, and a failure to train physicians to provide abortion services. Financial barriers remained significant. Where women were not covered by provincial funding, the charges ranged from $250 to $1,425.[57] Other barriers included partner coercion and parental consent requirements.

The *CARAL 2003 Report* also noted that hospital closings and the amalgamation of religious and non-sectarian hospitals further reduced the number of hospitals providing services.[58] Between 1997 and 1998 the number of Roman Catholic–operated hospitals grew by 11 per cent, while secular public facilities declined by 2 per cent. Of 127 hospital mergers between 1990 and 1998, half resulted in the elimination of all or some reproductive health services that had been available.[59]

CARAL's 2003 study presents a grim snapshot: only 17.8 per cent or 123 of all general hospitals in Canada provided abortion services. Prince Edward Island and Nunavut have neither hospitals *nor* clinics providing abortion services. Some provinces offered no *publicly funded* hospital-based abortion services.[60] The number of hospitals providing abortions varied widely from province to province.[61] Manitoba, New Brunswick, and Saskatchewan fund hospital abortions but provide no funding for clinic abortions.[62]

Quebec and Nova Scotia provide hospital abortions and partial clinic funding. Alberta, British Columbia, Ontario, and Newfoundland fund both hospital and clinic abortions. Provinces place caps on the number of abortions performed.[63] Even where hospitals do provide services, barriers are significant, ranging from requiring physician referrals – two physicians in New Brunswick – to waiting times of as much as six weeks.[64] Many hospitals imposed gestational limits.[65] Two hospitals required abortion to be used only after other alternatives had been considered, or only as a 'last resort.'

Hospitals that do offer services provided false, misleading, or inadequate information to women who inquire about the availability of services. Misinformation or deliberately misleading information was being given out by some doctors[66] and by some hospital switchboard operators.[67] One woman in New Brunswick was told by her family physician that he would no longer provide family medical care if she obtained an abortion. The limited availability of family physicians in the province makes this a serious threat.

In Alberta, British Columbia, Ontario, and Newfoundland – provinces that fund both hospital and clinic abortions – and Quebec, which provides broad hospital and Centres Locaux de Services Communautaires (CLSC)–based services, barriers remain significant. In other provinces, Prince Edward Island in particular, barriers remain impenetrable. We cannot conclude that all women who would choose to terminate their pregnancies are able to do so. We only know that in 1990, 91,476 women were able to access abortions,[68] and that in 2000 that figure had dropped slightly from a high in 1997 of 111,526 to 105,669.[69] It may be that fewer women now experience unsustainable pregnancies. More likely, women are unable to terminate pregnancies in accordance with their own needs and aspirations. In the absence of accessible health care services and accurate health care data, federal and provincial women's health policy is built on fairytales.

Abortion and Women's Health

Despite the continuing impediments to affordable and timely access, 105,669 Canadian women had an abortion in 2000; two-thirds in hospitals and the balance in clinics.[70] Abortion is essential health care. The federal government recognizes abortion as a 'medically necessary' health care service and thus one which should be publicly funded in accordance with the *Canada Health Act* (CHA).[71] All provinces and territories recognize that abortion is 'medically necessary' care, but many nonetheless limit their funding to specified parameters which often render access illusory, result in constitutionally impermissible delay, or require women to leave their home provinces. Under the CHA,[72] to qualify for federal funding provincial health care services must be accessible, universal, portable, comprehensive, and publicly administered. The CHA effectively prohibits private financing for 'medically required' physician services or 'medically necessary' hospital services. Failure to define these key terms encourages the provinces to impose the various barriers described earlier.

Despite the federal government's recognition that abortion is medically necessary, it has displayed a profound lack of attention to abortion as a health care issue. Funding arrangements under the CHA reflect the division of powers between the provincial and federal governments.[73] Thus, any serious attempt to ensure that provinces provide accessible abortion services, without extra costs paid by the user or charged by the service provider, requires the federal government to insist that the provinces comply or to impose penalties on the provinces for failing to do so.[74] Generally, the federal government has been reluctant to impose even the minimal penalties required by the provisions of the CHA. Because abortion is a medically necessary health care service, extra billing and user charges associated with it are the subject of mandatory (dollar for dollar) penalties under the CHA. However, the federal government has never demonstrated willingness to impose harsher penalties on provinces which fail to comply with the principles of Canadian health care. The provinces have been willing to forgo the minimal funds that the federal government has withheld, rather than to address the issue of privatized health care services generally or abortion in particular.[75] Given the highly politicized nature of health care services generally and abortion in particular, this is not likely to change.

Not surprisingly therefore, a recent motion designed to further undermine abortion was phrased as a query about medical necessity. Introduced in the House of Commons in October 2003, the motion called on the Standing Committee on Health to 'fully examine, study and report to Parliament on: (a) whether or not abortions are medically necessary for the purpose of maintaining health, preventing diseases or diagnosing or treating an injury, illness or disability; and [on] (b) the health risks for women undergoing abortions compared to women carrying their babies to full term.'[76] The motion was defeated 139 to 66.

The lack of attention is further demonstrated by the failure of Health Canada to consider sex and gender as determinants of health until very recently. [77] In 1999 Health Canada commissioned an Advisory Committee Report to redress this oversight.[78] In 2000 the Committee recommended collection of data specific to barriers to health care, including occupation, socioeconomic status, student status, educational level, work and child care, as well as time, distance and availability of services.[79] The Committee concluded '[t]here is no leadership in the area of abortion at the federal level ...'[80] In 2003, Health Canada issued a *Women's Health Surveillance Report*[81] containing specific chapters on sexual health, contraception, and perinatal care, but no new data on access to abortion. Instead, it repeated previously published teen pregnancy and abortion rates, recommended improvement in pregnancy prevention, and noted (again) the insufficient data available for analysis. The 2003 Statistics Canada *Health Indicators Report* provided information that was not disaggregated by gender.[82]

In 2001 Roy Romanow headed a Royal Commission to determine the future of health care. In the 392-page *Romanow Report*, the word 'abortion' appears only once, in a string reference to for-profit clinic service provision.[83] Even the gender critique of the *Romanow Report*, published by the National Coordinating Group on Health Care Reform and Women,[84] offered no discussion specific to abortion. It did note that the *Romanow Report* failed to take women's health needs into account and failed to discuss reproductive health services.[85] In contrast, a recent major American report on women's health used access to an abortion provider as one of four indicators of access to health care and identified unintended pregnancies as a 'Key Health Condition' indicator for women.[86]

Romanow did recognize the increasing privatization of health care and raised concerns about the use of independent facilities to deliver privatized services:[87] 'Early in my mandate, I challenged those advocating radical solutions for reforming healthcare – user fees, medical savings accounts, de-listing services, greater privatization, a parallel private system – to come forward with evidence that these approaches would improve and strengthen our health care system. *The evidence has not been forthcoming* ... There is no evidence these solutions will deliver better or cheaper care, or improve access (except, perhaps, for those who can afford to pay for care out of their own pockets).'[88]

Although privatization is not the only barrier to abortion services in Canada, clinic-based abortions constitute a striking and early example of privatized parallel health care. Furthermore, privatized abortion services have been offered on a number of models, in some cases at the same clinic location. Some women pay the entire cost of the procedure; others pay a supplemental fee while the provincial health plan funds the basic fee. In some cases the service occurs at public expense in a private clinic, in others the clinic itself is fully publicly funded. These various models of service delivery have changed over time, in part in response to the regime of legal regulation applicable. Privatization is often seen as the appropriate response to delays endemic to the public delivery of health care services. Yet abortion, the sine qua non of the need for timely care, has not been assessed as a subject of privatized care. It is deeply regrettable that abortion, both publicly and privately funded, was not evaluated in the search for evidence of the benefits and deficits of privatization and that this available demonstration of the impact of privatization on women was not studied.

Arguably, it is women who have the least to gain from for-profit private parallel systems.[89] Women lack autonomous household income, have fewer financial resources, are less likely to have health coverage through paid work, have fewer pension resources and are more likely to be poor. A study of even the limited information already available regarding abortion clinics would have provided invaluable information on the impact of privatization. Ironically, access to abortion services is so compromised in the public sector that private clinics have increased access for some women in some provinces – mainly women with financial resources – who are disproportionately white, middle class, educated women living in urban areas. Romanow's commitment to public health care is important for women, but his failure to address an important location of privatization, and its race-, gender- and class- specific impact is unacceptable. A careful study of the delivery of abortion services in Canada might well have provided information of value to Canadian women concerned about access to health care at the same time as it provided Romanow with important evidence concerning the impact of privatization on service delivery.

The Limits of Law

In Canada, access to publicly funded health care is widely acknowledged as a primary value of the Canadian state. Women, too, are entitled to health care. Access to health care includes access to repro-ductive health care, including therapeutic abortion.[90] The second gen-eration of reports on access to abortion mapped the broad range of barriers to women's access and provided disturbing detail on the de-gree of discriminatory conduct and of serious malpractice by hospital employees and medical practitioners.

Some barriers are endemic to accessing health care services generally, and will exist regardless of the organization of service delivery as public or private. However, barriers to abortion differ in dramatic ways from barriers to health care services generally. While all health care services are more difficult to access for rural or northern residents, abortion is characterized by a need for care within strict time limits. While access to sophisticated services requiring tertiary-care hospitals, specialists, and technology always is easier for those who live in urban environments, abortion is a procedure that can easily and safely be performed as day surgery outside of a hospital and should be available without the need to travel or to endure long waits for scarce urban specialists. While obtaining health care generally is more difficult for those not fluent in the dominant language, familiar with institutions and comfortable with professionals, abortion is the most stigmatized of health care services. While certain health care is not 'medically neces-sary' and must be purchased privately, cosmetic surgery or in vitro fertilization, for example, abortion is basic health care, recognized as 'medically necessary' by all provinces, but for which some women must pay. While access to some health care is rationed for reasons of cost or therapeutic appropriateness, abortion is denied for reasons of inappropriate political expediency or provider morality. While concern over delays in cardiac or cancer care engage political attention and generate fundraising initiatives and public-private partnerships, con-cern over abortion is considered political poison. The *CARAL 2003 Report* detailing diminished necessary health care for women, scandal-ously provided and scandalously withheld, received not a single press report.[91]

Individual service providers, doctors, nurses, reception staff in hospi-tals, and others, deliberately place obstacles in the way of women seeking services. Health care professionals, who withhold a diagnosis of pregnancy, threaten to withdraw services, fail to provide women with appropriate referrals, delay access, misdirect women to anti-choice organizations, or provide punitive treatment, commit medical malprac-tice.[92] Doctors who do so breach the provisions of the Canadian Medical Association's *Code of Ethics* prohibiting discrimination on the basis of gender, marital status, and medical condition.[93] They violate the CMA policy on matters related to induced abortion, including the obligation to provide counselling and early diagnosis without delay or refer the patient elsewhere, and to provide abortion services in accordance with specified standards of care.[94] They breach their obligations to provincial licensing bodies, giving rise to actionable conduct arguably subject to disciplinary action.[95] Other health care professionals have similar obligations, breach of which would violate their professional codes of conduct. While self-regulation of the medical and related health care professions is understood to be in the public interest, there is no evidence that any formal complaint has been filed against any doctor for failure to respond to the health care needs of a pregnant woman requiring information.[96] Instead, at least one provincial regulatory body, the College of Physicians and Surgeons of New Brunswick, recently issued a member's policy directive that seems to contradict the positions of both the CMA and the College of Obstetricians and Gynaecologists of Canada.[97] In a *Guideline* entitled *Moral Objections* the College advised: 'Council also feels that, while it is not an obligation to do so, it is preferred practice for physicians who have ... objections [to abortion] to refer the patient to another where such objections may not arise. Nevertheless, if the physician feels even that is unacceptable, Council does view it as an acceptable alternative for the physician to provide information, *upon the patient's request*, regarding resources which may be directly accessible to the patient'[98] (emphasis added).

Not only does this position appear to contradict the *Code of Ethics* but, in placing the obligation on the patient to ask for information, it contradicts the obligations imposed by the principles of informed consent.[99] Because abortion is not just a health care service denied but a health care issue denied, it has been and continues to be, at best, a site of political posturing[100] and professional indifference and, at worst, of manipulation and violence.[101] The failure of professional organizations and of legislatures to insist that medically necessary services be provided in a professional and non-discriminatory manner should shock us. Instead, individual women are left to bear the lack of access, privately, in stigmatized silence.

Earlier litigation strategies resulted in the removal of legal barriers at the federal and the provincial levels. Obstacles imposed at the federal level through *Criminal Code* prohibitions and by provincial legislation have been held unconstitutional. The decision in *Morgentaler* freed woman from criminal sanctions for pursuing an abortion. Provincial barriers imposed following *Morgentaler* generally were found to be a usurpation of federal criminal law powers, rather than a violation of *Charter* protections.[102] New challenges to the lack of access to services and to the requirement that women pay for abortion are pending in Quebec,[103] Manitoba,[104] and New Brunswick.[105] Other legal challenges will follow.

Subsequent *Charter* litigation has made some progress toward defining a right to health care in some circumstances.[106] Evolving jurisprudence imposes liability on hospitals for breach of the *Charter* in certain cases. *Charter* entitlement to *meaningful non-discriminatory access* to health care services was affirmed by *Eldridge v. B.C. (AG)*.[107] Health care services funded by the federal government and offered by the provinces may be limited, but such limitations must comply with *Charter* principles.[108] Continued government funding of provincial health plans by both federal and provincial governments in the light of these well- and oft-documented barriers to abortion, condones[109] *Charter* violations by delegated decision-makers, suggesting government liability for *Charter* breach. It is likely that a decision to remove abortion services from the list of 'medically necessary' services would violate *Charter* protections under section 7 and section 15.[110] Federal or provincial government-imposed civil restrictions that effectively deny access, or that augment delay, increase risk, and interfere with freedom of conscience and that specifically discriminate against women are all impermissible infringements of sections 2, 7, and 15 of the *Charter*, requiring demonstrable justification under section 1.[111]

In *Eldridge* the Supreme Court of Canada recognized that in providing medically necessary services, hospitals carry out specific government objectives[112] and are therefore subject to *Charter* requirements.[113] The Court held that health care services offered in such a way as to render them fundamentally inaccessible, breached *Charter* guarantees where the group affected could claim protection under section 15(1).[114] Failure to provide, or grossly insufficient provision of, medically necessary hospital or clinic services, unjustifiable delays arising from quotas, unreasonably limited surgical time for such services or other barriers arising from politically motivated rather than medically justifiable criteria, arguably violate section 7 provision for protection of life, health, and security of the person, section 2 protection of freedom of conscience, and section 15 prohibition on discrimination in health care.

Such barriers organize care necessary to women differently from care needed by men, and particularly impact on specifically protected groups of women.[115] Discriminatory delivery of medically necessary health services needed only by women is clear sex discrimination.[116] Where discriminatory delivery of medically necessary services disproportionately impacts racialized, immigrant, aboriginal, and poor women it violates section 15 protections on grounds of race and citizenship. There is evidence of discrimination on other enumerated and analogous grounds.

In *Auton*[117] the British Columbia Court of Appeal recognized that where the only effective treatment for autism was not provided by the province, and lack of access would have a profound and irremediable effect on children in need of treatment, funding could be ordered. In support of their reasons they relied on prohibitions against age and disability discrimination in section 15 of the *Charter*, as well as on obligations assumed by Canada as a signatory to the U.N. *Convention on the Rights of the Child*.[118] While the Supreme Court of Canada disagreed on appeal, additional cases are before the courts challenging this view.[119] In *Jane Doe 1 v. Manitoba*[120] the trial court upheld a class action on behalf of women who, in light of the six- to eight-week waiting period for a publicly funded hospital based abortion, choose a privately paid clinic abortion. The plaintiffs argued that because only women access abortions services, legislative restrictions on access violate section 15 of the *Charter* and 'imposes an unfair burden on women by forcing them to pay for medical services to be received in a safe and timely fashion as distinct from the rest of the population.'[121] They also argued breach of section 2(a) and of section 7. Relying on *Morgentaler*, Oliphant, J., found a violation of sections 2(a) and 7 to be: '[L]egislation that forces women to have to stand in line in an overburdened, publicly funded health care system and to have to wait for a therapeutic abortion, a procedure that provably must be performed in a timely manner, is a gross violation of the right of women to both liberty and security of the person ...'[122] An appeal has been filed by the Province.

Forced pregnancy has a long-term and pervasive impact on the lives of women who are precluded from terminating pregnancies they are unable to support. International obligations inform *Charter* analysis. Canada and the provinces[123] have obligations to ensure women's equality with regard to health care under the *Convention on the Elimination of All Forms of Discrimination against Women* (the *CEDAW Convention*).[124]

Thus, where no services are provided, as in Prince Edward Island, or in provinces where services are so limited as to be virtually unavailable in any meaningful way,[125] section 15 liability may well be engaged.

Conclusion

Despite legal victories, twenty-five years after the *Badgley Report* and fifteen years after *Morgentaler*, the insufficient and abusive provision of abortion services continues to violate women's equality protections under Canada's *Charter of Rights and Freedoms*. We have documented evidence of federal indifference to, and provincial defiance of *Morgentaler*. We have detailed reports of multiple gatekeepers, provider malpractice, and delays by professionals and governments that increase risk. We have descriptions of interference with women's constitutional rights to security of the person, equality, and freedom of conscience. We know that some women – aboriginal, disabled, racialized, rural, poor, immigrant, and young – bear an even greater share of the burden of justice denied. The reality for women without the economic and other resources to access available abortion services is that *Charter* protections are rhetorical at best. *Charter* expertise has grown significantly. Women's access to abortion has failed to keep pace. Despite *Charter* protections, access to abortion services has proved elusive at best for Canadian women.[126] The costs, delays, and lack of public funding to advance further legal challenges to inadequate services, and the limited impact of the victories that have been achieved, suggest that it is women who will continue to bear law's limitations despite their right to law's protection. For women who find themselves pregnant, access delayed is justice denied.

NOTES

I wish to thank the Social Sciences and Humanities Research Council for providing financial support for this project and Ms Tasha Yovetich for her excellent research assistance.

1 Canada, *Report of the Committee on the Operation of the Abortion Law* (Ottawa: Minister of Supply and Services [MSS] Canada, 1977) (Chair: Robin Badgley) at 17 [*Badgley Report*].
2 R.S.C. 1970, c. C-34.

3 *R. v. Morgentaler*, [1988] 1 S.C.R. 30 [*Morgentaler*].

4 Between 1900 and 1972 there were 1,793 persons in Canada who were charged with procuring or attempting to procure an abortion, 64.4% were convicted. See *Badgley Report supra* note 1 at 68 for detailed figures.

5 See Janine Brodie, Shelley A.M. Gavigan, and Jane Jenson, *The Politics of Abortion* (Toronto: Oxford University Press, 1992); Gail Kellough, *Aborting Law: An Exploration of the Politics of Motherhood and Medicine* (Toronto: University of Toronto Press, 1996).

6 *Criminal Code*, R.S.C. 1970, c. C-34, section 251. The same omnibus revisions removed the previous criminal prohibition on the distribution of contraception and information on family planning.

7 *Badgley Report, supra* note 1 at 27. The Terms of Reference were to conduct a study to determine whether the procedure provided in the *Criminal Code* for obtaining therapeutic abortions 'is operating *equitably* across Canada' (emphasis added).

8 *Ibid.* at 25.

9 *Badgley Report, supra* note 1 at 29. Between 1962 and 1966 abortion was the leading cause of death, accounting for 19.7% of deaths for women in Ontario; deaths from self-induced or illegal abortions dropped from 12.3 per year in 1958–69 to 1.8 in 1970–74.

10 *Ibid.* at 32.Two-thirds of hospitals performing abortions required spousal consent. Some required spousal consent even where the woman was separated or divorced and required the consent of the biological father if the woman was unmarried.

11 *Ibid.* at 30. 'If equity means the quality of being equal or impartial, then the criteria used by hospital therapeutic abortion committees across Canada were inequitable in their application and their consequences for induced abortion patients.'

12 *Ibid.* at 31. The Committee considered non-military hospitals only.

13 In 1981 U.S. data indicated that the risk of complications doubled from 2 per thousand to 4 per thousand women where abortions were performed at between 8 and 12 weeks' gestation, rising to 17 per thousand women at 17 weeks' gestation. Death rates, while generally low, increased by 40 to 60% per week for each week of delay after 8 weeks. Frederick S. Jaffee, Barbara L. Lindheim, and Phillip R. Lee, *Abortion Politics* (New York: McGraw-Hill, 1981). Canadian data published in 1977 showed complication rates of 1.6 per thousand women at 9–12 weeks, rising to 16 per thousand women at 17–20 weeks. *Badgley Report, supra* note 2 at 299. See also Surinder Wadhera and Cyril Nair, 'Early Complications of Legal Abortions, Canada, 1975–1979' (1984) 37 World Health Statistics Quarterly

84, which shows an increase in complications as a function of gestational age and a risk eleven times greater after 13 weeks' gestation; and Roy. G. Smith, James A. Palmore, and Patricia G. Steinhoff, 'The Potential Reduction of Medical Complications from Induced Abortion' (1978) 15 Int. J. Gynaecol. Obstet. 337, which indicates that complications after abortion are five times higher when performed at 13–16 weeks' gestation rather than during the first trimester.

14 Nationally 20.1% were extra-billed, although in Alberta 91.6% of women were extra-billed. Extra-billing for abortion services was significantly higher than extra billing for other services, e.g., extra billing generally was 2.9% for medical services in Nova Scotia, while for abortion services it was 44.8%. In some cases the provinces imposed extra payments that violated provincial health insurance regulations. *Badgley Report, supra* note 1 at 393.

15 *Ibid.* at 405.

16 As would Chantal Daigle fourteen years later. *Tremblay v. Daigle,* [1989] 2 S.C.R. 530.

17 The *Badgley Report* noted that there had been no detailed reviews by the provinces of the *Criminal Code* committees, the guidelines used, decisions made, or complications associated with abortion or childbirth. *Supra* note 1 at 22.

18 Ontario Ministry of Health (OMH), *Report on Therapeutic Abortion Services in Ontario,* prepared by Marion Powell (Ottawa: MSS, 1987) [*Powell Report*].

19 *Ibid.* at 28.

20 *Ibid.* at 29.

21 *Ibid.* at 30. She speculated that the procedures that were used, although increasing the complication rates, comported with what the billing codes recognized by the province.

22 'This Committee violates one of the most cherished principles in the practice of medicine, namely that physicians should never make medical decisions without seeing the patient. And, unlike in a court of law, the patient in question has no grounds for appeal from its decision. The TAC is an insult to both those who favour and oppose abortion and is one of the greatest examples of malpractice this nation has ever seen.' K. Walker, 'Who's Guilty, Morgentaler or Us?' *Pro-Choice News* (Summer 1986) 8–9, cited in *Powell Report, supra* note 18 at 28.

23 Pregnant women are most often threatened with loss of health care when there is a political dispute between doctors and the provinces with regard to provincial funding arrangements.

24 *The Politics of Abortion, supra* note 5 at 30. In that period a number of

institutions called on the federal government to remove all references to abortion from the *Criminal Code*, among them the United Church of Canada, the National Council of Women, the Canadian Medical Association, Status of Women Canada, and the Committee on Medical Care and Practice of the Ontario Medical Association.

25 *Canadian Charter of Rights and Freedoms*, Part I of the *Constitution Act, 1982*, being Schedule B to the *Canada Act 1982* (U.K.), 1982, c.11.

26 *Morgentaler, supra* note 3 at 30. See also the discussion by Robert Kouri, 'Achieving Reproductive Rights: Access to Emergency Oral Contraception and Abortion in Quebec,' this volume.

27 *Ibid.* at para. 33.

28 *Ibid.* at para. 26.

29 *Ibid.* at para. 28.

30 *Ibid.* at paras. 30–1.

31 *Ibid.* at paras. 43–4.

32 *Ibid.* at para. 46.

33 *Ibid.* at para. 50.

34 *Ibid.* at paras. 89–91, 98–100, 103–4, 108, 1111, 115, 117, 121, 143–147, and 151.

35 'At the most basic, physical and emotional level, every pregnant woman is told by the section that she cannot submit to a generally safe medical procedure that might be of clear benefit to her unless she meets criteria entirely unrelated to her own priorities and aspirations. Not only does the removal of decision-making power threaten women in the physical sense; the indecision of knowing whether an abortion will be granted inflicts emotional stress. Section 251 clearly interferes with a woman's bodily integrity in both a physical and emotional sense. Forcing a woman, by threat of criminal sanction, to carry a foetus to term unless she meets certain criteria unrelated to her own priorities and aspirations, is a profound interference with a woman's body and thus a violation of security of the person.' *Ibid.* at para. 24.

36 *Ibid.* at para. 245.

37 *Ibid.* at paras. 94–6.

38 *Ibid.* at para. 204.

39 *Ibid.*: 'When, however, as the evidence would indicate, many more would seek abortions on a basis far wider than that contemplated by Parliament, any system would come under stress and possibly fail. It is not without significance that many of the appellants' clients did not meet the standard set or did not seek to invoke it and that is why their clinic took them in.'

40 *An Act Respecting Abortion*, 34th Parliament, 2nd Session, 1989.

41 *British Columbia Civil Liberties Association v. British Columbia (A.G.)* (1988), 24 B.C.L.R. (2d) 189 (S.C.).

42 *Lexogest Inc. v. Manitoba (A.G.)* (1993), 101 D.L.R. (4th) 523 (Man.C.A.).

43 *Morgentaler v. New Brunswick (A.G.)* (1995), 121 D.L.R. (4th) 431 (N.B.C.A.).

44 *R. v. Morgentaler*, [1993] 3 S.C.R. 463.

45 *Morgentaler v. P.E.I. (Minister of Health and Social Services)* (1996), 139 D.L.R. (4th) 603 (P.E.I.C.A).

46 *Ontario (A.G.) v. Dieleman* (1994), 20 O.R. (3d) 229.

47 S.B.C. 1995, c.-35.

48 OMH, Task Group of Abortion Service Providers, *Report on Access to Abortion Services in Ontario* (Toronto: Queens Park, 1992) [*Report on Access*].

49 Ministry of Health, Abortion Services Review Committee, *Report of the Abortion Services Review Committee* (Yellowknife, NWT, 1992) [*NWT Report*]; Department of Health, *Status Report: Implementation Plan for Recommendations of the Abortion Services Review Committee* (Yellowknife, NWT, 1993).

50 *NWT Report* at 27. Unstated but implicit in the report is that the services were being provided in a racist manner to members of the aboriginal community. Women were repeatedly described by the doctors providing the services as 'stoic' and therefore not needing pain relief that was standard medical practice elsewhere.

51 *Ibid.* at 10.

52 British Columbia, Minister of Health and Minister Responsible for Seniors, *Realizing Choices: Report of the British Columbia Task Force on Access to Contraception and Abortion Services* (Victoria: Minister of Health, 1994).

53 *Ibid.* at 10: 'Because they are poor, some women are pressured by health care workers and other service providers to have an abortion, or to consent to sterilization.' At 12: 'Those (women with disabilities) who do become sexually active may be coerced into accepting the forms of contraception which service providers consider to be most appropriate, including sterilization.' At 14: 'First Nations women report many, many examples of poor treatment from judgmental and unsupportive doctors and other health care professionals. They may be pressured to use long-term forms of contraception against their wishes, or to have an abortion. Women have been told that they are incapable of parenting, and that they will always be poor.'

54 A privately funded lobby group that supports reproductive choice.

55 Nancy Bowes, Varda Burstyn, and Andrea Knight, *Access Granted, Too Often Denied: A Special Report to Celebrate the 10th Anniversary of the Decriminalization of Abortion* (Ottawa: Canadian Abortion Rights Action League, 1998) [*CARAL 1998 Report*]; CARAL, *Protecting Abortion Rights in Canada: A*

Special Report to Celebrate the 15th Anniversary of the Decriminalization of Abortion (Ottawa: CARAL, 2003) [*CARAL 2003 Report*]. See also, 'Women Face Varying Rules on Abortion,' *Globe and Mail*, 29 January 1998, A4, and Kouri, in this volume, at section entitled 'Abortion: A Right Compromised by Restricted Access.'

56 In July 2000 the B.C. Women's Equality Minister Joan Smallwood stated that statistics from the Ministry of Health showed a 20% decline in providers since 1994, the year that Dr Romalis was shot. *CARAL 2003 Report.*

57 *CARAL 2003 Report, supra* note 55 at 7.

58 *Ibid.* at 8. Peterborough Civic Hospital converted its Women's Health Centre to an independent facility when it signed a shared services agreement with St Joseph's Health Centre. The hospital also stopped providing free emergency contraception. In 1998 Wellesley Hospital in Toronto, which had provided abortions, was closed and its services transferred to St Michael's Hospital; the latter does not perform abortions or vasectomies, nor does it provide free condoms or contraceptive counselling. The merger resulted in the loss of 1,000 abortions per year.

59 Childbirth by Choice Trust, *Abortion in Canada Today: The Situation Province-by-Province* (Toronto: author, 2003) available www.caral.ca/uploads/Province%20by%20province%202003.doc (accessed 6 September 2005).

60 A 1996 study also reported that the number of Canadian hospitals offering abortion services had declined. The study is reported in Raymond Tatalovich, *Canadian-American Public Policy: The Abortion Controversy in Canada and the United States*, vol. 25 (Maine: University of Maine, 1996).

61 *CARAL 2003 Report, supra* note 55 at 71. The proportion of provincial hospitals providing abortion services is: Yukon (50%), Northwest Territories (67%), Nunavut (0%), British Columbia (22%), Alberta (5%), Saskatchewan (3%), Manitoba (4%), Ontario (23%), Quebec (35%), Prince Edward Island (0%), New Brunswick (7%), Nova Scotia (10%), and Newfoundland and Labrador (14%). Only 25 hospitals have written policies on abortion.

62 There is also a free-standing private clinic in Fredericton. *Ibid.* at 24.

63 For example, the number of abortions at the Kensington Clinic in Calgary is restricted to 1,500 procedures per year allegedly because of financial constraints. The number of second trimester (after 12 weeks) procedures funded by the Calgary Regional Health Authority is limited to two per week unless they are for women who reside north of Red Deer and are unable to obtain later terminations in Edmonton. This means that women from central and northern Alberta have better access to Calgary-based

services than do women from the Calgary region. Women who are out of province or do not qualify for health care insurance also have quicker access since they are not part of the imposed quota. See *supra* note 59.

64 Of the 59 hospitals that responded to a question concerning waiting time after contact, 19 could perform an abortion within 24 hours of intake, 40 within 48 hours, 22 in one to two weeks, 8 within two weeks, 6 in three weeks, and 2 in four weeks. In some instances the waiting period was as long as six weeks. See *CARAL 2003 Report, supra* note 55 at 6.

65 Two hospitals performed abortions up to 10 weeks' gestation, 24 up to 12 weeks, 9 up to 14 weeks, 4 up to 15 weeks, 4 up to 16 weeks, 9 up to 20 weeks, and 2 up to 23 weeks. Five hospitals left it to the doctor to decide. Saskatchewan has only two hospitals that provide abortion services, and the gestational cut-off is 12 weeks. 'In Saskatoon, with two visits to a doctor required before a woman receives "permission" to have an abortion, medical services are layered, in effect, functioning more as barriers than as conduits to information and services.' *Ibid.* at 38.

66 'Anti-choice doctors were noted for lying about abortion services, claiming that there was not enough time to do the abortion or that a hospital might not provide services after eight weeks. ... [A]nti-choice physicians were identified as refusing to refer women to an abortion provider and sometimes delaying appointments for tests until the pregnancy was too advanced to be eligible for the procedure.' *Ibid.*

67 Fifteen hospitals referred the caller to an anti-choice agency, 16 hung up without providing an adequate referral. *Ibid.* at 12.

68 Of those 71,222 were in hospitals.

69 Live births dropped slightly between a comparable period from 338,295 in 1998–9 to 331,522 in 2002–3. Statistics Canada, *Births and Birth Rate,* available at www.statcan.ca/english/Pgdb/demo04a.htm (accessed 6 September 2005).

70 Of these 63,535 were performed in hospitals; 41,919 in clinics. Statistics Canada, 'Induced abortions by area of report and type of facility performing the abortion, Canada, provinces and territories, annual (number)' (Table 106–9005), http://cansim2.statcan.ca/cgi-win/cnsmcgi.exe?Lang= E&RootDir=CII/&ResultTemplate=CII/CII___&Array_Pick=1&ArrayId= 1069005 (accessed 8 April 2004). The figures for 1990 were 71,222 hospital abortions and 20,354 clinic abortions for a total of 91,456.

71 In 1995 Federal Health Minister Diane Marleau said that provinces must pay the full cost of abortions at clinics or face deductions from federal transfer payments under the *Canada Health Act* (*CHA*). In the *CHA Annual Report, 2000–2001,* Health Minister Anne McLellan noted that the federal

government was working with territorial and provincial governments to ensure the funding of clinic abortions. The *CHA Report* added that the government had met with provincial counterparts in New Brunswick, that information sharing with New Brunswick continued and that outstanding issues also existed with regard to Prince Edward Island, Quebec, and Manitoba, http://www.hc-sc.gc.ca/medicare/Documents/CHA0001.pdf (accessed 6 September 2005). In the *2001–2002 CHA Annual Report*, Minister McLellan reported that $39,000 in transfer payments had been withheld from Nova Scotia for failure to pay the full facility fee to the Morgentaler Clinic in Halifax. Nova Scotia has made it clear that it is willing to forgo the revenue rather than comply. *Report on CHA, 2001–2002*, http://www .hc-sc.gc.ca/medicare/Documents/CHA0102.pdf (accessed 6 September 2005).

72 *Canada Health Act*, R.S.C. 1985, c. C-6.

73 See Colleen M. Flood, 'The Anatomy of Medicare,' in Jocelyn Downie, Timothy Caulfield, and Colleen Flood (eds.), *Canadian Health Law and Policy*, 2nd ed. (Toronto: Butterworths, 2002) at 1.

74 Penalties for user charges or for extra billing must be imposed. Greater penalties may be imposed. To date the federal government has not demonstrated the will to do so. See Flood, ibid. at 26–31; the *CHA Annual Report, 2001–2002*, at 11, and reports of prior years to the same effect; Auditor General of Canada, *Report of the Auditor General of Canada – 2002 Status Report*, chap. 3. 'Information that the Department provided to us shows that none of the investigations of potential non-compliance initiated since 1999 has been related to the criteria of the CHA. All new investigations reported to us have dealt with the provisions of the CHA, that is, user charges and extra-billing. The fact that there are no investigations related to the criteria of the CHA raises some questions (see para. 3.45), available at www.org.bvg .gc.ca/domino/reports.nsf/a1b15d892a1f761a852565c40068a492/efea (accessed 8 April 2004).

75 See the chart of annual deductions from funds transferred to the provinces and territories: in *Exhibit 3.6 Annual deductions from Canada Health and Social Transfer, by province and territory*, available at www.oag-bvg.gc.ca/ domino/reports.nsf/html/20020903xe06.html (accessed 8 April 2004).

76 Canada, House of Commons, 37th Parliament, 2nd Session, No. 131, 1 October 2003, at 1079. Breitkreuz (Yorkton-Melville) / Casson (Lethbridge). Also the Protection of Conscience Project proposed legislation: *An Act to Ensure Protection of Conscience in the Provision of Medical Services*, available at http://www.consciencelaws.org/ (last accessed 8 April 2004). *Silent No More in Canada* is a website to counter the New Brunswick complaint

brought by Dr Morgentaler, available at www.theinterim.com/2004/
feb/02silentnomore.html (accessed 6 September 2005). For a pro-choice
initiative, see *Clarification.ca: Ask me about my abortion*, available at
www.clarification.ca/ (accessed 8 April 2004).
77 In 1998 the Hon. Monique Bégin chaired the Advisory Committee on
Women's Health Surveillance (ACWHS).
78 Canada, ACWHS, *Women's Health Surveillance: A Plan of Action for Health
Canada* (Ottawa: Health Canada, 2000), http://www.hc-sc.gc.ca/pphb-
dgspsp/publicat/whs-ssf/pdf/whs0200.pdf (accessed 8 April 2004).
79 *Ibid.* at 89.
80 *Ibid.* at 97. See at 96: 'Abortion data have been collected and reported to
Statistics Canada/CIHI, but this reporting is very limited in terms of
variables and is even more limited in the reporting from clinics in terms
of variables and number of clinics supplying information.' The time lag
between data collecting and reporting was also noted. The *Statistical Report
on the Health of Canadians*, prepared by the Federal, Provincial and Territorial Advisory Committee on Population Health (Ottawa: Health Canada,
1999) did contain a separate chapter on therapeutic abortions, setting out
the information derived from Statistics Canada data collection.
81 Health Canada, Population and Public Health Branch, *Women's Health
Surveillance Report: A Multidimensional Look at the Health of Canadian Women*
(Ottawa: author, 2003), http://secure.cihi.ca/cihiweb/dispPage.jsp?cw_
page=PG_29_E&cw_topic=29&cw_rel=AR_342_E (accessed 8 April 2004).
The report noted the following biases in the health system: narrow focus –
concentration on reproductive processes leading to overmedicalization;
grouping of women with men in assessing disease and treatment consequences; exclusion of women from policy-making, research, medical
specialties, and power. British Columbia, Ontario, and the Atlantic provinces have also produced women's health reports, as has the National
Women's Law Center (NWLC) in the United States. See B.C., Women's
Health Bureau, *Provincial Profile of Women's Health: A Statistical Overview of
Health Indicators for Women in British Columbia* (Ottawa: Health Canada,
2000); D.E. Stewart *et al.*, *Ontario Women's Health Status Report* (Toronto:
Centre for Research in Women's Health and Institute for Clinical Evalua-
tive Sciences, 2002); R. Colman, *Women's Health in Atlantic Canada: A
Statistical Portrait* (Halifax: Maritime Centre of Excellence for Women's
Health, 2000); NWLC, *Making the Grade on Women's Health: A National and
State-by-State Report Card* (Washington, DC: National Women's Law Center, 2000).
82 Statistics Canada, *Health Indicators*, no. 2 (November 2003), http://www
.statcan.ca/english/freepub/82-221-XIE/01103/toc.htm (accessed

12 November 2003). Stroke and heart attack are not desegregated, for example, although caesarean section and vaginal birth following caesarean were used as indicators of health system performance, as were hysterectomy readmission rates. Prostatectomy readmission rates also were tracked. More recently, see Rebecca Sutherns, Marilou McPhedran, and Margaret Haworth-Brockman, *Rural, Remote and Northern Women's Health Policy and Research Directions*, (Ottawa: Centres of Excellence for Women's Health, 2004), http://www.pwhce.ca/pdf/rr/RRN_Summary_CompleteE .pdf (accessed 8 September 2005).

83 'In terms of direct health care services, the precise number of for-profit facilities delivering direct health care services is unknown. One estimate in 1998 ... suggested that there were 300 private for-profit clinics in Canada delivering many diagnostic and therapeutic services formerly provided in hospitals, including abortions, endoscopies, physiotherapy, new reproductive technologies and laser eye surgeries. In addition, there are a growing number of small private for-profit hospitals or stand-alone clinics in some provinces providing more complex surgeries, some requiring overnight stays.' See Canada, Commission on the Future of Health Care in Canada, *Building on Values: The Future of Health Care in Canada – Final Report*' (Saskatoon: Commission on the Future of Heath Care in Canada, 2002) (Chair: Roy Romanow) [*Romanow Report*].

84 Canadian Women's Health Network, National Coordinating Group on Health Care Reform and Women, *Reading Romanow: The Implications of the Final Report of the Commission on the Future of Health Care in Canada for Women* (Winnipeg: Centre for Health Studies, 2003), www.cewh-cesf.ca/ healthreform/index.html (accessed 8 April 2004) [*Reading Romanow*].

85 'The Report fails to discuss the critical role reproductive health services, such as fertility control, access to abortion, the prevention and treatment of sexually transmitted infections and maternity care play in primary health care for women.' See *Reading Romanow, supra*, note 84 at 53. More appropriately, the *Ontario Women's Health Status Report* contained a specific chapter on abortion: see Stewart *et al., supra,* note 81 at 178.

86 NWLC, *supra*, note 81 at 14, 124, 197.

87 'The Commission is strongly of the view that a properly funded public system can continue to provide the high quality services to which Canadians have become accustomed. Rather than subsidize private facilities with public dollars, governments should choose to ensure that the public system has sufficient capacity and is universally accessible.' *Romanow Report, supra* note 83 at 9.

88 *Ibid.*

89 See *Reading Romanow, supra* note 84 at 3, 9; Esyllt Jones and Ana St Croix

Rothney, *Women's Health and Social Inequality*, www.policyalternatives.ca (accessed 8 September 2005).

90 'Reproductive health is a state of complete physical, mental and social well-being and not merely the absence of disease or infirmity, in all matters relating to the reproductive system and to its functions and processes. Reproductive health therefore implies that people are able to have a satisfying and safe sex life and that they have the capability to reproduce and the freedom to decide if, when and how often to do so.' UN, Department of Public Information, *Platform for Action and Beijing Declaration. Fourth World Conference on Women, Beijing, China, 4–15 September 1995* (New York: UN, 1995), para. 94.

91 For more recent press coverage see Peter Wilson, 'Canadians for Choice Is Taking on the Fight for Access to Hospital Abortions,' *Globe and Mail*, 6 May 2004.

92 Doctors, hospitals and other health care providers are subject to provincial human rights codes requiring them to provide medical services in a non-discriminatory manner. See *Korn v. Potter*, (1996) 134 D.L.R. (4th) 437 . Where colleges have been made aware of ongoing concerns they may be liable for failure to respond to complaints. See *McClelland et al. v. Stewart et al.* (2003), 229 D.L.R. (4th) 342 (B.C.S.C.) See also *Finney v. Barreau du Quebec*, [2004] S.C.J. No. 31.

93 Canadian Medical Association, *Code of Ethics*, ss. 7, 8, http://www.cma.ca/cma/common/displayPage.do?pageId=/staticContent/HTML/N0/l2/working_on/review.htm (accessed 12 July 2003).

94 Canadian Medical Association, *Induced Abortion*, http://www.cma.ca/cma/common/displayPage.do?pageId=/staticContent/HTML/N0/l2/where_we_stand/1998/12-15.htm (accessed 17 March 2002). The CMA position also states that abortion should be uniformly available and that all costs should be covered by health insurance.

95 Some governing colleges have specific policies on abortion. No formal complaint appears ever to have been made. See also the chapter by Joanna Erdman & Rebecca Cook in this volume. On the limits of self-regulation of the medical profession see Linette McNamara, Erin Nelson, and Brent Windwick, 'Regulation of Health Professionals' in Downie *et al.*, *supra*, note 73 at 55; Bernard M. Dickens, 'Informed Consent' in ibid. at 129, 148; Sanda Rodgers, 'Health Care Providers and Sexual Assault: Feminist Law Reform?' (1995) Can. J. of Women and the Law 159.

96 The websites of provincial colleges governing physicians and surgeons all were searched. As well, telephone inquiries were made to all provincial colleges governing physicians and surgeons in May 2004.

97 'The Society of Obstetricians and Gynaecologists of Canada (SOGC) has supported a woman's right to choose safe abortion services.' SOGC Policy Statement No. 124, March 2003, http://www.sogc.org/sogcnet/sogc_docs (accessed 8 September 2005).

98 College of Physicians and Surgeons of New Brunswick, Guideline #8, Bulletin, November 2002, http://www.cpsnb.org/english/Guidelines/guidelines-9.html (accessed 8 April 2004). It appears that the College intended that this policy clarify an obligation to provide information to the patient if she so requested. Arguably, it achieves the contrary. Telephone interview with College Registrar, 13 May 2004.

99 See Dickens, *supra* note 95 at 129, and Erdman and Cook, in this volume. See also *Eldridge v. British Columbia (Attorney General)*, [1997] 3 S.C.R. 624 at para. 70 on the interrelationship of consent and *Charter* protections.

100 For recent examples dating to the 2004 federal election campaign see the following items in the *Globe and Mail*: Jill Mahoney, 'Conservative Critic Wants New Abortion Rules: Urges Mandatory Third-Party Counselling,' 1 June 2004; Jeff Sallot, 'Abortion Creeps Back on to Political Agenda,' 2 June 2004; Jill Mahoney and Brian Laghi, 'Harper Stands by MP in Abortion Furor,' 2 June 2004; Margaret Wente 'Abortion: The Tories' other Flashpoint,' 3 June 2004; Joseph Arvay and others, Open letter to Stephen Harper 'Can We Trust You, Sir, to Defend the Charter?' 5 June 2004; Christie Blatchford, untitled, 5 June 2004; 'Abortion and Politics,' 7 June 2004; John Ibbitson, 'Abortion a Moot Debate,' 8 June 2004; Canadian Press, 'Martin Picks at Harper on Abortion,' 8 June 2004; Barbara McAdorey, 'Counselling is Already Mandatory,' 9 June 2004; Steven Crane, Kim Lunman, and Drew Fagan, 'Bishop Lashes Martin for Abortion Stand: Liberal Leader's "moral conscience" a "source of scandal" Calgary prelate says,' 9 June 2004. See http://www.globeandmail.ca/servlet/Page/document/hubsv3/tgamHub?hub=Search&query=abortion (accessed 6 September 2005).

101 Despite a Policy Statement by the Society of Obstetricians and Gynaecologists of Canada supporting non-surgical medical abortion using anti-progestins and prostaglandins, medical abortions using methotrexate and misoprostol are available on a severely limited basis, and RU-486 has not been approved for use in Canada, although it is available in Europe. Much political posturing has occurred in response to the opening of legal, free standing clinics by Dr Morgentaler. See the references to *Hansard* in *R. v. Morgentaler, supra*, note 44 at para. 57 seq. Other less well-known examples abound. In 1991, the Saskatchewan College of Physicians and Surgeons (CPSS) passed a by-law to allow

clinic-based abortions. The Saskatchewan government refused to approve the by-law. The same year, Conservative Premier Grant Devine challenged provincial funding for hospital abortions though a plebiscite in the provincial election. Newly elected NDP Premier Romanow responded to the results of the plebiscite with a legal opinion that abortion services could not be de-insured as a matter of constitutional law. In 1996, the CPSS ruled that medical abortions can be performed outside of hospitals but, contradicting its earlier position, decided that surgical abortions may be performed only in hospitals. In 1999, the Alberta College of Physicians and Surgeons (CPSA) determined that non-surgical medical abortions using methotrexate and misoprostol should be restricted to a clinic or hospital approved to perform surgery.

102 See Sanda Rodgers, 'Misconceived: Reproduction, Women's Equality and the Failure of the Supreme Court of Canada' in Sheila McIntyre and Sanda Rodgers, eds., *Diminishing Returns: Inequality and the Canadian Charter of Rights and Freedoms* (Toronto: Irwin Law, 2006).

103 *Association pour l'accès à l'avortement v. Procureur général du Québec*, [2003] J.Q. no. 13752. See Kouri at note 43 seq., in this volume.

104 *Jane Doe 1 v. Manitoba*, [2004] M.J. No. 456 [*Jane Doe 1*].

105 Tracey Thorne, 'NB, Morgentaler Head to Court over Abortion Payments' (2002) 167: 11 Cdn. Med. Assn. J. 1277.

106 See *Chaoulli c. Québec (Procureur général)*, [2005] S.C.C. 35. For a discussion see Martha Jackman, this volume. See also Colleen M. Flood, Kent Roach, and Lorne Sossin, *Access to Care, Access to Justice: The Legal Debate over Private Health Insurance in Canada* (Toronto: University of Toronto Press, 2005).

107 *Eldridge, supra* note 99 at 624.The *Eldridge* decision is an excellent example of the limits of successful *Charter* litigation in actually delivering those victories. See CAD Chat, a publication of the Canadian Association of the Deaf (CAD), 'Failure to Comply with the Supreme Court's 1997 Eldridge Decision Slaps Deaf and Disabled Communities (1999) 11 CAD Chat 2; Ontarians with Disabilities Act ODA Committee, 'Members Statements in the Ontario Legislature re: ODA Legislation,' 10 April 2000, http://www.odacommittee.net/hansard44.html (accessed 8 April 2004); CAD, 'Health Care: The Eldridge Decision,' 20 April 2004, http://www.cad.ca/english/resources/pp_health_care.htm (accessed 8 April 2004).

108 *Eldridge, supra* note 107 at paras. 20, 29.

109 Knowing disregard of discriminatory conduct by agents of public institutions in provision of public services has been held to violate provincial human rights codes, see *Ross v. New Brunswick School District No. 15,*

[1996] 1 S.C.R. 825. There is little doubt after *Eldridge* that hospitals are public services bound to respect section 15 of the *Charter.*

110 See Donna Greschner, Discussion Paper No. 20, 'How Will the Charter of Rights and Freedoms and Evolving Jurisprudence Affect Health Care Costs?' *Romanow Report, supra* note 83 at 8; Martha Jackman, 'The Implications of Section 7 of the *Charter* for Health Care Spending in Canada,' ibid., and 'The Application of the Canadian Charter in the Health Care Context' (2000) 9:2 Health Law Rev. 22, at 25. For cases that deny *Charter*-based claims to health care, see *Ontario Nursing Home Association v. Ontario* (1990), 72 D.L.R. (4th) 166 at 177; *Brown v. British Columbia (Minister of Health)* (1990), 66 D.L.R. (4th) 444 (B.C. S.C.) at 467–9; *Cameron v. Nova Scotia,* [1999] N.S.J. No. 297 (N.S.C.A.) at para. 160. For additional cases that arguably recognize a claim that the *Charter* can support a right to health care, see *Sawatzky v. Riverside Health Centre Inc.,* [1998] M.J. No. 506 (Man.Ct.QB); *R. v. Parker,* [2000] O.J. No. 2787 (Ont. C.A.); *Chaoulli, supra* note 106. See also Erdman and Cook, in this volume.

111 See *Morgentaler, supra* note 44. Wilson, J. relied on s. 2 protections as well as section 7. In *Winnipeg v. D.F.G.,* [1997] 3 S.C.R. 925 and in *Dobson v. Dobson,* [1999] 2 S.C.R. 753, the Supreme Court of Canada was attentive to a pregnant woman's autonomy of decision-making with regard to her own life and health. However, the decision of the Court was based on private tort law principles rather than expressly on *Charter* protections. See also, *Rodriguez v. British Columbia (Attorney General),* [1993] 3 S.C.R. 519; Erdman and Cook, this volume.

112 'The structure of the *Hospital Insurance Act* reveals, therefore, that in providing medically necessary services, hospitals carry out a specific governmental objective. The *Act* is not ... simply a mechanism to prevent hospitals from charging for their services. Rather, it provides for the delivery of a comprehensive social program. Hospitals are merely the vehicles the legislature has chosen to deliver this program ... [I]n decades ... health care, including that generally provided by hospitals, has become a keystone tenet of governmental policy.' *Eldridge, supra* note 99 at para. 50.

113 '[T]he Charter applies to private entities in so far as they act in furtherance of a specific governmental program or policy. In these circumstances, while it is a private actor that actually implements the program, it is government that retains responsibility for it.' *Eldridge,* ibid., at para. 42; see also para. 44.

114 To date the Court has not clearly addressed the possibility that the *Charter* may impose affirmative duties on governments to take positive action, although this possibility has not been foreclosed. Such an affirmative

duty arguably would include providing effective access to abortion. See *McKinney* per Wilson, J.: 'it is not self-evident to me that government could not be found to be in breach of the Charter for failing to act' (at 412); *Haig v. Canada*, [1993] 2 S.C.R. 995 at 1038, per L'Heureux-Dubé, J.; *Eldridge, supra* note 99 per LaForest, J., at para. 73.

115 Rebecca J. Cook, Bernard M. Dickens, and Mahmoud F. Fathalla, *Reproductive Health and Human Rights* (New York: Oxford University Press, 2003) at 351. See also, UN, Department of Public Information, *supra* note 90 at paras. 114, 132, 135; Committee on the Elimination of Discrimination against Women (CEDAW) Pt. III, chap. 6, s. 2, para. 11.

116 *Janzen v. Platy Enterprises Ltd.*, [1989] 1 S.C.R. 1252.

117 *Auton (Guardian ad litem of) v. British Columbia (Attorney General)*, [2004] 3 S.C.R. 657, [2004] S.C.C. 78.

118 [1992] Can. T.S. No. 3.

119 Unlike Greschner (this volume), in my view the recent Supreme Court decision in *Auton* erodes rather than strengthens *Charter* values. Most recently in *Wynberg v. Ontario*, Kiteley, J., ordered the province to provide treatment for autism. [2005] O.J. No. 1228.

120 *Jane Doe 1, supra* note 104.

121 *Ibid.* at para. 36

122 *Ibid.* at para. 78.

123 *Supra*, note 117 at 441.

124 UN, *Convention on the Elimination of All Forms of Discrimination against Women* (New York: United Nations, 1979). See generally Cook *et al., supra,* note 115; see also Erdman and Cook, this volume.

125 Accessibility changes so quickly from province to province that it is hard to identify those provinces with the greatest formal barriers to service. At this time they include New Brunswick, which requires the consent of two doctors, and Manitoba, where there is a six-week wait for a hospital-based abortion and clinic services require private payment. Informal barriers are even more difficult to quantify. See text at *supra* note 63 seq.

126 For a discussion of the barriers see Greschner, *supra*, note 110 at 19; Radha Jhappan, 'Introduction: Feminist Adventures in Law,' in Radha Jhappan, ed., *Women's Legal Strategies in Canada* (Toronto: University of Toronto Press, 2002); Sheila McIntyre, 'Feminist Movement in Law: Beyond Privileged and Privileging Theory,' in ibid. at 42; Sheilah L. Martin, 'Abortion Litigation,' in ibid. at 335.

6 Protecting Fairness in Women's Health: The Case of Emergency Contraception

JOANNA N. ERDMAN AND REBECCA J. COOK

It is estimated that 50 per cent of pregnancies in Canada are unintended.[1] Approximately 24 per cent of these pregnancies end in abortion.[2] In 2002 Canadian women obtained 105,154 induced abortions.[3] Abortion is now the most common outcome for teenage pregnancies. For every 100 live births for women aged 15–19 in 2002, there were 125 abortions.[4] Statistics from Alberta also reveal that abortions among younger women are performed later in pregnancy.[5] Sanda Rodgers describes well the increasing difficulty that women, and especially adolescents, have in obtaining access to abortion services in an affordable and timely manner (see chapter 5, this volume) and that undoubtedly contributes to the trend towards having abortions later in a pregnancy. Long waiting lists, the lack of trained providers, lack of funding or simply lack of services, and hospital policies result in significant access barriers.[6] These barriers are multiplied for women living in rural communities.[7] Only 17 per cent of hospitals in Canada provide abortion services.[8]

Unintended pregnancy and abortion entail physical, emotional, social, and economic risks for women. Unintended pregnancy is associated with higher maternal morbidity, a greater risk of depression, maternal and child abuse, and social and economic hardships. Adolescent pregnancy carries an increased risk of obstetrical complications and premature delivery. As compared with adolescents who postpone having children, young women with unintended births are more likely to terminate their schooling and to require social assistance. Abortion, although safe and effective, is a medically and psychologically invasive procedure. Only some provincial and territorial governments fully fund abortion services performed in both hospitals and private clinics. In all other provinces and territories, women must pay themselves in whole or in part for the service.[9]

A key strategy for decreasing the rate of unintended pregnancy, and thereby the need for abortion, is to reduce barriers to access to contraceptives. The broader objective is to ensure that women in all social groups have equal and reasonable access to the resources necessary for the realization of their sexual and reproductive health.

Emergency contraception (EC) offers an enormous potential as the only contraceptive method that can be used *after* sexual intercourse to prevent unintended pregnancies and reduce the need for abortion services.[10] The World Health Organization describes EC as 'contraceptive methods that can be used by women in the first few days following unprotected intercourse to prevent an unwanted pregnancy.'[11] EC is a form of contraception intended for occasional use, such as in cases of unprotected intercourse, contraceptive failure, or sexual assault.

The most effective method of EC consists of two 0.75 mg doses of the progestrin levonorgestrel administered 12 hours apart and initiated within 72 hours after intercourse. When correctly used, this method prevents 89 per cent of expected pregnancies.[12] Its effectiveness, however, depends on how quickly women obtain the product after unprotected or inadequately protected intercourse. If taken within the first 24 hours, levonorgestrel prevents 95 per cent of pregnancies that would have otherwise resulted. If taken more than 49 hours after intercourse, the regimen prevents only 58 per cent of expected pregnancies.[13] Levonorgestrel thus exhibits a significant downward gradient in efficacy as the time between intercourse and use increases.[14] As a consequence of this narrow window of effectiveness, the International Consortium for Emergency Contraception explains that EC 'entail[s] unique service delivery issues, such as the need to ensure rapid access to the method to maximize efficacy.'[15]

Since 2000, levonorgestrel has been available in Canada as a prescription drug under the brand name of Plan B™. On 19 April 2005, in an effort to facilitate women's timely access to EC, Canada joined more than thirty countries[16] that allow women to legally obtain levonorgestrel for use as EC without a prescription.[17] However, the deregulation of EC as a prescription drug will not necessarily result in its 'over-the-counter' (OTC) availability, such that it may be purchased without professional supervision at any retail outlet. Rather, once a drug is deregulated as a prescription product, provincial and territorial pharmacy regulatory authorities are responsible for determining the appropriate conditions for its sale. These authorities act in consultation with and on the recommendation of the National Drug Scheduling Advisory Committee (NDSAC) of the National Association of Pharmacy Regulatory Authorities (NAPRA).

In November 2001 NDSAC recommended that, following federal deregulation, levonorgestrel packaged and labelled for EC should require professional intervention from the pharmacist at the point of sale and be retained within an area of the pharmacy where there is no public access or opportunity for patient self-selection. The availability of a drug directly from pharmacists following an assessment of appropriateness and counselling on its proper use is referred to as 'behind-the-counter' (BTC) dispensing. Concurrent with Health Canada's deregulation of EC, NDSAC announced that, as of 19 April 2005, EC is to be dispensed BTC.[18]

BTC availability offers an important compromise: it allows EC to be more widely accessible, while ensuring some level of professional consultation and control. Given that pharmacies are conveniently located and open on evenings, weekends, and holidays, BTC availability of EC will increase women's access. Given their professional expertise, pharmacists are also considered to be well positioned to screen women to ascertain the appropriateness of EC treatment and to counsel them about the use and side effects of EC as well as about other contraceptive options.[19] The advantages of BTC dispensing are already recognized in three Canadian provinces. Prior to the federal deregulation of EC, British Columbia,[20] Quebec,[21] and Saskatchewan[22] provided pharmacists with the independent authority to prescribe and dispense EC.

BTC availability of EC concedes to a more restricted form of access than NDSAC or provincial and territorial pharmacy regulatory authorities could allow. Once deregulated by Health Canada, EC could be available OTC, but retained within an area of the pharmacy supervised by a pharmacist. This form of availability would allow women to consult with health professionals if they choose to do so. It would not, as with BTC availability, oblige women to submit to assessment by a pharmacist and consultation in order to access EC. This mandatory requirement for professional intervention reduces, and in certain circumstances prohibits, reasonable access to EC. It compromises women's privacy, increases out-of-pocket costs, and creates potential barriers because of pharmacists' exercise of their right to conscientious objection. The barriers to access imposed by BTC availability are justified only if safety and efficacy concerns about the administration of EC necessitate some form of professional consultation and control. Evidence demonstrates that this is not the case; women can safely and effectively self-diagnose, self-select, and self-administer EC.

Donna Greschner (Chapter 2, this volume) examines the benefits of evidence-based decision-making. The purposes of this chapter are to demonstrate the lack of evidence-based grounds for requiring pharmacist assessment and consultation and to examine the extent to which such unnecessary intervention by pharmacists unfairly impedes women's reasonable access to EC. BTC availability of EC demonstrates that regulations concerning the place and conditions of sale for contraceptives inhibit women's safe and effective access to essential reproductive health care.

More broadly, this case study reveals that fairness in health care requires more than the mere availability of services. A fair health care system recognizes the distinctive needs of all the patients it serves and delivers care in a manner responsive to those needs. These needs include the medical, psychological, social, and economic needs of all users of the health care system.[23] Access to reproductive health care should be equitable, responsive to diversity, and not limited because of discrimination based on gender, age, socio-economic status, or geographic location.[24] If reproductive health care is to be effectively available, health care systems must account for the distinctive barriers that women face in obtaining access to care.

A fair health care system also requires mechanisms that enable citizens to hold their governments accountable for decisions that are inequitable and unresponsive to the distinctive needs of women. Human rights law, both constitutional and international, is an important mechanism of accountability to ensure fairness in the availability of and access to reproductive health care. The final section of this chapter demonstrates that the denial of fair access to EC is not merely poor health care policy. It is a denial of women's basic human rights. Professional controls that unfairly impede women's safe and effective access to EC violate the *Canadian Charter of Human Rights and Freedoms*[25] and contravene Canada's obligations under the *Convention on the Elimination of All Forms of Discrimination against Women (CEDAW Convention)*.[26]

'Behind-the-Counter' (BTC) Availability: Evidence-Based Decision-Making?

The decisions of highly specialized regulatory agencies are generally treated with great deference.[27] Courts, and other institutions of legal review, are understandably unwilling to turn themselves into 'academ[ies] of science,'[28] and substantively second-guess expert assessments. Nevertheless, all policy decisions, including those of a scientific nature, are subject to meaningful legal review and must be supported by evidence. A decision that lacks a logical relationship between the grounds of the decision and the premises shown to be true is an arbitrary and therefore, patently unreasonable, decision.[29]

On 19 April 2005, Health Canada amended the *Food and Drug Regulations*[30] to remove levonorgestrel from Part II of Schedule F when indicated for use as EC. Schedule F lists chemical substances intended for human use that require a prescription to be sold in Canada. The amendment came into force following a 75-day consultation process, which began on 22 May 2004 with the publication in Part I of the *Canada Gazette* of the proposed regulatory amendment accompanied by a Regulatory Impact Analysis Statement (RIAS).[31] The RIAS discussed the benefits and costs of the proposed regulation and provided reasons as to the preferability of deregulation compared with other available options. It also explicitly responded to concerns and considerations that had been raised during stakeholder consultations. In June 2003 Health Canada distributed a consultation letter to provincial and territorial deputy ministers of health, registrars of provincial medical and pharmacy associations, and professional health and consumer associations, as well as other stakeholders, soliciting their comments on the proposed deregulation of EC.[32] The publication of the proposed regulation and the RIAS thus served an important accountability function. It rendered transparent the evidence and considerations upon which Health Canada based its decisions with respect to the prescription status of EC.

As explained in the RIAS, Health Canada's proposal to deregulate EC followed an extensive review of the clinical evidence and safety data submitted by the Canadian distributor of Plan B™, Paladin Labs, Inc.[33] Health Canada assessed the received evidence and data against prescribed factors to determine whether safety and efficacy concerns necessitated prescription controls. These factors include undesirable or severe side effects, the presence of a dependence or abuse potential, and whether EC requires individual instructions or direct practitioner supervision. Most importantly, Health Canada assessed whether levonorgestrel possessed a high level of risk relative to its expected benefits.

Health Canada recognized that there is a 'long history of safe and effective use of levonorgestrel as an EC.'[34] The average risk of pregnancy after a single act of unprotected intercourse is approximately 8 per cent. EC reduces the risk of pregnancy on average by 89 per cent.[35] In other words, for every 100 episodes of unprotected intercourse without use of EC, there would be an average of eight pregnancies. EC reduces this to an average of one pregnancy.

Health Canada determined that '[o]ccasional use of levonorgestrel for emergency contraception is safe for virtually all women.'[36] Studies report only minimal side effects, most commonly nausea, breast tenderness, lower abdominal pain, fatigue, headache, heavier or lighter menstrual bleeding, dizziness, and diarrhea.[37] Severe symptoms, if they occur, are usually managed with painkillers. No deaths, suicides, or other serious consequences of an acute overdose of EC have been reported.[38] Even regular postcoital use is not associated with serious or lasting adverse events. Pregnancy or abortion places women at significantly greater medical risk than brief use of EC.[39]

There are no contraindications to the use of EC, even for women who have problems with long-term hormonal contraception.[40] Pregnancy is a listed contraindication because, like all contraceptives, EC will not work if a woman is pregnant. Studies that have examined births to women who inadvertently continued to take oral contraceptives without knowing they were pregnant confirm that the treatment is not teratogenic.[41] Levonorgestrel does not increase the risk of ectopic pregnancy. In support of Health Canada's position, guidelines from the Society of Obstetricians and Gynaecologists of Canada (SOGC)[42] and the American College of Obstetricians and Gynecologists (ACOG)[43] do not require a pregnancy test before EC treatment.

Furthermore, EC carries no abuse potential that is likely to lead to harmful non-medical use. This is in part because other methods of contraception are more effective than repeated use of EC and the side effects, although temporary and not serious, deter frequent use or overuse. Studies demonstrate that making EC more widely available does not increase risk-taking in contraceptive use.[44] In fact, women who are most diligent about ongoing contraceptive use are those most likely to seek EC.[45] While women provided with EC in advance of need are more likely to use it, they are neither more likely to use it repeatedly nor abandon longer-term contraception.[46] Moreover, experience in countries where EC is already available without a prescription demonstrates that women have not 'abused' its availability.[47]

On the basis of its review, Health Canada decided that '[a]s measured against the factors for listing drugs on Schedule F ... maintaining levonorgestrel 0.75 mg on Schedule F is not appropriate. The benefits of more timely access to levonorgestrel as an EC outweigh any theoretical risks.'[48]

The RIAS also suggested that Health Canada's decision was partially based on the assurance that once deregulated as a prescription product, EC would be available BTC. Health Canada does not have the jurisdiction to decide the conditions and place of sale of non-prescription drugs. This task falls to provincial and territorial pharmacy regulatory authorities and NDSAC.[49] NDSAC is a subgroup of NAPRA, an umbrella association that represents the registrars of provincial colleges of pharmacy.[50] NAPRA was established to align provincial regulations and ensure that the conditions for the sale of drugs are consistent across the country.[51]

In November 2001 NDSAC recommended that, following deregulation, 'levonorgestrel ... packaged and labelled for emergency contraception ... would meet the requirements for Schedule II status.'[52] Schedule II drugs require professional intervention from the pharmacist at the point of sale, with attention given to communication about the symptoms or condition to be treated, the possible side effects or drug interactions, and the selection of an appropriate drug. The drugs must also be retained within an area of the pharmacy where there is no public access or opportunity for patient self-selection.[53] Schedule II status is commonly referred to as BTC dispensing.

In both the June 2003 consultation letter and the May 2004 proposed regulation, Health Canada supported NDSAC's recommendation, which stated: 'Given their expertise and accessibility when access to other health professionals is limited, pharmacists are well positioned to play a major role in increasing women's access to emergency contraception and in providing counselling about contraceptive options.'[54] In December 2004 NDSAC confirmed that its recommendation for Schedule II would be final upon Health Canada deregulating and approving the final labelling requirements for EC.[55] There is no evidence that the committee held any further consultations as to the appropriate conditions for the sale of EC prior to its announcement that '[a]s of April 19, 2005, [the same day as Health Canada's deregulation of EC came into force] levonorgestrel, in oral dosage units of 0.75 mg packaged and labelled for emergency contraception (Plan B), has moved to Schedule II.'[56]

Although an extensive review preceded Health Canada's decision to remove prescription controls for the sale of EC, it does not appear that prior to endorsing NDSAC's recommendation Health Canada conducted a similarly thorough review respecting the need for intervention by pharmacists. Nor does it appear that NDSAC, prior to making its recommendation, extensively reviewed whether safety and efficacy concerns require pharmacist assessment and consultation. If either agency did undertake a significant review, they have failed to disclose the nature of evidence considered during their review.

The November 2001 minutes of the NAPRA meeting state that during a brief twenty minutes, 'the Committee heard a presentation from representatives of the four co-sponsoring agencies of the request for Schedule II status for Plan B emergency contraception.'[57] The Committee agreed that 'levonorgestrel ... packaged and labelled for emergency contraception ... would meet the requirements for Schedule II status, after applying Factors 1, 2, 8, and 9.'[58] Similar to the review performed by Health Canada, NDSAC assessed levonorgestrel against prescribed factors to determine whether safety and efficacy concerns necessitated BTC restrictions. Factor 2 states that a Schedule II drug 'must be readily available under exceptional circumstances when a prescription is not practical.'[59] Health Canada similarly recognized that 'timely access to levonorgestrel is important for it to be effective as an EC.'[60] A prescription requirement jeopardizes women's health by decreasing or delaying the use of EC. Not all women can miss work or afford the transportation and childcare costs associated with obtaining and filling a prescription within 72 hours of unprotected intercourse. Pharmacies, however, are conveniently located and open on evenings, weekend and holidays. While this factor supports the deregulation of EC as a prescription drug, it does not necessitate BTC restrictions. OTC distribution would likewise render EC readily available under exceptional circumstances when a prescription is impractical.

In 2001, when NDSAC first assessed EC, it did not have the benefit of considering the clinical evidence and safety data submitted by Paladin Labs to Health Canada, nor of Health Canada's review of the evidence and its consultation with stakeholders. Moreover, at that time, the evidence on the safety and efficacy of OTC distribution of EC did not exist in the scientific literature. In both December 2004 and April 2005, when NDSAC confirmed and implemented its recommendation, the Committee chose not to reassess its recommendation in light of the voluminous consultations and medical and social science studies that had emerged since 2001. This evidence, however, establishes the safety and effectiveness of OTC distribution as measured against Factors 1, 8, and

9 of Schedule II. It demonstrates that the sale of EC does not warrant pharmacist intervention.

Factor 9 requires that a Schedule II drug '[be] a new ingredient for self-medication and monitoring by the pharmacist is necessary to facilitate observation and reporting of any unexpected event.'[61] This factor does not pertain to EC. Rather, as confirmed in the RIAS that accompanied Health Canada's proposed regulation, '[l]evonorgestrel as a component of oral contraceptive products has been widely used as a prescription drug in women for several decades.'[62] The oral contraceptive pill is arguably the most extensively studied medication in the history of pharmaceuticals.[63] Moreover, given that an identical dose of hormones would be used in OTC dispensing of EC as is currently used in the prescription regimen, existing efficacy data that justify prescription distribution of EC directly apply to OTC distribution.[64]

Factor 1 requires that the 'initial need for a drug is normally identified by the practitioner, in addition chronic, recurrent, or subsequent therapy must be monitored by the pharmacist.'[65] A woman is best positioned to identify when she has had unprotected intercourse. In fact, all health practitioners must themselves rely on women to diagnose the need for EC. Only a woman's recognition that she has had unprotected sexual intercourse will lead her to seek EC. Although a pharmacist could dissuade a woman from unnecessarily using the product when she is at particularly low risk of conception, there is no medical reason for doing so. Even if the risk of pregnancy is not high, a woman may wish to reduce her risk for non-medical reasons.[66] Recurrent use is also not associated with serious or lasting adverse events. In the RIAS, Health Canada noted that '[f]ollow-up of patients is generally not required unless there is a delay in the return of menstrual period.'[67] Delay of menses and the need to seek follow-up care can be addressed in product labelling.

Pursuant to Factor 8, 'use of the drug requires reinforcement or an expansion of the directions for use, through pharmacist-patient dialogue.'[68] This factor is contradicted by medical evidence. Individualized instruction and direct supervision of EC are unnecessary as the treatment is identical for all women.[69] In this respect, EC is simpler to administer than many medications currently availability OTC, which require tailored dosages based on patient characteristics or therapeutic response.[70]

Recent studies confirm that as long as credible information about EC is provided at the point of sale, women can safely and effectively self-

administer it. A study evaluating women's comprehension of a prototype OTC label for EC found that 97 per cent of participants understood
that the first pill should be taken within 72 hours or as soon as possible
after intercourse.[71] More than 93 per cent understood that the product is
indicated for the prevention of pregnancy after unprotected sex, that it
does not prevent HIV or AIDS, and that women who are already pregnant should not use the drug. A second study, evaluating whether
women use EC appropriately and safely when it is dispensed OTC,
indicated that nearly all participants used the product safely without
professional evaluation and counselling.[72] In both studies, vulnerable
groups, such as the young, minority women, or less-educated women,
were not substantially less likely than others to use the product incorrectly. It is noteworthy that permitting OTC distribution of EC would
not prevent women from having contact with health care providers, if
they choose to do so.[73] NDSAC's Schedule III is intended for drugs that
'are suitable for self-selection, but may pose risks for certain groups of
people.'[74] These drugs are 'to be sold from the self-selection area of the
pharmacy, operated under the direct supervision of the pharmacist.'[75]
This distribution mechanism provides for professional guidance in a
less intrusive manner.

Authoritative evidence thus confirms that women can effectively
self-diagnose, self-select, and self-administer EC. The lack of evidence
supporting pharmacist assessment and consultation reveals that for EC,
the question of availability is more than simply a scientific risk assessment. It is well recognized that '[t]he more an issue is in the public eye,
the more expert judgments are likely to be influenced unconsciously by
pre-existing policy preferences or by supposedly unrelated factors such
as media presentations, the opinion of colleagues or friends, or even the
emotional overtones of certain words used in the debate.'[76] In the
context of controversial issues, decision-makers may camouflage policy
decisions as science to evade political, legal, and institutional accountability.[77] Without law tempering science, there is a risk that relatively
unaccountable scientific experts will effectively overstep the legitimate
bounds of their disciplines and exclude important social and legal
values from policy decisions.[78]

Pharmacist Intervention: Unfair Barrier to Access?

Decision-makers cannot blind themselves to the realities that underlie
their decisions, nor to the implications that result from their decisions.
The manner in which reproductive health care is made available to

women, for example, the conditions of sale for contraceptives, dramatically affects women's access to such care. Effective access requires more than the mere availability of services. If reproductive health care is to be effectively available, a health care system must recognize the distinctive needs of women in accessing care and deliver care in a manner responsive to those needs.

The General Recommendation on *Women and Health*, developed by the Committee on the Elimination of Discrimination against Women (CEDAW Committee),[79] requires that health policies address the health of women from the perspective of women's needs. This Recommendation also recognizes that the distinctive factors that differ for women include not only biological but also socioeconomic and psychosocial factors.

The provision of health care services in a manner that recognizes and accommodates the distinctive needs of all the patients it serves is a requirement of a fair health care system. Fairness requires that health care be delivered with the philosophy of 'the right services, the right provider, the right time and the right place.'[80] The fairness of a policy, therefore, cannot be evaluated simply on its face. To appreciate the true impact of BTC distribution of EC, it is necessary to investigate the extent to which pharmacist intervention reduces, and in certain circumstances prevents, women's access to *ostensibly* available services. This investigation requires that pharmacist intervention be assessed against the socioeconomic and psychosocial characteristics distinctive to women, especially those belonging to vulnerable and disadvantaged groups, in obtaining access to health care.

The Barrier of Affordability

A fair health care system ensures that reproductive health care services are affordable for all, including socially disadvantaged groups. Poverty among women is unacceptably high, particularly among single mothers, Aboriginal women, and immigrant and refugee women. In the case of single-parent mothers, the poverty rate is 42 per cent. For single mothers aged 25 years or younger, the poverty rate is 74 per cent.[81] The average economic cost of an unintended pregnancy is $1,289.[82] The average cost of an abortion is $618.[83] In some provinces, women seeking timely access to abortion services must pay themselves in whole or in part for the service. Greater availability of EC has the potential to significantly reduce the costs of birth control for women.

At present, under the Medicare system all provinces reimburse physicians for their consultation with those requesting EC. The remaining cost to the patient for a single package of Plan B™ is approximately $16.00 plus the dispensing fee charged by the pharmacy.[84] In provinces where pharmacists may prescribe EC, the consultation fee for the assessment and counselling ranges from $15 to $45. Unlike physician consultations, only some provincial and territorial health plans will cover pharmacists' counselling fees and only in some circumstances. In other provinces and territories, patients may be required to pay the consultation fee, the cost of medication, and the pharmacy distribution fee.[85] If EC were to be distributed OTC, the private cost for consultation with a pharmacist is removed.

The Barrier of Conscientious Objection

Some pharmacists are morally opposed to providing emergency contraception. In most provinces and territories, pharmacists are allowed to refuse to dispense medication for moral reasons. Pharmacists who will not dispense a drug are obliged as a matter of professional ethics and law to refer women to another pharmacist or health facility where EC can be readily obtained.[86] This principle accords with the human rights standard articulated in the CEDAW Committee's General Recommendation on *Women and Health*. It provides that when health professionals refuse to provide services on the basis of conscience, 'measures should be introduced to ensure that women are referred to alternative health providers.'[87]

A refusing pharmacist places a disproportionately heavy burden on economically disadvantaged women in small towns or rural areas where there may only be a few pharmacists within reach.[88] Even where referral services are available, refusing pharmacists create barriers, which women may be unwilling to confront when accessing care. Subjecting women to the potential of moral confrontations with pharmacists is unfair when pharmacist intervention is unnecessary for the safe administration of EC. Policy-makers ought to be sensitive to the anxiety that women are likely to experience from judgmental attitudes and the impact that such disapproval may have on women's ability to make informed choices about their contraceptive needs.

The Barrier of a Lack of Privacy

A fair health care system is respectful of women's privacy. The CEDAW Committee's General Recommendation on *Women and Health* recognizes that while 'lack of respect for the confidentiality of patients will affect both men and women, it may deter women from seeking advice and treatment and thereby adversely affect their health.'[89] In acknowledgment of this fact, Health Canada recommends that the 'least *invasive* intervention that is appropriate and effective should be used in delivering health care.'[90]

Pharmacist intervention may dissuade women from seeking EC where assessment and consultation questionnaires require them to reveal their reasons for requiring EC. For example, the informed consent form for EC in British Columbia requires women to state whether their exposure to unintended pregnancy was the result of unprotected intercourse or birth control failure.[91] Many women are uncomfortable disclosing such personal information.

EC is an extremely valuable preventive therapy for adolescent pregnancy. Studies show that girls aged 15–19 are more likely than older women not to plan intercourse and to use contraception intermittently or not at all.[92] Because of concerns about privacy and confidentiality, however, adolescents are hesitant to seek EC. Adolescents fear judgment and parental notification.[93] Evidence indicates that a majority of adolescent patients do not discuss the option of EC in advance with their physicians.[94] Mandated consultation with a pharmacist is unlikely to lessen adolescents' reluctance to seek care. Most pharmacies do not have areas where a pharmacist can hold a private discussion. Recent studies indicate that pharmacists feel unprepared to address adolescent reproductive and sexual health concerns.[95] Even among pharmacists trained to provide EC, many reported having inadequate training to deal with parental inquiries about the provision of EC to children.[96]

The Barrier of Paternalism

Mandated pharmacist intervention is justified on the basis that pharmacists can screen patients and counsel them on the inappropriateness of recurrent EC use and the prevention of sexually transmitted infections. Health Canada recommended that 'additional [pharmacist] counselling could provide information on the options for ongoing contraception and the correct use of chosen method(s) of contraception.'[97] These justifications for pharmacist intervention reveal an underlying fear that if EC is too easily available, women, especially young women, will be more promiscuous and more likely to engage in unprotected sex. Encouragement of promiscuous sex, it is argued, will only contribute to a rise in pregnancy, abortion, and sexually transmitted infections. Mandatory pharmacist intervention guards against frequent usage, and thus mitigates incentives for irresponsible sexual activity.

There is no evidence to support the claim that increased access to EC leads women to abandon traditional contraception methods[98] or encourages adolescents to engage in promiscuous sex.[99] In most cases, the need for EC arises from a woman's recognition that her ongoing or regular contraceptive method may have failed. This is supported by evidence that women who are diligent about ongoing contraceptive use are those most likely to seek EC.[100] Even if EC did adversely affect regular contraceptive use, women are entitled to know and choose from all safe and effective options.[101]

Clinical practice guidelines of the SOGC state that the provision of EC is the standard of care for victims of sexual assault.[102] The guidelines also recommend that 'hormonal EC ... be considered for any woman wishing to avoid pregnancy, who presents within 5 days of unprotected or inadequately protected sexual intercourse.'[103] Practitioners thus provide substandard care where they fail to offer EC as an option, or fail to refer patients to places where EC is available. Failure to disclose EC as an option renders a patient's consent to treatment uninformed, and it may therefore result in professional discipline or legal sanction.[104]

The concordance of these guidelines suggests that there is no legitimate reason why a victim of sexual assault should receive the option of EC, but a woman who voluntarily opts to have unprotected sexual intercourse should not. Effective access to preventive care should not be denied on the basis of voluntary versus forced sexual intercourse. Seeking to deter unsafe sexual behaviour through a quasi-punitive delivery of health care is a direct violation of a woman's right to make informed choices. A fair health care system recognizes and protects free and informed decision-making. The use of EC represents a responsible and informed decision by a woman seeking to prevent an unintended pregnancy, and it should be respected as such.

Legal Accountability for Unfair Barriers to Access

A health care system that recognizes the distinctive needs of women in accessing care, and delivers care in a manner responsive to those needs, is not simply the mark of a fair health care system. It is a legal entitlement. The law of human rights, both constitutional and international, is an important mechanism that enables citizens to hold their governments accountable for health care decisions that are inequitable or unresponsive to the needs of women.

All government decisions are subject to meaningful legal review. Human rights obligations flow down the chain of statutory authority and apply to regulatory decisions and policies that depend for validity on statutory authority.[105] In *Baker v. Canada (Minister of Citizenship and Immigration)*,[106] the Supreme Court of Canada confirmed that all 'discretion must be exercised in accordance with the boundaries imposed in ... the principles of the rule of law ... the fundamental values of Canadian society, and the principles of the *Charter*.'[107] Provincial and territorial pharmacy regulatory authorities, responsible for deciding the conditions and place of sale of a drug, are therefore subject to constitutional obligations.

It is an unreasonable regulatory policy to require women to submit to a pharmacist assessment and consultation to access EC when authoritative evidence confirms that women can safely and effectively self-diagnose, self-select, and self-administer. It is also an unfair regulatory policy to unnecessarily impede women's effective access to EC and to thereby subject women to an increased risk of unintended pregnancy and abortion. The purpose of the following analysis is to demonstrate that regulatory policies that unreasonably and unfairly deny women access to essential reproductive health care violate women's security of the person, contrary to section 7 of the *Charter*, and contravene the principle of substantive equality under section 15(1) of the *Charter* and Article 12(1) of the *CEDAW Convention*. Neither *Charter* infringement is saved by section 1.

Security of the Person

EC is only effective if used within 72 hours after intercourse. It is most effective when used within the first 24 hours following intercourse. Any delay increases the chance of pregnancy. Unintended pregnancy carries costly physical, emotional, social, and economic risks for women. A woman who cannot access EC within the required time frame but wishes to terminate the resulting pregnancy must resort to an abortion, a procedure that carries greater physical risk and emotional distress than EC.

Conditioning the availability of EC on pharmacist counselling decreases its timely availability and thereby increases the rates of unintended pregnancy and abortion. As a consequence, unnecessary pharmacist intervention infringes a woman's physical and psychological integrity, contrary to section 7 of the *Charter*. Section 7 guarantees everyone 'the right to life, liberty and security of the person and the right not to be deprived thereof except in accordance with the principles of fundamental justice.'[108]

In *R v Morgentaler*,[109] the Supreme Court of Canada struck down the criminal prohibition on abortion unless authorized by a committee of three doctors. The procedural aspects of the provision were held to violate section 7 of the *Charter*. It was recognized that 'state interference with bodily integrity and serious state-imposed psychological stress ... constitute a breach of security of the person.'[110] The majority of the Court held that the legislative provision effectively denied every pregnant woman access to a 'safe medical procedure ... unless she meets criteria entirely unrelated to her own priorities and aspirations.'[111] Justice Beetz confirmed that a 'pregnant woman's person cannot be said to be secure if, when her ... health is in danger, she is faced with a rule ... which precludes her from obtaining effective and timely medical treatment.'[112]

The unnecessary requirement for pharmacist intervention similarly endangers a woman's health by precluding her from obtaining timely preventative care. In *Morgentaler*, the Court accepted that unnecessary delay caused by procedural mechanisms profoundly affects women's physical and emotional well-being.[113] First, the Court noted that delay in obtaining an abortion results in the use of different techniques that carry an increased physical risk. The failure to render EC in a timely manner similarly compels women to utilize services that carry a relatively increased physical risk, such as abortion. Second, the Court noted that women suffer psychological harm as a consequence of delay.[114] When pregnancy is prevented through EC, women avoid the more emotionally challenging experience of having to decide whether or not to terminate a pregnancy. This is especially true for victims of sexual assault. An unreasonable delay in access to care after forced sexual intercourse prolongs a woman's victimization by failing to protect her against further psychological and physical consequences of the assault.

A legislative scheme that arbitrarily limits the right of a woman to deal with her body as she chooses violates the principles of fundamental justice. A scheme is arbitrary if it bears no relation to the objective that lies behind the legislation.[115] Since women can effectively self-diagnose, self-select, and self-administer EC, a regulation that requires women to consult a pharmacist prior to obtaining EC impedes access to essential reproductive care without furthering the objectives that lie behind the regulation.

Substantive Equality under the Charter and the CEDAW Convention

Discrimination on grounds of sex is prohibited under the *Charter* and by human rights treaties to which Canada is a party. Canada is therefore obligated to eliminate all forms of discrimination against women. A health care system that unfairly denies women access to essential reproductive health care on the basis of sex violates the principle of substantive equality and constitutes discrimination under both Section 15(1) of the *Charter* and Article 12(1) of the *CEDAW Convention*. Section 15(1) provides that '[e]very individual is equal before and under the law and has the right to equal protection and equal benefit of the law without discrimination and, in particular, without discrimination based on ... sex, age ... or physical disability.'[116] Article 12(1) of the *CEDAW Convention* requires that member states 'take all appropriate measures to eliminate discrimination against women in the field of health care in order to ensure, on a basis of equality of men and women, access to health care services, including those related to family planning.'[117]

In *Eaton v. Brant County Board of Education*,[118] the Supreme Court outlined two principal objects underlying the guarantees of non-discrimination and substantive equality.

The first objective is to eliminate 'discrimination by the attribution of untrue characteristics based on stereotypical attitudes relating to immutable conditions such as race or sex.'[119] In *Andrews v. The Law Society of British Columbia*,[120] the Supreme Court held that it is discriminatory to draw a distinction on the basis of wrongly attributed personal characteristics, 'which has the effect of imposing burdens, obligations or disadvantages ... not imposed on others, or which withholds or limits access to opportunities, benefits, and advantages available to other members of society.'[121]

The second objective is to obligate governments to 'account [for] the true characteristics of [a] group which act as headwinds to the enjoyment of society's benefits and to accommodate them.'[122] In *Law v. Canada (Minister of Employment and Immigration)*,[123] the Supreme Court of Canada confirmed that government action that is insensitive to the needs, capacities, and merits of different individuals, and fails to account for the context underlying those differences, violates the principle of substantive equality.[124] The CEDAW Committee's General Recommendation on *Women and Health* advises that women's biological differences respecting pregnancy and its prevention should be accommodated in ways that adequately reflect those differences.[125] The needs of different subgroups of women, such as adolescents or victims of sexual assault, should also be accommodated according to their respective differences.[126]

In *Law*, the Supreme Court affirmed that the paramount goal of substantive equality is respect for the innate and equal dignity of every individual without distinction on the basis of a listed or analogous ground under Section 15(1), including sex.[127] Substantive equality posits 'a society in which all persons enjoy equal recognition at law as human beings or as members of Canadian society, equally capable and equally deserving of concern, respect and consideration.'[128]

Unwarranted professional controls perpetuate gender stereotyping and fail to account for the distinctive needs of women in accessing care. BTC availability of EC does not recognize women as equal members of society, equally capable and equally deserving of concern, respect, and consideration. Rather, conditioning access to essential reproductive health on unnecessary professional intervention treats women as less worthy than others on the basis of their sex.

Imposition of Disadvantage, Stereotyping, or Social Prejudice
In *Law*, the Court held that human dignity is 'harmed by unfair treatment premised upon personal traits or circumstances which do not relate to individual needs, capacities or merits.'[129] In *Gosselin v. Quebec (Attorney General)*,[130] the Court further explained that 'a law that imposes restrictions or denies benefits on account of presumed or unjustly attributed characteristics is likely to deny essential human worth and to be discriminatory.'[131]

Authoritative evidence demonstrates that as measured against Factors 1, 8, and 9 of Schedule II, EC does not warrant pharmacist intervention. The lack of evidence supporting NDSAC's recommendation leads one to question the basis upon which the Committee was nevertheless prepared to propose, and Health Canada prepared to accept, BTC availability for EC. Was EC assessed against considerations other than those factors prescribed for Schedule II? If so, why was EC treated differently from other drugs?

Given the historic patterns of discrimination against women in relation to their sexual and reproductive health, and the fact that EC is indicated for a condition related to women's sexuality and reproduction, a strong presumption is raised that the decision respecting the appropriate conditions for the sale of EC was motivated or perpetuated by the very same discriminatory views. In *Gosselin*, the Court recognized pre-existing disadvantage as a key marker of discrimination and marginalization. The Court stated that '[h]istoric patterns of discrimination ... often indicate the presence of stereotypical or prejudicial views that have marginalized its members and prevented them from participating fully in society. This, in turn, raises the strong possibility that current differential treatment of the group may be motivated by or may perpetuate the same discriminatory views.'[132]

As a class, women of reproductive age, and particularly the subclasses of adolescents and economically disadvantaged women, have historically been and continue to be subject to stereotypes and generalizations in the provision of sexual and reproductive health care. Control over women's bodies and minds has historically not been their own. Women were and continue to be viewed as incapable of responsibly engaging in sexual intercourse and deciding the course of their reproductive care. Their choices were and continue to be unreasonably questioned, verified, and approved by male partners, health professionals, and the state. In *Morgentaler*, Justice Wilson expressly recognized that the former abortion committees in essence asserted that a 'woman's capacity to reproduce is not to be subject to her own control. It is to be subject to the control of the state.'[133]

Pharmacist intervention in the distribution of EC is suspect given the pre-existing generalization or stereotype that women are incapable of making informed decisions about their sexual behaviour and medical care. The requirement for pharmacist assessment and consultation is at least partially premised on the belief that, with increased access, women will irrationally forgo regular and more effective forms of contraception. Stereotypical assumptions about women's tendency towards promiscuous sexual behaviour and the mismanagement of their sexual health have clearly influenced this concern. Provider intervention also appears to rely on the misassumption that women cannot recognize or administer treatment to prevent an unplanned pregnancy without supervision. It is thus not the drug that is unsafe or ineffective, but the administering patient. Barriers to access are erected on the basis of women's wrongly perceived personal characteristics.

In *Law*, the Court recognized that government conduct that imposes disadvantage, stereotyping, or social prejudice violates essential human dignity and freedom.[134] Human dignity, the Court continued, concerns 'physical and psychological integrity and empowerment.'[135] These are the components of autonomous action. Health care policy based on stereotypical grounds deprives women of equal respect for their human dignity by lessening their autonomy. The *CEDAW Convention* explicitly acknowledges that substantive equality requires governments to provide health care in a manner 'consistent with the human rights of women, including the rights to autonomy ... informed consent and choice.'[136] In *Morgentaler*, Justice Wilson similarly recognized that the right to autonomously decide whether to 'reproduce or not to reproduce ... is properly perceived as an integral part of modern woman's struggle to assert *her* dignity and worth as a human being.'[137]

The indignity of refusing women reasonable access to EC is most accurately described as a denial of women's autonomous choice to reproduce. When access to EC is conditioned on pharmacist assessment and consultation, women are not free to make informed choices about their sexual and reproductive health. They are deprived the power to define and direct their lives, as well as the capacity to shape their identity as a human beings.

Insensitivity to the Needs, Capacities, and Merits of Women

In *Andrews*, the Supreme Court held that the 'accommodation of differences ... is the essence of true equality.'[138] The purpose of section 15(1) is not only to prevent stereotypes or generalizations that harm human dignity, but also to enhance the equal dignity of every individual by enacting policies and laws that are 'sensitive to the needs, capacities and merits of different individuals.'[139] Under Article 12(1) of the *CEDAW Convention*, Canada is similarly obliged 'to ensure [that] access to quality health care services ... are delivered in a way that ensures that a woman gives her fully informed consent, respects her dignity, guarantees her confidentiality and is sensitive to her needs and perspectives.'[140]

When regulatory authorities determine the conditions of availability for a drug intended only for women, but fail to consider the distinctive needs, capacities and merits of women, they are acting in a discriminatory manner. Such failure suggests that women's health – and its protection and promotion – is not as important as the health of others. When women are precluded from equally participating in and benefiting from a supposed universal health care system, they are devalued as members of society, equally deserving of respect and consideration.

By subjecting women to unnecessary pharmacist intervention, the regulatory authorities have failed to recognize the distinctive socioeconomic and psychosocial needs of women in accessing EC. They have structured the availability of a therapeutic treatment for women in a manner that precludes the real possibility of women using that treatment. If regulatory authorities had considered the distinctive needs and capacities of women, the barriers of BTC availability, which include affordability, conscientious objection, lack of privacy, and paternalism, would have been identified. To the extent that government authorities have failed to do so, the regulatory policy is discriminatory on the basis of gender, age, and socioeconomic status.

It is sometimes argued that the adverse effects suffered by women in accessing health care stem not from the imposition of a burden by government regulation, but from women's existing social and economic disadvantages that the state neither created nor exacerbated. Section 15(1), it is claimed, does not oblige governments to implement programs to alleviate disadvantages that exist independently of state action. In *Eldridge v. British Columbia (Attorney General)*,[141] the Supreme Court of Canada held that such a distinction between state-imposed and pre-existing disadvantages 'bespeaks a thin and impoverished vision of s. 15(1). It belies this Court's equality jurisprudence.'[142] Although it is true that women's access to EC is not impeded by the method of availability per se, governments are nevertheless obliged to account for the distinctive disadvantages that affect women's capacity to access EC. This is the very thrust of a substantive theory of equality. Governmental activity does not escape constitutional scrutiny simply because it is facially neutral. On the contrary, it is the very 'neutrality' of the policy, its unresponsiveness to the factual realities of women's lives, that renders it discriminatory.

Demonstrable Justification in a Free and Democratic Society

The unfair denial of effective access to emergency contraception is not demonstrably justified in a free and democratic society, and thus cannot be saved by section 1 of the *Charter*. BTC availability of EC fails the *R. v Oakes* test.[143] While the objectives of drug regulations, safety and efficacy, can be of sufficient importance to override constitutionally protected rights, in the circumstances of EC, the means to achieve these objectives are neither reasonable nor demonstrably justified. A regulation that requires women to consult a pharmacist prior to obtaining

EC – or any other drug – when there is no scientific or medical reason to do so, is arbitrary. Moreover, given evidence that confirms the safety and effectiveness of self-administration with proper product labelling, the regulations do not minimally impair women's rights. Last, the barriers to access imposed by BTC availability outweigh any benefit provided by pharmacist controls.

Conclusion

A health care system is an outgrowth of the political culture, and the social and moral values of the society it serves. If Canada is to remain a society dedicated to the equitable treatment of all persons, all levels of governments must remain conscious of human rights values in the organization and distribution of health care. The primary objective of Canadian health care policy cannot merely be the protection, promotion, and restoration of the physical and mental well-being of residents. It must also be the *fair* protection, promotion, and restoration of health. A fair health care system requires, at a minimum, that all individuals have reasonable access to the health care that is related to their basic needs. Women's lack of fair access to EC is part of a larger injustice of obstacles women face in accessing health care. Governments must attend astutely to the differential impact of all health care policies, identifying opportunities to maintain and improve women's fair access to the health care system. As noted by the B.C. Supreme Court in *R v. Lewis*,[144] 'Health care has fundamental value in our society. A woman's right to access health care without unnecessary loss of privacy and dignity is no more than the right of every Canadian to access health care.'[145]

NOTES

1 S. Dunn and E. Guilbert, 'SOCG Clinical Practice Guidelines: Emergency Contraception' (2003) 131 J. Obstet. Gynaecol. Can. 673 at 674 ['SOGC Clinical Practice Guidelines'].

2 Statistics Canada and Canadian Institute for Health Information, 'Pregnancy Outcomes by Age Group' (October 2004), http://www.statcan.ca/english/Pgdb/hlth65a.htm (accessed 6 March 2005).

3 Statistics Canada and Canadian Institute for Health Information, 'Induced Abortions by Age Group' (February 2005), http://www.statcan.ca/english/Pgdb/health43.htm (accessed 6 March 2005).

4 Statistics Canada and Canadian Institute for Health Information, 'Induced Abortions per 100 Live Births' (February 2005), http://www.statcan.ca/english/Pgdb/health42d.htm (accessed 6 March 2005).

5 For women less than 19 years of age, induced abortions were performed most often between 9 and 12 weeks gestation. Women aged 25 to 44 were more likely to have induced abortions at less than 9 weeks. Reproductive Health Report Working Group, *Alberta Reproductive Health: Pregnancies and Births 2004* (Edmonton: Alberta Health and Wellness, 2004), http://www.health.gov.ab.ca/resources/publications/pdf/reproductive04 .pdf (accessed 6 March 2005) at 29 and Table A9.

6 See Rodgers, this volume; Childbirth by Choice Trust, *Abortion in Canada Today: The Situation Province-by-Province* (Toronto: Childbirth by Choice Trust, 2003), http://www.caral.ca/uploads/Province%20by%20province%202003.doc (accessed 6 March 2005); and Canadian Abortion Rights Action League (CARAL), *Protecting Abortion Rights in Canada: A Special Report to Celebrate the 15th Anniversary of the Decriminalization of Abortion* (Ottawa: Canadian Abortion Rights Action League, 2003), http://www.caral.ca/uploads/caralreporti.pdf> (accessed 6 March 2005).

7 L. Eggertson, 'Abortion Services in Canada: a Patchwork Quilt with Many Holes' (2001) 164:6 Can. Med. Assoc. J. 847.

8 CARAL, *supra* note 6.

9 Nova Scotia, Quebec, and the Yukon only partially fund clinic abortions, and patients are required to pay the facility an amount ranging from $200 to $750. The New Brunswick provincial government entirely refuses to fund medically unnecessary abortions. *Childbirth by Choice, supra* note 6.

10 EC acts before implantation, and is therefore not an abortifacient. EC will not dislodge a pre-existing implanted embryo. See D.A. Grimes and E.G. Raymond, 'Emergency Contraception' (2002) 137:3 Ann. Intern. Med. 180 at 181.

11 World Health Organization (WHO), *Emergency Contraception: A Guide for Service Delivery* (Geneva: WHO, 1998), http://whqlibdoc.who.int/hq/1998/WHO_FRH_FPP_98.19.pdf (accessed 6 March 2005) at 7.

12 D.A. Grimes *et al.*, 'Randomised Controlled Trial of Levonorgestrel versus the Yuzpe Regimen of Combined Oral Contraceptives for Emergency Contraception' (1998) 352:9126 Lancet 428 at 431 ['Levonorgestrel v. Yuzpe Regimens'].

13 *Ibid.*

14 *Ibid.* See also C. Westhoff. 'Emergency Contraception' (2003) 349:(19) N. Eng. J. Med. 1830 at 1831.

15 International Consortium for Emergency Contraception, *Emergency Contra-*

ceptive Pills: Medical and Service Delivery Guidelines, 2nd ed. (Washington: International Consortium for Emergency Contraception, 2003), http://www.cecinfo.org/files/Guidelines per cent202nd per cent20editione.pdf (accessed 6 March 2005).

16 EC is available without a doctor's prescription in 30 countries, including the United Kingdom, France, Belgium, Sweden, and Norway. D. Grimes, 'Switching Emergency Contraception to Over-the-Counter Status' (2002) 347:11 N. Engl. J. Med. 846 at 846 ['Switching EC'].

17 Health Canada, News Release 2005-25, 'Minister Dosanjh Announces Regulatory Changes to Allow Levonorgestrel 0.75 mg (Plan B) to Be Sold without a Prescription' (20 April 2005), http://www.hc-sc.gc.ca/english/media/releases/2005/2005_25.html (accessed 25 April 2005). An amendment to the *Food and Drug Regulations*, C.R.C., c. 870 permitting levonorgestrel 0.75 mg to be sold without a prescription came into force on 19 April 2005. The amendment was published in Part II of the *Canada Gazette* on 4 May 2005. See Regulations Amending the Food and Drug Act Regulations (1272-Levonorgestrel) SOR/2005-105 April 19, 2005, Vol 139, No. 9, http://canadagazette.gc.ca/partII/2005/20050504/html/sor/05-e.html#avis (accessed 21 August 2005).

18 NDSAC, *Drug Schedules Notice Board*, http://www.napra.org/docs/0/92/111.asp (accessed 25 April 2005).

19 In preparation for BTC dispensing of EC, the Canadian Pharmacists Association has developed screening and counselling guidelines. See CPhA, 'CPhA (CPhA) Takes Action: Emergency Contraception,' http://www.pharmacists .ca/content/about_cpha/Whats_Happening/CPhA_in_Action/emerge_ contra.cfm (accessed 6 March 2005).

20 In October 2000 the lieutenant governor of British Columbia amended the *Prescribed Health Care Profession Regulation*, B.C. Reg. 354/2000 to allow trained and certified pharmacists to dispense EC without a prescription. On 2 April 2001, the regulatory change was granted statutory authority with the passage of Bill 8, *Emergency Contraceptive Access Act*, S.B.C. 2001, c. 11. A recent study found that allowing pharmacists to prescribe and distribute EC in B.C. increased the number of EC prescriptions in that province by increasing access through extended hours of operation of pharmacies and the higher number of locations from which EC could be obtained. See J.A. Soon et al., 'Effects of Making Emergency Contraception Available without a Physician's Prescription: A Population-Based Study' (2005) 172:7 Can. Med. Assn. J. 878.

21 Section 17(6) of the *Pharmacy Act*, R.S.Q., c. P-10 permits pharmacists to dispense EC OTC, provided a training certificate has been issued to the

pharmacist pursuant to a regulation under para. o of s. 94 of the *Professional Code* (c. C-26).

22 Under the *Pharmacy Amendment Act, 2003,* S.S. 2003, c. 8, the Council of the Saskatchewan College of Pharmacists can create bylaws permitting pharmacists to prescribe drugs consistent with their scope of practice. Under this authority, pharmacists may independently dispense EC.

23 Health Canada, 'Certain Circumstances: Issues in Equity and Responsiveness in Access to Health Care in Canada' (Ottawa: Health Canada, 2001), http://www.HealthCanada-sc.gc.ca/hppb/healtHealth Canadaare/pdf/circumstances.pdf (accessed 6 March 2005).

24 Health Canada, *Report from Consultations on a Framework for Sexual and Reproductive Health* (Ottawa: Health Canada, 1999), http://www.HealthCanada-sc.gc.ca/hppb/srh/pubs/report/ (accessed 6 March 2005) ['Health Canada Framework'].

25 Part I of the *Constitution Act*, 1982, being Schedule B to the *Canada Act 1982* (U.K.), 1982, c.11.

26 Adopted 18 Dec. 1979, G.A. Res. 34/180, U.N. GAOR 34th Sess. (entered into force 3 Sept. 1981).

27 See generally, *Canadian Union of Public Employees, Local 963 v. New Brunswick Liquor Corporation,* [1979] 2 S.C.R. 227, 97 D.L.R. (3d) 417.

28 Canadian courts have used this phrase to express their reluctance to enter scientific debates. Sexton J.A. employed this term in *Inverhuron and District Ratepayers' Assn. v. Canada (Minister of the Environment)* (2001), 273 N.R. 62 at para. 36 (F.C.C.A.), aff'g (2001) 39 C.E.L.R. (N.S.) 13 (F.C.T.D.).

29 See *Caiwaw v. Pacar of Canada Ltd.*, [1989] 2 S.C.R. 983.

30 C.R.C., c. 870.

31 *Regulations Amending the Food and Drug Regulations (1272 – Levonorgestrel)*, Notice, C. Gaz. 2004.1.Vol. 138, No. 21, http://canadagazette.gc.ca/partI/2004/20040522/html/regle1-e.html#avis (accessed 6 March 2005) [*Canada Gazette* – Part 1].

32 Letter from R.G. Peterson, Director General (Therapeutic Products Directorate), 'Re: Amendment to the Food and Drug Regulations – Schedule 1272 (Deletion of Levonorgestrel, When Indicated for Use as an Emergency Contraceptive, from Schedule F of the Food and Drug Regulations)' (16 June 2003).

33 Paladin Labs., Press Release, 'Paladin Announces Submission to Health Canada for Non-Prescription Status for Plan B™ (8 March 2002), http://www.paladin-labs.com/press_Release_archives/2002_03_08.html (accessed 6 March 2005).

34 *Canada Gazette* – *Part 1, supra* note 31.

35 *Levonorgestrel v. Yuzpe Regimens, supra* note 12 at 431.
36 *Canada Gazette – Part 1, supra* note 31.
37 D. Grimes, E. Raymond, and B. Scott Jones, 'Emergency Contraception Over-the-Counter: The Medical and Legal Imperatives' (2001) 98:1 Obstet. Gynecol. 151 at 152 ['Medical and Legal Imperatives'].
38 *Ibid.*
39 A. Glasier, 'Safety of Emergency Contraception' (1998) 53:5 J. Amer. Med. Women's Assn. 219 at 221.
40 WHO, *Medical Eligibility Criteria for Contraceptive Use,* 3rd ed. (Geneva: WHO, 2004), http://www.who.int/reproductive-health/publications/MEC_3/mec.pdf (accessed 6 March 2005).
41 See M.B. Bracken, 'Oral Contraception and congenital Malformations in Offspring: A Review and Meta-analysis of the Prospective Studies' (1990) 76 Obstet. Gynecol. 552; P. Simpson, 'Spermicides, Hormonal Contraception and Congenital Malformations' (1990) 6 Adv. Contracept. 141.
42 *SOGC Clinical Practice Guidelines, supra* note 1 at 677.
43 American College of Obstetricians and Gynecologists (ACOG), *Emergency Oral Contraception: ACOG Practice Guidelines No. 25* (Washington: ACOG, 2001).
44 A. Glasier and D. Baird, 'The Effects of Self-Administering Emergency Contraception' (1998) 339:1 N. Engl. J. Med. 1 at 4 ['Effects of Self-Administration'].
45 See E. Kosunen, S. Sihvo, and E. Hemminki, 'Knowledge and Use of Hormonal EC in Finland' (1997) 55 *Contraception* 153.
46 'Effects of Self-Administration,' *supra* note 44 at 4. See also S. Rowlands. 'Repeated Use of Emergency Contraception by Younger Women in the UK' (2000) 26:3 Br. J. Fam. Plann. 138.
47 See E. Aubeny, 'Can Hormonal Emergency Contraception (EC) Be Available without Medical Prescription?' (2000) 5:1 Eur. J. Contracept. Reprod. Health Care 41.
48 *Canada Gazette – Part 1, supra* note 31.
49 The supply of health goods and services is the exclusive jurisdiction of provincial and territorial governments pursuant to their jurisdiction over the establishment, maintenance, and management of Hospitals [s. 91(7)], property and civil rights [s. 92(13)], and matters of a local or private nature [91(16)] under the *Constitution Act,* 1867 (U.K.), 30 and 31 Vict. C.3, reprinted in R.S.C. 1985, App. II, No. 5.
50 Member pharmacy regulatory authorities include the Alberta College of Pharmacists, the College of Pharmacists of British Columbia, the Government of Northwest Territories, Manitoba Pharmaceutical Association, New

Brunswick Pharmaceutical Society, Newfoundland Pharmaceutical Society, Nova Scotia College of Pharmacists, Pharmacy Services Division of the Canadian Armed Forces, Prince Edward Island Pharmacy Board, the Saskatchewan College of Pharmacists, and the Yukon Government.

51 Provincial implementation of the NDSAC model differs across Canada. In Manitoba, New Brunswick, Ontario, and Nova Scotia, the provincial governments have adopted the NDSAC model ('scheduling by reference'). Provincial legislation delegates regulatory power to the respective Colleges of Pharmacy to amend drug schedules in accordance with NDSAC recommendations. Prince Edward Island is expected to pass similar legislation. Newfoundland and Labrador, Saskatchewan, and British Columbia have adopted the NDSAC system, but have not delegated regulatory authority to their respective colleges. Alberta has not adopted the national drug scheduling system, but generally follows NDSAC recommendations. Quebec has no plans to adopt the national model.

52 NDSAC, *Minutes from National Drug Scheduling Advisory Committee: Request for Non-Prescription Status for Plan B* (3–4 Nov. 2001), http://www.napra.org/docs/0/92/116/122/128.asp (accessed 6 March 2005) [NDSAC *Minutes*].

53 NAPRA, *Outline of National Drug Schedules*, http://www.napra.ca/docs/0/92/112/154/139.asp#schII (accessed 6 March 2005) [*Outline of National Schedules*].

54 *Canada Gazette – Part 1*, *supra* n31 and Peterson, *supra* n33.

55 NDSAC *Minutes ... Correspondence re: Plan B Schedule Status* (12–13 December 2004), http://www.napra.ca/pdfs/drugsched/0412minutes.pdf (accessed 6 March 2005).

56 NAPRA, *Drug Schedules Notice Board*, http://www.napra.org/docs/0/92/111.asp (accessed 25 April 2005).

57 NDSAC *Minutes, supra* n52. The sponsoring agencies were the SOGC, the CPA, CanReg Inc., and Women's Capital Corporation.

58 *Ibid.*

59 NAPRA, *Outline of the Scheduling Process: Factors for Schedule II*, http://www.napra.ca/docs/0/92/112/154/140.asp#factII (accessed 6 March 2005) [*Schedule II Factors*].

60 *Canada Gazette – Part 1*, *supra* note 31.

61 *Schedule II Factors, supra* note 59.

62 *Canada Gazette – Part 1, supra* note 31.

63 'Medical and Legal Imperatives,' *supra* note 37 at 152.

64 *Ibid.*

65 *Schedule II Factors, supra* note 59.

66 C. Ellerston et al., 'Should Emergency Contraceptive Pills Be Available without Prescription?' (1998) 53:5 J. Amer. Med. Women's Assn. 226 at 227.
67 *Canada Gazette – Part 1, supra* note 31.
68 *Schedule II Factors, supra* note 59.
69 Ellerston, *supra* note 64.
70 'Medical and Legal Imperatives,' *supra* note 37 at 152.
71 E.G. Raymond, S.M. Dalebout, and S.I. Camp, 'Comprehension of a Prototype Over-the-Counter Label for an Emergency Contraceptive Pill Product' (2002) 100:2 Obstet. Gynecol. 342.
72 E.G. Raymond, P. Chen, and S.M. Dalebout, '"Actual Use" Study of Emergency Contraceptive Pills Provided in a Simulated Over-the-Counter Manner' (2003) 102:1 Obstet. Gynecol. 17.
73 'Switching EC,' *supra* note 16 at 847.
74 *Outline of National Schedules, supra* note 53.
75 *Ibid.*
76 H. Brooks, 'The Resolution of Technically Intensive Public Policy Disputes' (1984) 9:1 Science, Technology and Human Values 39 at 40.
77 W.E. Wagner, 'The Science Charade in Toxic Risk Regulation' (1995) 95 Colum. L. Rev. 1613 at 1617.
78 J.D. Fraiberg and M.J. Trebilock, 'Risk Regulation: Technocratic and Democratic Tools for Regulatory Reform' (1998) 43 McGill L.J. 835 at para 26.
79 CEDAW, General Recommendation 24, Women and Health (Article 12), CEDAW/C/1999/I/W.G.II/WP.2/Rev.1, http://www.un.org/womenwatch/daw/cedaw/recommendations/recomm.htm#recom24 (accessed 6 March 2005) ['General Recommendation'].
80 Health Canada Framework, *supra* note 24.
81 National Council on Welfare, *Poverty Profile 2001* (Ottawa: Minister of Public Works and Government Services Canada, 2004) at 44 and 107, online: <http://www.ncwcnbes.net/htmdocument/reportpovertypro01/PP2001_e.pdf> (accessed 6 March 2005).
82 J. Trussell et al., 'Cost Savings from Emergency Contraceptive Pills in Canada' (2001) 97:5 (Part 1) Obstet. Gynecol. 789 at 791.
83 *Ibid* at 789–90.
84 *Ibid.*
85 In British Columbia, pharmacies contract with the Ministry of Health's third party prescription payment plan to be paid a $15 counselling fee for pharmacist-initiated EC prescriptions. Pharmacies without a contract set their own price (usually $25), which is paid by the patient. The provincial drug insurance plans in Quebec and Saskatchewan pay pharmacists $15 for the counselling component of a pharmacist-initiation EC prescription. See also Robert Kouri (chapter 6, this volume).

86 R.J. Cook, B.M. Dickens, and M.F. Fathalla, *Reproductive Health and Human Rights: Integrating Medicine, Ethics and Law* (Oxford: Oxford University Press, 2003) at 291–2; J. Cantor and K. Baum, 'The Limits of Conscientious Objection – May Pharmacists Refuse to Fill Prescriptions for Emergency Contraception?' (2004) 351:19 N. Eng. J. Med. 2008 at 2011.

87 'General Recommendation,' *supra* note 79 at para. 11.

88 *Cantor, supra* note 84 at 2010.

89 General Recommendation, *supra* note 79 at para. 12(d).

90 Health Canada Framework, *supra* note 24.

91 The informed consent form used by pharmacists dispensing EC OTC in British Columbia requires patients to identify whether their need for EC results from the failure of a birth control method or unprotected inter-course. Pharmacists retain the form on file for three years. College of Pharmacists of British Columbia, *Informed Consent for Emergency Contraception*, http://www.bcpharmacists.org/resources/pdf/Info_Cons_for_ ECP.pdf (accessed 6 March 2005).

92 See C.E. Lindberg, 'Emergency Contraception for Prevention of Adolescent Pregnancy' (2003) 28:3 MCN Am. J. Matern Child Nurs. 199; P.J.A. Hillard, 'Oral Contraceptive Non-compliance: The Extent of the Problem' (1992) 8:1 Adv Contracep. 13.

93 C.R. Kartoz, 'New Options for Teen Pregnancy Prevention' (2004) 29:1 MCN Am. J. Matern. Child Nurs. 30 at 30; see also D.A. Reddy, R. Fleming, and C. Swain, 'Effect of Mandatory Parental Notification on Adolescent Girls' Use of Sexual Health Care Services' (2002) 288 JAMA 710; K.W. Wilson and J.D. Klein, 'Health Care and Contraceptive Use among Adolescents Reporting Unwanted Sexual Intercourse' (2002) 156:4 *Arch. Pediatr. Adolesc. Med.* 341.

94 See D.B. Langille and M.E. Delaney, 'Knowledge and Use of Emergency Postcoital Contraception by Female Students at a High School in Nova Scotia' (2000) 91:1 Can. J. Public Health 29 at 31.

95 See S.D. Sommers et al., 'The Emergency Contraception Collaborative Prescribing Experience in Washington State' (2001) 41 J. Am. Pharm. Assoc. 60.

96 L.A.E. Conard et al., 'Pharmacists' Attitudes toward and Practices with Adolescents' (2003) 157:4 *Arch. Pediatr. Adolesc. Med.* 361 at 361. See also Kouri, *supra* note 83.

97 *Canada Gazette Notice, supra* note 31.

98 R.A. Jackson *et al.*, 'Advance Supply of Emergency Contraception: Effect on Use and Usual Contraception – A Randomized Trial' (2003) 102:1 Obstet. Gynecol. 8 at 12, 13.

99 See M.A. Gold, A. Schein, and S.M. Coupey, 'Emergency Contraception:

A National Survey of Adolescent Health Experts' (1997) 29:1 Fam. Plann. Perspect. 5. Another study demonstrates that educating teens about EC does not increase their sexual activity levels or use of the drug, but increases their knowledge about proper administration of EC. See A. Graham et al., 'Improving Teenagers Knowledge of Emergency Contraception: Cluster Randomized Controlled Trial of a Teacher-Led Intervention' (2002) 234:7347 Br. Med. J. 1179.

100 Kosunen, *supra* note 45.
101 Ellerston, *supra* note 64 at 228.
102 *SOGC Clinical Practice Guidelines, supra* note 1 at 676.
103 *Ibid.*
104 *Reibl v. Hughes* (1980), 114 D.L.R. (3rd) 1 (S.C.C.) following *Cobbs v. Grant* (1972) 8 Cal.3d 229, 242 [104] Cal.Rptr. 505, 502 P.2d 1, as applied in *Kathleen Brownfield v. Daniel Freeman Marina Hospital* (1989) 208 Cal. App 3d 405, 412, 413 (failure to adequately disclose EC as an option within 72 hours of unprotected intercourse, when a skilled practitioner would have provided such information, can justify an award of damages for negligence if the woman demonstrates that she suffered injury and would have otherwise taken that option).
105 P. Hogg, *Constitutional Law of Canada*, looseleaf, 3rd ed. (Toronto: Carswell, 1992) at 34-8.3–34-9.
106 [1999] 2 S.C.R. 817.
107 *Ibid.* at para. 56.
108 *Charter, supra* note 24 at section 7.
109 [1988] 1 S.C.R. 30 [*Morgentaler*].
110 *Ibid.* at para 20.
111 *Ibid.* at para 22.
112 *Ibid.* at paras. 83 and 84.
113 *Ibid.* at para 23.
114 *Ibid.* at para 28.
115 See *Rodriguez v. British Columbia (Attorney General)*, [1993] 3 S.C.R. 519 at 619, McLachlin J. (in dissent).
116 *Charter, supra* note 24 at section 15(1).
117 *CEDAW Convention, supra* note 26 at art. 12(1).
118 [1997] 1 S.C.R. 241 [*Eaton*].
119 *Ibid.* at para. 67.
120 [1989] 1 S.C.R. 143 [*Andrews*].
121 *Ibid.* at para. 37.
122 *Eaton, supra* note 118 at para. 67.
123 [1999] 1 S.C.R. 497 [*Law*].

124 *Ibid*. at para. 53.

125 'General Recommendation,' *supra* note 79 at para. 6.

126 *Ibid*. at paras. 9–12.

127 *Law, supra* note 123 at para. 51.

128 *Ibid*.

129 *Ibid*. at para. 51.

130 [2002] 4 S.C.R. 429.

131 *Ibid*. at para. 37.

132 *Ibid*. at para. 30.

133 *Morgentaler, supra* note 109 at para. 243.

134 *Law, supra* note 123 at 51.

135 *Ibid*. at para. 53; citing Lamer C.J. in *Rodriguez, supra* note 115 at 554.

136 'General Recommendation,' *supra* note 79 at para. 31.

137 *Morgentaler*, supra note 109 at para. 240.

138 *Andrews, supra* note 120 at 169.

139 *Law, supra* note 123 at para. 53.

140 'General Recommendation,' *supra* note 79 at para. 22.

141 [1997] 3 S.C.R. 624.

142 *Ibid*. at para. 73.

143 [1986] 1 S.C.R. 103.

144 (1996), 139 D.L.R. (4th) 480.

145 *Ibid*. at 509.

7 Achieving Reproductive Rights: Access to Emergency Oral Contraception and Abortion in Quebec

ROBERT P. KOURI

Although controversies relating to access and allocation of services are encountered in virtually all facets of health care, in Quebec they are particularly evident in matters relating to contraception and abortion. The social, economic, and to a somewhat lesser extent, political ramifications surrounding the provision of these services influence policies affecting the reproductive rights of the individual. The two preceding chapters examine access to emergency contraception and to abortions. This chapter reviews access to both in Quebec.

In a paper made public on 26 February 1996, the Quebec Ministry of Health and Social Services set out the priorities and strategies for government policy in matters of family planning.[1] Rather than being a radical departure from previous policies, which have tended to be piecemeal and sectoral, it advocated continuity but with an emphasis on new challenges arising from certain sociological phenomena including the increased incidence of sexually transmitted diseases and the ever-present problem of adolescent pregnancy.[2] The constant increase in the number of voluntary terminations of pregnancy for women of all ages as well as regional disparities in the availability of abortion services were also matters of concern.[3]

Accordingly, the government set out a two-pronged approach: on the one hand it proposed to increase the availability and utilization of contraception and, on the other, to reduce the number of abortions in the second trimester. With regard to contraception, it sought to reduce to less than 15 per thousand the pregnancy rate for adolescents under 17 years of age, and, more generally, to respond to a need for contraceptive methods better adapted to the specific circumstances of young women.[4]

As for voluntary terminations of pregnancy, it was felt that the services offered should answer the requirements of women in a manner commensurate with their particular situation, more specifically, as they relate to teenagers, women members of cultural minorities, or women from backgrounds characterized by deprivation. A more explicit goal was to reduce by one-third the number of second-trimester abortions generally and to cut the rate of terminations by half for women under twenty years of age.[5] The obvious danger, of course, is that it will be easier for the government to fulfil its goal of reducing abortion rates through underfunding and underprovision of abortion services rather than through reducing the demand for abortions by ensuring better access to emergency oral contraception (EC).

Although these policies were generally received with approval, two criticisms have been voiced by the Quebec Council on the Status of Women (Conseil du Statut de la Femme). The Council felt that the government's paper failed to address the key issue of the costs incurred by women in obtaining contraception and abortion services. Moreover, the government's position alluded to the problem of regional disparities in the provision of services only in very general and non-committal terms. The Council noted in this regard that certain administrative regions offered no abortion services at all within their territories, and only five regions out of sixteen provided terminations of pregnancy after a gestational age of 14 weeks.[6]

Mindful of the orientations put forward by the government, the purpose of this chapter is to examine first, whether the strategies adopted in Quebec are likely to adequately provide emergency oral contraception, and second, to discuss whether timely abortion services are sufficiently available to women in all regions of Quebec.

Improved Access to Emergency Oral Contraception: An Essential Element of Reproductive Autonomy

Traditionally, the prescription of medication has been a prerogative of physicians and dentists.[7] However, to render emergency contraception more readily available throughout the Province of Quebec, the College of Physicians requested that legislation be adopted allowing pharmacists to prescribe the so-called 'morning-after pill.' The Quebec government proceeded first by Order- in-Council, 23 August 2001, and adopted a *Regulation Respecting the Acts Contemplated in Section 31 of the Medical Act which May Be Done by Classes of Persons other than Physicians*.[8] The Regulation allows pharmacists to 'prescribe medication' required for the purpose of emergency oral contraception provided that 'the act is done by a pharmacist who holds a certificate delivered by the Ordre des pharmaciens du Québec attesting to his [or her] successful completion of the training requirements. The pharmacist shall personally fill the prescription.'[9] A concomitant regulation,[10] adopted under the *Professional Code*,[11] obliges all pharmacists to undertake this training except, inter alia, those whose moral convictions are opposed to the utilization of emergency oral contraception. The course, which lasts thirty-two hours, includes social, pharmacotherapeutic, clinical, ethical, and legal aspects of EC.[12]

The promulgation of this regulation was something of a stopgap measure, given the perceived urgency of ensuring readily accessible emergency contraception throughout the province. A more permanent legislative solution was found when, on 14 June 2002, the National Assembly adopted Bill 90, *An Act to Amend the Professional Code and Other Legislative Provisions as Regards the Health Sector.*[13] Under its terms, the *Pharmacy Act*[14] was amended to allow pharmacists to '[prescribe and personally dispense] emergency oral contraception medication provided a training certificate has been issued to the pharmacist by the Order pursuant to a regulation under paragraph o of section 94 of the Professional Code.'[15]

Although this innovative approach[16] to a persistent social dilemma appears to have ameliorated the problem of accessibility, there remain a number of barriers to access, not the least of which is the problem of confidentiality. For example, in order to prescribe the medication, the pharmacist must conform to the standards and protocols established by the Order of Pharmacists,[17] which require that in addition to dispensing the medication the pharmacist take a case history and provide counselling to the patient. The counter where prescriptions are filled is not an appropriate place to perform this service and pharmacists, although encouraged to provide a special area offering a modicum of privacy in which to hold the consultation, are hardly likely to undertake the expense required to do so. Thus, there is the problem (identified by Erdman and Cook in chapter 6) that women will still be deterred from seeking EC because of the requirement to be counselled first by a pharmacist.

Another area of difficulty relates to fear on the part of young women, in particular, that pharmacists might reveal to their patients or to others that they have obtained EC. Quebec law allows minors aged 14 years of age or more to consent alone to care required by their state of health; the person having parental authority is to be advised only when the minor remains in a health or social service establishment for more than 12 hours.[18] But two situations can compromise the basic duty of confidentiality. The first pertains to the provision of care by a pharmacist in a non-hospital milieu. In cases of treatment administered in an institution governed by the *Health Services and Social Services Act*,[19] section 21 requires that the holder of parental authority be entitled to access to a minor's health record. Such institutions include local community service centres, hospital centres, child and youth protection centres, residential and long-term care centres, and rehabilitation centres. The only exception to section 21 is the situation where the minor is 14 years of age or over and, having been consulted by the institution, he or she expressly refuses to allow his or her record to be communicated to the parent, and the institution determines that communication of the record will or could be prejudicial to the minor's health. This right of parental access is even more evident in cases where EC is provided by a pharmacist in private practice because, under the *Professional Code*, parental right of access is restricted only when the pharmacist determines that disclosure of the record would likely cause serious harm to the client or to a third party.[20] As a general rule, one could hazard the opinion that parental wrath would probably not meet this standard. Interestingly enough, the *Professional Code* seems at odds with the *Code of Ethics of Pharmacists*,[21] since communication of a record can be refused under the latter if, in fact, there is good reason to believe that this communication could be detrimental to the patient. One could argue that the stricter standard set out in a general law such as the *Professional Code* should prevail over a standard established by mere regulation.

Granted, it is highly unlikely that parents would think to consult their child's pharmaceutical record, since they would not be informed that EC had been provided. However, the system is not foolproof in that, should the medication be paid for under a private group insurance plan[22] that is in the parents' name, the insurance company would normally forward the receipts to the parents.[23]

A similar situation may arise out of the *Youth Protection Act*[24] when circumstances 'provide reasonable grounds to believe that the security or development of a child is considered to be in danger within the meaning of subparagraph g of the first paragraph of section 38 [referring to victims of sexual abuse].'[25] In cases of abuse, the Director of Youth Protection must be advised, and any inquiries would inevitably be brought to the parents' attention. Indeed, as a matter of policy, patient confidentiality could, in fact, be compromised by an investigation. While properly stating that the rights of the child are paramount, the *Youth Protection Act* also declares that the primary responsibility for the child rests with the parents.[26] Accordingly, there is a duty to keep parents fully informed.[27] Even when applying urgent measures that could include removing the child from his or her present environment, both the child and the parents must be consulted.[28] The purpose of the consultation is 'to obtain the opinion of the child and the parents on the necessity of applying urgent measures and on the type of measures to be applied.'[29]

There are further barriers to access by Quebec women to emergency postcoital contraception. The first relates to the payment of professional fees. If the service is provided by a physician in private practice, at a hospital or at a local community service centre, the government will assume the cost. If a pharmacist provides the same service, his or her fees for the consultation, generally in the area of $45 excluding the cost of the medication itself, must be paid by the patient. The new legislation thus gives with one hand and takes with the other. Since the efficacy of EC depends upon the rapidity with which it is administered,[30] clearly it is far easier for women to get to a pharmacist than to seek an appointment with a physician or to wait in an emergency room. However, only women with the necessary financial means will, in fact, be able to pay for the pharmacist's services. As a means of circumventing this problem, women are often advised to obtain a physician's prescription in advance as a precautionary measure so it is readily available in case of need.[31] Surely, however, sound government policy would result in the removal of all financial barriers for women to access emergency contraception.

When recourse to EC is unavailable or undertaken outside the window of opportunity,[32] one must contemplate surgical or medical abortion.

Abortion: A Right Compromised by Restricted Access

Since the Supreme Court of Canada's decisions in *R. v. Morgentaler*[33] and *Tremblay v. Daigle*,[34] the most pressing issues in Quebec relate to the questions of access to abortion services and the limitations to access caused by distance, waiting times, and out-of-pocket payments. The 1998 *Morgentaler* judgment relied in part on the *Charter* argument that section 251 of the *Criminal Code*[35] contained restrictions and procedures seriously contravening women's rights to abortion. But the Court did not address the question whether there exists a right to publicly funded abortion services.[36] As a result, the issue of accessibility has not been truly resolved in Quebec.[37] The unavailability of services in more remote areas of the province clearly constitutes a barrier for women who live in those areas. However, even in urban centres, the constraints on hospitals and on local community service centres, which are required by law[38] to not incur deficits, have limited the availability of abortion services.[39] As a result, a lack of financial resources has created unacceptable delays, placing women before the Hobson's choice of going on a waiting list or of taking recourse to a privately funded clinic. At the time of writing, thirty-nine hospitals and local community service centres, representing 34.8 per cent of all institutions actually provide abortion services in the Province of Quebec. (The Canadian Abortion Rights Action League [CARAL] points out that this represents the highest percentage of hospitals and related institutions in Canada for any jurisdiction in Canada.)[40] Yet more than a third of all abortions in Quebec are performed in private clinics where women must pay for a portion of the costs of the treatment provided.[41] Indeed, under the *Health Insurance Act*,[42] only the physician's actual fees in private clinics are reimbursed; the patient must pay all other expenses. Consider that, in Quebec, in 2003, 26,920 therapeutic abortions by dilatation and curettage were performed, of which between 8,000 and 10,000 were performed in private clinics.[43] There is clearly a de facto two-tiered system in place in Quebec.

Another factor that skews the whole picture of availability involves the eligibility rules as applied by various institutions. In certain areas of the province, a person may get an abortion up to 20 weeks of gestation. Other establishments will provide this service only up to 12, 13, 14, or perhaps 16 weeks of gestation. In areas adjacent to Montreal or Sherbrooke, for example, it is possible for women to have access to institutions willing to perform later-term abortions. But for women in remoter areas where the cut-off point is set earlier, a trip to an urban centre becomes unavoidable. Here also, regional disparities in the level of services offered are a source of hardship and unfairness.

To deal with the inequities inherent in the system, a group called Association pour l'accès à l'avortement[44] (the Association) recently applied for, and was granted the right to bring a class action on behalf of 'all women covered by the Quebec Health Insurance Plan who disbursed a sum of money in order to obtain an abortion in the Province of

Quebec.'[45] The suit is grounded on the violation of four statutes, including the *Health Insurance Act* (HIA), the *Canadian Charter of Rights and Freedoms*,[46] the Quebec *Charter of Human Rights and Freedoms*,[47] and the *Canada Health Act* (CHA).[48] More particularly, it is alleged that a termination of a pregnancy is an insured service under the *Health Insurance Act*. Yet more than 30 per cent of all abortions are performed in private clinics. Since the sums paid by the Régie de l'assurance maladie du Québec for professional fees and expenses are quite modest, these clinics require that their patients pay a portion of the costs to be able to maintain services.[49] The action also alleges that the Government of Quebec is in violation of sections 7, 15, and 28 of the *Canadian Charter*,[50] sections 1, 6, and 10 of the *Quebec Charter*,[51] and section 7 of the *Canada Health Act*,[52] which guarantees universality, comprehensiveness, and accessibility. In addition to the fees actually disbursed by each patient, the Association seeks reimbursement by the government of the sum of $250 for trouble and inconvenience in addition to $500 per person in exemplary damages,[53] along with costs and interest. It has been estimated that damages in this suit on behalf of 100,000 women could total to $50 million.[54]

It should be noted that the *Health Services and Social Services Act* provides that 'every person is entitled to receive ... health services and social services which are scientifically, humanly and socially appropriate.'[55] But section 13 of the Act expressly recognizes that the health care system operates under certain constraints requiring that this right be exercised 'within the framework of the legislative and regulatory provisions relating to the organizational and operational structure of the institution and within the limits of the human, material and financial resources at its disposal.'[56] It is also fair to state that the Government of Quebec does not, as a matter of policy,[57] seek to restrict access to abortion as an indirect means of advancing a particular moral point of view.[58] Indeed, the obvious restrictions to access that *do* exist are as a result of budgetary constraints. But while there is not direct or overt discrimination, the unintended consequence of governmental policies is discriminatory, as I will elaborate further below.

Without predicting the outcome of the Association's case, one can surmise nonetheless that certain grounds invoked by the plaintiffs offer a greater potential for success than others. Commencing with the *Canadian Charter* and the *Quebec Charter*, which can be examined together because of the similarity of the provisions invoked and their analogous application by the courts,[59] it should be pointed out that although

Morgentaler, through its application of section 7 of the *Canadian Charter*,[60] has freed women and their physicians from the threat of criminal sanctions, it remains in essence the acknowledgment of a 'negative' right to security from state interference in this type of decision. The cases decided since *Morgentaler* have generally failed to recognize the right to security as a positive constitutional right and failed to demand that governments offer and assume complete financial responsibility for certain services such as abortion.[61]

Many writers have expressed the opinion that there is no positive section 7 right to health care.[62] Marco Laverdière, for example, asserts that the right to security would be infringed only if government measures prevented a person from opting for a service the costs of which would normally be assumed by the patient.[63] In contrast, Martha Jackman has argued strongly (chapter 5, this volume, and elsewhere) that section 7 of the *Canadian Charter* does indeed guarantees a constitutional right to publicly funded health care.[64]

It is evident that the judicial debate on positive entitlement to health care under the *Canadian Charter* is far from resolved, at least for the moment. In *Auton (Guardian ad litem of) v. British Columbia (Attorney General)*,[65] Chief Justice McLachlin, writing on behalf of the Supreme Court of Canada, expressed the view that since section 7 was raised only 'fleetingly' in the submissions before the Court, there were insufficient grounds to conclude that the government of British Columbia had indeed infringed the petitioners' section 7 rights.[66] It remains to be seen whether the *Chaoulli* v *Québec (A.G.)*[67] case pending before the Supreme Court (also discussed by Jackman in chapter 5), will be seized upon by the Court as an opportunity to clarify its position on this issue.

Equality rights protected under section 15(1) of the *Canadian Charter* would seem to offer firmer grounds for the recognition of the right to free access to family planning services such as emergency contraception and abortion. The Supreme Court of Canada in *Eldridge v. British Columbia (A.G.)*[68] set out the elements of a violation of section 15(1), namely that because of a distinction drawn, the claimant has been denied equal benefit of the law, and this denial constitutes discrimination on one of the grounds mentioned in the *Canadian Charter*.[69] The Court also mentioned that any discrimination on the basis of pregnancy would necessarily entail discrimination on the basis of sex.[70] There would result a duty to take positive action to redress inequities suffered by disadvantaged groups only when they suffer undue hardship.[71] In writing the unanimous decision, Justice La Forest affirmed that the government failed to demonstrate that the refusal to provide sign language interpreters had to be tolerated to achieve the objective of limiting health care expenditures.[72]

Yet, in *Cameron*,[73] the Court of Appeal of Nova Scotia refused to order the Nova Scotia government to reimburse plaintiffs the costs of intracytoplasmic sperm injection procedures (needed so that a couple, the male partner being infertile, could conceive a child). While finding that there had been discrimination based upon infertility and a denial of equal benefit under the Health Care Insurance Plan,[74] it was held that this policy of refusing reimbursement was justified under section 1 of the *Canadian Charter*.[75]

More recently in *Auton*,[76] the Court of Appeal of British Columbia held that the failure of the Provincial Crown to provide intensive 'applied behavioural analysis' or 'intensive behavioural intervention' therapy to autistic children of preschool age was a form of discrimination on the basis of age and mental disability. The Court acknowledged that while government monies should be allocated by the legislature, this principle '[would] not always prevail when the issue is compliance with the Constitution.'[77] Accordingly, the failure to provide treatment to a child suffering from autism in the context of a universal health care program could not be justified by section 1 of the *Canadian Charter*.[78] In this regard, the Court of Appeal was able to distinguish from *Cameron* in that the claimants in that case had already received some government supported treatment, whereas in *Auton* no such treatment had yet been provided.[79] Nevertheless, the Supreme Court of Canada reversed the Court of Appeal and refused to recognize that a violation of section 15(1) of the *Canadian Charter* had indeed occurred, since the legislative scheme under scrutiny did not promise that funding would be provided for all medically required treatment. All that the legislation *did* promise was 'core funding' for services provided by medical practitioners with funding for non-core services left to the Province's discretion.'[80] The Court went on to state that even if the therapy in question were a benefit provided by law as a non-core benefit,[81] the petitioners would still have failed since, in relation to a comparator group including disabled persons or persons suffering a disability other than mental disability,[82] there had been no differential treatment in the provision of emergent and only recently recognized non-core therapy.[83]

In its suit, the Association pour l'accès à l'avortement also claims that the Government of Quebec has violated the terms of the *Canada Health Act* provisions relating to accessibility and universality.[84] Although the

Superior Court refused to grant a preliminary exception brought by the government requesting that an allegation invoking the principles of the CHA be struck, the Court *did* state that the claimant lacked standing to invoke the violation of this particular statute in order to obtain redress.[85] As Claire Farid properly points out, 'provincial compliance with the CHA [is] a political decision which does not impose enforceable legal obligations on the province.'[86]

Perhaps the best chance of success ultimately will rest upon the *Health Insurance Act*[87] and the regulation respecting its application,[88] which deals with 'insured services' including all services rendered by a physician that are 'medically required,'[89] as well as family planning services determined by regulation and furnished by a physician.[90] To claim reimbursement from the government, it should suffice for the patient to establish that abortion is a medically required service[91] and that this service has not been expressly excluded under the terms of the Act or its regulations.

In my opinion, the Supreme Court of Canada will be hesitent in opening the floodgates to litigation by acknowledging a positive right to health care under section 7 of the *Canadian Charter* because of the economic and political uncertainties inherent in a decision to this effect. The Court (*Auton* notwithstanding) will likely continue to be more amenable to entertaining a challenge based on the discriminatory manner in which the law is applied (that is, to hearing challenges under section 15). In this regard, the Quebec government's need to limit health care expenditures, which according to *Eldridge* could justify restricting access to certain services under section 1, would be unlikely to be a sufficient justification for unequal treatment of women in need of abortions performed in private clinics.[92] Given the consequences of imposing a financial burden on economically disadvantaged women seeking abortion, it is far from evident that this must be tolerated to achieve the objective of limiting costs, especially when the government already provides some funding to private clinics and depends upon their existence to fulfil a vital service. In this regard, the Manitoba Court of Queen's Bench's decision in *Jane Doe 1* v *Manitoba* [93] is of particular interest. The Court found in favour of two plaintiffs who, when faced with the choice of waiting several weeks to obtain an abortion as an insured service in a government-funded hospital, opted to undergo terminations without delay in a private clinic that was not funded by the province. In granting summary judgment, the Court held[94] that by delaying access to state-funded therapeutic abortions, the impugned legislation violated several of their *Canadian Charter* rights including freedom of conscience (s. 2(a)), the right to liberty and security (s. 7), and the right to equality (s. 15). It would appear that Justice Oliphant was influenced by the 'inconsistent policy of the Government'[95] according to which it would not assume the cost of abortions performed in privately run clinics unless the patient was on social assistance.

In addition to *Canadian Charter* challenges, there remains the possibility of actions in tort or civil liability being brought, as evidenced by the recent *Cilinger v. Centre hospitalier de Chicoutimi et al.*[96] case. Here authorization was granted to initiate a class action suit against twelve hospitals on behalf of women who had been or who are at present on a waiting list for more than eight weeks while awaiting radiology treatments for breast cancer. It should be noted, however, that an attempt to implead the Attorney General of Quebec as co-defendant was rejected by the Superior Court on the ground that decisions made by the government concerning the financing of hospitals were *décisions de politique*, or policy decisions, which would not engage the liability of the Crown.

Before concluding, any discussion of terminations of pregnancy would be incomplete without reference to chemically induced abortions and the saga involving RU 486 in Canada. In the latter part of 2000 Minister of Health Allan Rock approved a research protocol involving mifepristone along with misoprostol to evaluate the efficacy and safety of this type of abortifacient. Five hospital centres located in Vancouver, Winnipeg, Toronto, Quebec City, and Sherbrooke were designated to participate in the research project.[97] In September 2001 the clinical trials were suspended following the death from toxic shock syndrome of a 26-year-old woman while in her tenth week of pregnancy, who had been administered RU 486 seven days before her death. The woman had received the medication and had died at the Sherbrooke University Hospital Centre.[98]

It is paradoxical that clinical trials of this medication have been discontinued in Canada, when one considers that it has received general acceptance worldwide. Approved for use in many countries, including the United States, France, Britain, Sweden, Spain, Germany, Scandinavia, the Netherlands, Switzerland, countries of the former Soviet Union, and China, the 95.5 per cent efficacy of RU 486 when used within the first 7 weeks of gestation, coupled with the low morbidity and mortality rates, appears to constitute a significant means of enhancing women's reproductive choice. The political response to the tragedy of the loss of one life in a research trial has imperiled the security and safety of thousands of other women in Canada who may have otherwise benefited from access to RU 486.

Conclusion

Since publication in 1996 by the Quebec Ministry of Health and Social Services of its policy paper on family planning,[99] certain trends in this area have become quite evident. The most striking statistics relate to the rates of termination of pregnancy, which continue to rise. According to comprehensive figures for 2003, in Quebec for every 100 live births, there were 40 terminations – 73,600 births and 29,429 abortions.[100] The abortion rate for teenagers appears to have remained constant, so the stated objective of reducing the rate of terminations by half for this group of women has obviously not been met. Moreover, criticisms by the Quebec Council on the Status of Women[101] of the Quebec government's report on family planning[102] have not yet been fully addressed by the province. The costs of abortion in private clinics have gone beyond a source of concern to become a source of litigation. Regional disparities in abortion services not been eliminated.

The strategy of allowing pharmacists to prescribe and dispense post-coital emergency contraception is an obvious step in the right direction, not only for reasons of accessibility but also from a financial point of view. Dealing expeditiously with the potential risk of an undesired pregnancy makes more sense from medical, economic, and social perspectives than waiting passively until the pregnancy is confirmed and a chemical or surgical abortion is performed. Yet, that pharmacists can charge a fee for the consultation prior to prescribing this medication may, in cases of economic hardship, constitute a disincentive for women to avail themselves of EC. Moreover, as Erdman and Cook point out in chapter 6 (this volume), if medical considerations were to so permit, an additional factor facilitating reproductive choice would be to approve the proposal by the Therapeutic Products Directorate to remove levonorgestrel from Schedule F of the Food and Drug Regulations and to grant it non-prescription status.[103]

The limited availability of certain abortion services in Quebec and the additional fees charged when provided by private clinics remain an ongoing source of unfairness. Unless a settlement is reached, a decision in the class-action suit of the Association pour l'accès à l'avortement against the Quebec government will undoubtedly constitute a precedent with repercussions extending beyond the borders of Quebec.

Although more generous funding is needed to truly ensure reproductive choice, it would be excessively simplistic to view a greater allocation of public spending as a panacea. Indeed, the problem for Quebec goes beyond merely the question of availability. Other considerations come into play that explain to some extent Quebec society's ambivalence regarding demographic considerations. First, as a number of (male) Quebec politicians have learned, there can be no retreat from the principle of reproductive choice even though the number of births in Quebec in 2003 was lower than it was in 1909.[104] Second, a rapidly aging population and the economic burden that imposes on future generations, as well as maintaining the vitality and presence of the French language in Canada and Quebec, remain constant preoccupations.[105] These tensions are reflected in the Quebec government's choice of policy and laws, which attempt to facilitate reproductive choice, while doing nothing to dismantle the many socioeconomic and geographic barriers to access to services.

NOTES

The writer would like to acknowledge the contribution of Sophie Brisson, student in the Master's program in health law and research assistant for the Groupe de recherche en droit de la santé de l'Université de Sherbrooke (GREDSUS). Any errors, of course, remain those of the author.

1 Quebec, Ministère de la santé et des services sociaux, *Orientations ministérielles en matière de planification des naissances* (Quebec: Ministère de la santé et des services sociaux, 1996) at 5.
2 *Ibid.* at 6.
3 *Ibid.* at 12.
4 *Ibid.* at 23.
5 *Ibid.* at 24.
6 Quebec, Conseil du statut de la femme, *Commentaires du Conseil du statut de la femme sur les Orientations ministérielles en matière de planification des naissances* (Quebec: Service de la production et de la diffusion, 1996) at 11, para. 2.1.1, 14–15, para. 2.2.1.
7 *Medical Act*, R.S.Q. c. M-9 ss. 19, 31, 43; *Dental Act*, R.S.Q. c. D-3, s. 34.
8 R.R.Q. 1981, c. M-9 r. 1.1 as am. by O.C. 964-01, 23 Aug. 2001, G.O.Q. 2001.II. 4862.
9 *Ibid.*, s. 3.

10 *Règlement sur les activités de formation obligatoire des pharmaciens pour la prescription des médicaments permettant une contraception orale d'urgence*, R.R.Q. 1981, c. P-10, r. 1.1 (in effect from 20 September 2001; there is no English version of this regulation) [*Règlement obligatoire*].

11 R.S.Q. c. C-26.

12 *Règlement obligatoire, supra* note 10, annex 1:

Éléments du contenu des activités de formation continue obligatoire pour la prescription de médicaments aux fins de la contraception orale d'urgence
1. Considérations sociales
2. Considérations pharmaco-thérapeutiques
3. Considérations cliniques
   – l'anamnèse
   – le processus décisionnel
   – les conseils
   – le monitorage
4. Considérations éthiques
5. Considérations légales.

13 2d. Sess., 36th Leg., Quebec, 2002 (assented to 14 June 2002), S.Q. 2002, c. 33.

14 R.S.Q. c. P-10 s. 17(6).

15 *Supra* note 11, s. 94(o) provides in part that the Bureau of a professional order may, by regulation 'determine the continuing education activities or the framework for continuing education activities, in which the members or a class of members of the order are required to take part, in accordance with the terms and conditions fixed by resolution of the Bureau.'

16 Inspired by a similar initiative in British Columbia; see Reproductive Health Technologies Project, 'B.C. Women Gain Access to Emergency Contraception Directly from Pharmacists' (2000), www.rhtp.org/ec/ec_news/ec_2000_10_26.htm64.224.39.134/news_archives/news_ec_bcpharm.htm (accessed 22 Aug. 2005); B.C. Pharmacy Association, 'Pharmacists and the Emergency Contraceptive Pill' (2002), www.bcpharmacy.ca/pressroom/position_statements/BCPhA%20Stmt-Pharmacists%20%20ECP.Final.PDF (accessed 20 Aug. 2005).

17 The Quebec Order of Pharmacists, 'Norme 2001.01 Prestation des services reliés à la contraception orale d'urgence' (approved by the Bureau of the Order of Pharmacists of Quebec, Order of Pharmacists 1 Oct. 2001), http://www.opg.org/fr/normes_guides/pdf/122%20norme.doc (accessed 22 Aug. 2005).

18 According to *Civil Code of Quebec* S.Q., 1991, c. 64. s. 14 C.c.Q., '[c]onsent to

care required by the state of health of a minor is given by the person having parental authority or by his tutor' and 'A minor fourteen years of age or over, however, may give his consent alone to such care. If his state of health requires that he remain in a health or social services establishment for over twelve hours, the person having parental authority or tutor shall be informed of that fact.'

19 R.S.Q. c. S-4.2.

20 *Supra* note 11 at s. 60.5.

21 R.R.Q. 1981, c. P-10, r. 5, s. 3.07.01.

22 As provided for by *An Act Respecting Prescription Drug Insurance*, R.S.Q. c. A-29.01, s. 16. Under s. 15(4), if eligible persons are not covered by a group insurance contract or an employee benefit plan, they are provided coverage by the Régie de l'assurance maladie du Québec [Régis], a publicly administered plan.

23 Since the coverage would extend to their children under 18 years of age, *ibid.*, s. 18. See also Direction de Santé Publique, Régie Régionale de la Santé et des Services Sociaux de Québec, 'La contraception orale d'urgence (COU), quoi de neuf?' (2003) 15:4 Bulletin de Santé publique, special insert.

24 R.S.Q. c. P-34.1.

25 *Ibid.* at s. 39.

26 *Ibid.* at s. 2.2.

27 *Ibid.* at ss. 2.4, 5. According to s. 1(e), '"parents" means the father and mother of a child or, where applicable, any other person acting as the person having parental authority').

28 Ibid. at ss. 46(a), 47.

29 Quebec, Groupe de travail sur la révision du Manuel de référence sur la protection de la jeunesse, *Manuel de référence sur la protection de la jeunesse* (Quebec: Ministère de la santé et des services sociaux, 1998) at 176, para. 3.2 (translated by author;) it also states that the purpose of this consultation is to obtain their consent.

30 According to the Canadian Pharmacists Association (CPA), 'Emergency Contraception, Questions and Answers' (Ottawa: CPA, 2002) at 3, http://www.pharmacists.ca/content/about_cpha/whats_happening/cpha_in_action/pdf/CPhAECPQA.pdf (accessed 22 Aug. 2005), 'If progestin-only pills (Plan B) are given within the first 24 hours following unprotected intercourse, 95% of pregnancies that would have resulted are prevented. If progestin-only pills are given between 24-48 [*sic*] hours, they are 85% effective and if given between 48 to 72 hours post-coitus, 58% of potential pregnancies are prevented.' A copper-bearing intrauterine contraceptive

device can be used up to seven days after intercourse to prevent conception according to the Society of Obstetricians and Gynaecologists of
Canada (SOGC). See Victoria Davis and Shella Dunn, 'Emergency Postcoital Contraception' (2000) 92 SOGC Clinical Practice Guidelines, available at www.sogc.org/SOGCnet/sogc_docs/common/guide/pdfs/
ps92.pdf (accessed 22 Aug. 2005) also in (2000) 22:7 J. Soc. Obstet.
Gynaecol. Can. 544. See also the Position Statement of the Adolescent
Health Committee of the Canadian Paediatric Society, 'Emergency
Contraception' (2003) 8:3 Paediatrics and Child Health 181.

31 *Ibid.*

32 California Abortion and Reproductive Rights Action League, *Emergency
Contraception: The Resource Guide for California*, 2nd ed. (n.p., 2001) at 8.

33 [1988] 1 S.C.R. 30, rev'g (1985), 52 O.R. (2d) 253 (Ont. C.A.), aff'g (1984),
47 O.R. (2d) 353 (Ont. H.C.J.). [*Morgentaler*].

34 [1989] 2 S.C.R. 530, rev'g [1989] 27 Q.A.C. 81 (C.A.), rev'g [1989] R.J.Q.
1980 (Sup. Ct.).

35 R.S.C. 1985, c. C-46.

36 *Morgentaler, supra* note 33. See esp. Dickson C.J. at 57ff, Beetz J., at 90ff,
Wilson J. at 173ff.

37 Indeed, according to Claire Farid, 'Access to Abortion in Ontario: From
Morgentaler 1988 to the *Savings and Restructuring Act*' (1997) 5 *Health Law
Journal* 119 at 125: While the Court clarified that provisions like s. 251
could not be used to prevent women from having abortions, there was no
identification of a governmental responsibility to ensure that women were
in fact able to access this procedure.'

38 See *An Act to Provide for Balanced Budgets in the Public Health and Social
Services Network*, R.S.Q. c. E-12.0001, esp. s. 4: 'No public institution may
have a deficit at the end of a fiscal year.' In part, s. 11 provides: 'The
Minister may also ... issue, in respect of a public institution, a directive
concerning the management of its human, budgetary, physical or informa-
tional resources. The directive is binding on the institution from the date
fixed therein.' As possible sanctions in cases of non-compliance, s. 14 establishes the assumption of provisional administration of the institution
or placing institutional budgetary matters in the hands of a government-
appointed controller (it should be noted that this law has not been abro-
gated).

39 Anne St-Cerny, 'Trente ans après la première mobilisation des femmes
canadiennes et québécoises sur l'avortement' (2000) 21 Sans Préjudice ...
pour la santé des femmes 8, [*Sans Préjudice*] http://www.rqasf.qc.ca/
spa21.pdf (accessed 22 Aug. 2005).

40 Canadian Abortion Rights Action League (CARAL), 'Abortion in Canada Today: The Situation Province-by-Province,' (2003) http://www.caral.ca/uploads/Province%20by%20province%202003.doc (accessed 22 Aug. 2005).

41 Nathalie Parent, 'L'avortement, un droit toujours menace' (2001) 24 Sans Préjudice, http://www.rqasf.qc.ca/sp24/sp24_10.htm (accessed 22 Aug. 2005).

42 R.S.Q. c. A-29, s. 3: 'The cost of the following services rendered by a professional in the field of health are assumed by the Board on behalf of every insured person, in accordance with this act and the regulations: (a) all services rendered by a physician that are medically required ... (d) family planning services determined by regulation and furnished by a physician.'

43 Régie, 'Tableau 2.11 Nombre et coût des 50 actes chirurgicaux les plus coûteux par ordre décroissant du côut, rémunération à l'acte, médecine et chirurgie, 2003,' http://www.ramq.gouv.qc.ca/fr/statistiques/documents/2003/tab211.pdf (accessed 22 Aug. 2005).

44 *Association pour l'accès à l'avortement* v *Québec (A.G.)* (25 June 2003), Montreal 500-06-000158-028, B.E. 2003BE-770 (Sup. Ct.), Sévigny J. (Azimut) [*Association*]. It is interesting to note that the Association had applied to the Court so that the person representing the group may remain anonymous because of potential threats and a fear of violence. The Superior Court rejected the motion, stating that the acts of violence alluded to had taken place in Ontario and British Columbia, and nothing indicated that there was actual danger in Montreal or more generally in Quebec. Citing the public nature of trials and the administration of justice, it was held preferable to reject concealment of the representative's identity: *Re Association pour l'accès à l'avortement* (6 Feb. 2002), Montreal 500-05-069637-013, J.E. 2002-587 (Sup. Ct.) (Azimut), rev'd (19 April 2002), Montreal 500-09-011914-025, J.E. 2002-928 (C.A.) (Azimut). The Court of Appeal stated that there was sufficient danger to justify the order requested, especially since it would limit minimally the open and public nature of the proceedings.

45 Free translation of 'toutes les femmes bénéficiaires du régime public d'assurance maladie du Québec qui ont déboursé une somme d'argent pour obtenir un avortement dans la province de Québec,' *Association*, ibid. para. at 17.

46 Part I of the *Constitution Act, 1982*, being Schedule B to the *Canada Act 1982* (U.K.), 1982, c. 11 [*Canadian Charter*].

47 R.S.Q., c. C-12 [*Quebec Charter*].

48 R.S.C. 1985, c. C-6.

49 It should be noted that there have been agreements between the Regional Health and Social Services Board of Montreal and the Fémina and Morgentaler clinics covering the full costs but only for second-trimester abortions. See para. 25 of the *Requête introductive d'instance* in Association *pour*, supra n44. In an interesting manoeuvre, the Attorney General of Quebec attempted to impede these privately funded abortion clinics by arguing that if they unlawfully charged additional fees to patients for insured services, then the clinics themselves should reimburse their patients. This argument was rejected by the Superior Court since the action by the Association was not intended to establish that the private clinics had acted illegally. Even if, hypothetically, additional fees were paid contrary to law, it would be the duty of the Régie and not the Attorney General to recover any sums paid. See *Association pour l'accès à l'avortement v. Québec (A.G.)* (13 Feb. 2004), Montreal 500-06-000158-028, J.E. 2004-690 (Sup. Ct.), Bénard J., leave to appeal to C.A. refused (24 March 2004), Montreal 500-09-014309-041 (C.A.) (Azimut).

50 *Supra* note 46.

51 *Supra* note 47 at s. 1; 'Every human being has a right to life, and to personal security, inviolability and freedom.' Section 6 provides for the peaceful enjoyment of property: 'Every person has a right to the peaceful enjoyment and free disposition of his property, except to the extent provided by law.' Section 10 forbids discrimination: 'Every person has a right to full and equal recognition and exercise of his human rights and freedoms, without distinction, exclusion or preference based on race, color, sex, pregnancy, sexual orientation, civil status, age except as provided by law, religion, political convictions, language, ethnic or national origin, social condition, a handicap or the use of any means to palliate a handicap' and '[D]iscrimination exists where such a distinction, exclusion or preference has the effect of nullifying or impairing such right.'

52 *Supra* note 48.

53 Plaintiffs have utilized the expression 'exemplary damages' in their action in furtherance of a claim under s. 49 of the *Quebec Charter, supra* note 47. Although the expression 'exemplary damages' was utilized in the original version, it has been replaced by the term 'punitive damages.' As provided for by s. 49, punitive damages may be claimed in the case of an unlawful and intentional interference with any right or freedom recognized by the *Quebec Charter*.

54 Clairandrée Cauchy, 'Recours collectif autorisé pour les femmes qui ont dû payer pour un avortement' *Le Devoir* (27 June 2003) A2.

55 *Supra* note 19 at s. 5.

56 *Ibid.*, s. 13.
57 *Supra* note 1 at 7.
58 *R. v. Morgentaler* (1995), 122 D.L.R. (4th) 728 (P.E.I.S.C.).
59 See, e.g., *Quebec (Commission des droits de la personne et des droits de la jeunesse) v. Montréal (City of)*, [2000] 1 S.C.R. 665, L'Heureux-Dubé J. At 688: 'While there is no requirement that the provisions of the [*Quebec*] *Charter* mirror those of the *Canadian Charter*, they must nevertheless be interpreted in light of the *Canadian Charter*. Thus when a statutory provision is open to more than one interpretation, it must be interpreted in a manner consistent with the provisions of the *Canadian Charter*' (references omitted), aff'g [1998] R.J.Q. 688 (C.A.), rev'g (1995), 25 C.H.R.R. D/407 and D/412 (T.D.P.). See also *University of British Columbia v. Berg*, [1993] 2 S.C.R. 353 at 373, Lamer C.J.
60 *Supra* note 46.
61 See *Brown v. British Columbia* (1990), 66 D.L.R. (4th) 444 (B.C.S.C.) (refusal to fully subsidize the costs of AIDS medication); *Cameron v. Nova Scotia (A.G.)* (1999), 177 D.L.R. (4th) 611 (N.S.C.A.), aff'g (1999), 172 N.S.R. (2d) 227, leave to appeal to S.C.C. refused [1999] S.C.C.A. No. 531 [*Cameron* cited to D.L.R.] (refusal to assume the costs of fertility treatments outside the province); *Auton (Guardian ad litem of) v. British Columbia (Minister of Health)* [2004] S.C.R. 657, rev'g [2003] 1 W.W.R. 42, (2002) (C.A.), aff'g in part [2000] 8 W.W.R. 221 (B.C. Sup. Ct.) [Court of Appeal cited to B.C.L.R.]. See generally *Gosselin v. Québec (A.G.)*, [2002] 4 S.C.R. 429, McLachlin C.J. At 491: 'Nothing in the jurisprudence thus far suggests that s. 7 places a positive obligation on the state to ensure that each person enjoys life, liberty or security of the person. Rather, s. 7 has been interpreted as restricting the state's ability to *deprive* people of these' (emphasis in the original). However, the judge goes on to state at 491–2: 'One day s. 7 may be interpreted to include other obligations ... It would be a mistake to regard s. 7 as frozen, or its content as having been exhaustively defined in previous cases,' aff'g [1999] R.J.Q. 1033 (C.A.), aff'g [1992] R.J.Q. 1647 (Sup. Ct.).
62 For example, Brent Windwick, 'Health-Care and Section 7 of the Canadian Charter of Rights and Freedoms' (1994) 3 Health Law Review 20 at 22; Canadian Bar Task Force on Health Care, *What's Law Got to Do with It? Health Care Reform in Canada* (Ottawa: Canadian Bar Association, 1994) at 26; Claire Farid, *supra* note 37; Tamara Friesen, 'The Right to Health Care' (2001) 9 Health L. J. 205 at 213, 217; Patrice Garant, 'Vie, liberté, sécurité et justice fundamental,' in Gerald Beaudoin and Errol Mendes, *Charte canadienne des droits et libertés*, 3rd ed. (Montreal: Wilson and Lafleur, 1996)

at 442; Marco Laverdière, 'Le cadre juridique canadien et québécois relatif au développement parallèle de services privés de santé et l'article 7 de la Charte canadienne des droits et libertés' (1998–99) 29 R.D.U.S. 117 at 172.

63 Laverdière, *ibid.* at 192.

64 M. Jackman, 'The Regulation of Private Health Care under the *Canada Health Act* and the Canadian Charter' (1995) 6 Constitutional Forum 54 at 56.

65 *Supra* note 61.

66 *Ibid.* at paras. 64–7.

67 *Chaoulli v. Quebec (Attorney General)* (2005), 335 N.R. 25, J.E. 2005-1144, 2005 S.C.C. 35, rev'g [2002] R.J.Q. 1205 (C.A.), and [2000] R.J.Q. 786 (Sup. Ct.), which had rejected a motion for declaratory judgment in order to declare unconstitutional ss. 15 of the *Health Insurance Act*, *supra* note 42, and 11 of the *Hospital Insurance Act*, R.S.Q., c. A-29, prohibiting the reimbursement of insured services by private insurers, when these services are provided by physicians who do not participate in the Quebec health services regime.

68 [1997] 3 S.C.R. 524 (held that the failure to provide sign language interpreters to the hearing impaired seeking medical services was discriminatory), rev'g (1995), 7 B.C.L.R. (3d) 156 (C.A.), rev'g (1992), 75 B.C.L.R. (2d) 68 (Sup. Ct.) [*Eldridge*].

69 *Eldridge, ibid.* at para. 58.

70 *Ibid.* at para. 74. See also *Brooks v. Canada Safeway Ltd.*, [1989] 1 S.C.R. 1219, Dickson C.J. At 1242: ('In retrospect, one can only ask – how could pregnancy be *anything other than* sex discrimination? ... Discrimination on the basis of pregnancy is a form of sex discrimination because of the basic biological fact that only women have the capacity to become pregnant' (emphasis in original), rev'g (1986), 42: Man. R. (2d) 27, rev'g (1985), 38 Man. R. (2d) 192 (Q.B.), rev'g (1984), 6 C.H.R.R. D/2560 and D/2840.

71 *Eldridge, supra,* note 68 at para. 79.

72 Ibid. at para. 94.

73 *Cameron, supra* note 61. See also Barbara von Tigerstrom, 'Equality Rights and the Allocation of Scarce Resources in Health Care: A Comment on *Cameron v Nova Scotia*' (1999) 11:1 Constitutional Forum 30.

74 *Cameron, supra,* note 61 at 654, 662 (Chipman J.A.). While concurring in the result, Bateman J. felt that plaintiff's infertility was not a disability for which protection is offered under s. 15(1), *ibid.* at 676.

75 Chipman J.A. expressed the opinion that '[t]he policy makers require latitude in balancing competing interests in the constrained financial

environment. We are simply not equipped to sort out the priorities. We
should not second guess them, except in clear cases of failure on their part
to properly balance Charter rights of individuals against the overall
pressing objective of the scheme under the Act,' *ibid*. at 667. See also *ibid*.
at 664.

76 *Auton, supra* note 61.
77 *Ibid*. at para. 57
78 *Ibid*. at para. 59.
79 *Ibid*. at para. 66.
80 *Supra* note 61 at para. 35.
81 *Ibid*. at para. 47.
82 *Ibid*. at para. 55.
83 *Ibid*. at para. 58.
84 *Supra* note 35, ss. 7, 10, 12.
85 *Association* (13 Feb. and 24 March 2004), *supra* note 49 at para. 28.
86 Farid, *supra* note 37 at 141.
87 *Supra* note 42, ss. 1(a), 3(a), 3(d).
88 *Regulation Respecting the Application of the Health Insurance Act*, R.R.Q. 1981,
    c. A-29, r. 1, s. 34.2.
89 *Supra* note 42 at s. 3(a).
90 *Ibid*. at s. 3(d).
91 The *Canada Health Act Annual Report, 2000–2001*, alludes to certain difficul-
    ties relating to abortion services that are considered medically necessary,
    Health Canada, *Canada Health Act Annual Report, 2003–2004* (Ottawa:
    Travaux Publics et Services Gouvernementaux, 2001) at 8–10, http://
    www.hc-sc.gc.ca/medicare/Documents/LCSRA0001.pdf (accessed
    28 Aug. 2004).
92 *Eldridge*, supra note 68 at para. 94.
93 [2004] M.J. No. 456 (Q.B.) (Q.L.).
94 *Ibid*. at paras. 79–80.
95 *Ibid*. at para. 77.
96 (29 March 2004), Montreal 500-06-000116-000, J.E. 2004-697 (Sup. Ct.),
    Bishop J. (Azimut) (rectified 29 Mar. 2004) [*Cilinger*]. The Court applied the
    criteria elaborated by the Supreme Court in *Just v. British Columbia*, [1989]
    2 S.C.R. 1228, and stated that policy decisions can only be attacked if they
    were made in bad faith or were manifestly unreasonable (*manifestement
    déraisonnables*). Evidence in the present case did not establish prima facie
    that one of these alternatives was present, *Cilinger, ibid*. at paras. 110–21.
    See also a somewhat similar case in *Stein v Tribunal Administratif du
    Québec*, [1999] R.J.Q. 2416 (Sup. Ct.), Cohen J. (stated in a judgment on

Motion for Judicial Review that three cancellations of an operation for the removal of cancerous liver lesions and making the patient wait for surgery more than twelve weeks since discovery of the lesions was 'irrational, unreasonable and contrary to the purpose of the Health Insurance Act which is designed to make necessary medical treatment available to all Quebecers,' at 2421–2; the patient sought and obtained experimental treatment in the U.S. and was seeking reimbursement).

97 Anne St-Cerny and Nathalie Parent, 'Le point sur l'avortement par medicaments' (2002) 27 Sans Préjudice 7, available at www.rqasf.qc.ca/sp27/sp27_07 .htm (accessed 22 Aug. 2005).

98 A more detailed report of this case may be found at Christian Sinave et al., 'Toxic Shock Syndrome Due to *Clostridium sordelli*: A Dramatic Postpartum and Postabortion Disease' (2002) 35 Clinical Infectious Diseases 1441.

99 *Supra* note 1.

100 Institut de la statistique du Québec, 'Interruptions volontaires de grossesse, rapport pour 100 naissances, taux IVG pour 1 000 femmes, hystérectomies, ligatures, vasectomies, réanastomoses et vasovasostomies, Québec, 1971–2003' (Quebec: author, online 2005), http://www.stat.gouv .qc.ca/donstat/societe/demographie/naisn_deces/naissance/415.htm (accessed 22 Aug. 2005); Institut de la statistique du Québec, 'Naissances et taux de natalité, Québec, 1900–2003' (Quebec: author, online 2005), http://www.stat.gouv.qc.ca/donstat/societe/demographie/naisn_deces/ naissance/401.htm (accessed 22 Aug. 2005).

101 Quebec, Conseil du statut de la femme, *supra* note 6.

102 Quebec, Ministère de la santé et des services sociaux, *supra* note 1.

103 J. Erdman and R. Cook (chapter 5, this volume). This would happen by placing the listed drug in question on Schedule 2, which means that it could be dispensed by the pharmacist after a consultation with the patient. See CPhA, *supra* note 30 at 1.

104 There were 77,144 births in 1909 in comparison to 73,600 in 2003. See Institut de la statistique Québec, *supra* note 100.

105 Indeed, according to l'Institut de la statistique du Québec, unless circumstances change, there will be negative population growth as of 2021. Institut de la Statistique du Québec, 'Premier bilan des nouvelles perspectives démographiques du Québec, 2001–2051,' http://www.stat.gouv.qc.ca/ salle-presse/communiq/2004/fevrier/fev0402a.htm (accessed 22 Aug. 2005). The report states: 'Pour contrecarrer la voie tracée par ces décès anticipés, il faudrait que le nombre annuel de naissances, qui est actuellement de 74 000, s'élève graduellement pendant 30 ans pour dépasser le

nombre de 100 000, et qu'il s'y maintienne. En d'autres termes, il faudrait atteindre, d'ici là, une fécondité d'au moins deux enfants par femme (in order to reverse the trend arising from these anticipated deaths, the annual birth rate, which is presently at 74,000, would have to gradually increase over the next 30 years to more than 100,000 and then remain stable. In other words, between now and then, a birth rate of two children per woman would have to be attained)' (translated by author).

PART THREE

Access for the Vulnerable:
Case Studies from Aboriginal
Health and Mental Health

8 Jurisdictional Roulette: Constitutional and Structural Barriers to Aboriginal Access to Health

CONSTANCE MACINTOSH

Aboriginal peoples have a unique relationship with the government of Canada that is characterized, among other things, by a complex legislative and constitutional regime. Because this regime has developed in an uneven and fractured fashion, it has resulted in jurisdictional confusion and policy vacuums regarding many aspects of Aboriginal peoples' lives.[1] One such aspect is the governance of matters relating to health. The experience of the reserve communities of Grassy Narrows and White Dog are illustrative of how jurisdictional divisions complicate health governance. The river system, lake, and fish, upon which these communities had relied for sustenance, over the course of several decades became contaminated with mercury-laden effluent from pulp and paper operations. The communities' efforts to force environmental clean-up were continually frustrated by administrative barriers. Although the operations that were producing the effluent did eventually put antipollution measures into effect, the 300-mile-long river system in question is expected to remain contaminated for several generations.[2]

Canada's Royal Commission on Aboriginal Peoples assessed what had transpired in Grassy Narrows and White Dog and found that, as a result of jurisdictional divisions, the health governance system had completely failed these communities. The Commission concluded that '[t]he combination of federal responsibility for public health on reserve and provincial responsibility for environmental protection and the regulation of industry off-reserve (where the problem originated) left the communities with no defined authority to appeal to or work with.'[3] The Royal Commission found the communities were further hampered as they lacked political power to overcome 'the inertia of governments and industry.'[4] Instead, they faced a kind of jurisdictional roulette, trying to guess where the ball would finally come to rest.

Had the environmental problem been fully contained within an Indian reservation – and so on federal land – the federal governance structure would likely have been engaged, resulting in the dispatch of an environmental health officer. However, as there is no legislative or program mechanism currently in place to *remedy* environmental problems on reserves, there is no budget line to cover any associated costs.[5] As a result, a special submission and plan would have had to be made to the Treasury Board.[6]

Improving Aboriginal health requires engaging with how these jurisdictional and legislative divides underlie, shape, and govern the healthcare landscape. In this chapter, I identify and explore these divides.

The Health Status of Aboriginal Peoples in Canada

The poor status of Aboriginal health is well documented. In 1996, the Royal Commission described the health of Aboriginal people in Canada as in a 'crisis.'[7] In 2000, the *Kirby Report* characterized it as a 'national disgrace,'[8] and in the 2002 *Romanow Report*, the health status of Aboriginal people was described as 'simply unacceptable.'[9] Romanow concluded that '[t]he reasons for this are complex and relate to a number of different factors, many of which have less to do with health and more to do with social conditions.'[10] This conclusion is supported by data regarding rates of infectious disease, the prevalence of which often reflects broader social and economic factors, such as overcrowded housing.[11] Compared to the general population, First Nations people suffer: three times the rate of pertussis, seven times the rate of chlamydia, twelve times the rate of hepatitis A among their children,[12] eight to ten times the rate of tuberculosis, and twenty times the rate of shigellosis.[13] And, although Aboriginal peoples constitute only 3 per cent of Canada's population, more than 10 per cent of persons with AIDS/HIV in Canada are Aboriginal.[14] Upon encountering such data, one might assume that Aboriginal health is unfunded. To the contrary, Aboriginal health needs are the subject of a vast amount of funding and research.

In 2003 the federal budget included $2.2 billion for Aboriginal and Northern initiatives that target the broad determinants of health, including housing, education, culture, water, and sewage. It also committed $1.3 billion over five years specifically to health programs for First Nations and the Inuit, and this included a stable funding base for the Non-Insured Health Benefits Program and community health programs, a comprehensive nursing strategy, capital investments, and a national immunization strategy.[15]

Despite the influx of money, the disparity persists and it will continue to persist until further steps are taken. One step would involve developing an understanding of the sources and consequences of the jurisdictional divisions and barriers to Aboriginal access to health care.

Jurisdictional Divides: Jurisdiction over Indian Health

A key jurisdictional division regarding responsibility for Aboriginal health is entrenched in the *Constitution Act, 1867*.[16] Under this instrument, the federal government is assigned jurisdiction over 'Indians, and Lands reserved for the Indians,'[17] while provinces are considered to have been assigned jurisdiction over health.[18] So who has jurisdiction, and thus governance responsibilities, over the *health* of '*Indians*'? Further uncertainty results from the implementation of section 88 of the *Indian Act*, which expressly provides that provincial laws of general application are applicable to Indians.[19] Such legislation could obviously include health matters.

Jurisprudence regarding whether labour relations in on-reserve health facilities are regulated federally or provincially has tested this governance question, but so far provided little guidance on the broader question of jurisdiction over Aboriginal health. This is in part because the test for assessing whether a provincial law is one of 'general application' asks the oblique question of whether the law affects 'Indians' or impedes 'Indianness.'[20]

In *Westbank First Nation v. British Columbia (Labour Relations Board)*,[21] the Court found that labour relations in a long-term care facility, which was both owned and operated by a First Nation, were within provincial jurisdiction. Key facts supporting this finding were that less than one-third of the current residents were Aboriginal and that the population served by the facility had been extended to include the surrounding non-Aboriginal community. The First Nation appealed this finding and argued that the percentage of Aboriginal versus non-Aboriginal residents varied and that they had broadened the user-base to keep the facility economically viable, that is, so Aboriginal people could continue to be served by an Aboriginal facility.[22] On appeal, the decision was upheld.[23] Although the appellate court agreed that the ratio of Aboriginal to non-Aboriginal residents was not relevant, the facility's broad community-based mandate rendered the facility insufficiently 'Indian' to fall within federal jurisdiction.[24]

The Federal Court came to a different conclusion in *Sagkeeng Alcohol Rehabilitation Centre Inc. v. Abraham*.[25] This action involved employees of a drug addiction rehabilitation centre that was located on a Manitoba reserve and funded by Health Canada. Here the Court found that the question of jurisdiction was answered through reference to the 'nature of the operation,' which the Court found was 'a form of health care service designed and operated to meet the needs of its Indian beneficiaries.'[26]

A conceptual difficulty that emerges in comparing these decisions is that, arguably, the facility in *Westbank* would have *originally* had sufficient 'Indianness' to fall within federal jurisdiction. As the court found that the ratio of residents was not relevant, the facility would have continued to remain under federal jurisdiction despite accepting non-Aboriginal residents if it had not formally *acknowledged* this practice. It seems to defy common sense that the facility lost its 'Indianness' – and so changed the jurisdiction under which it operated – as an unintended consequence of a decision designed to ensure that an Aboriginal-owned and -operated facility could continue to serve Aboriginal people.

Section 88 aside, health qua health can and does fit within either jurisdictional envelope. Although the majority of the Supreme Court of Canada in *Schneider v. The Queen* found that 'general jurisdiction over health matters is provincial,' they also determined that the *Constitution Act, 1867*, allowed for limited federal jurisdiction 'ancillary to the express heads of power in section 91.'[27] Justice Estey, in his concurring reasons, characterized health as quite flexible, and requiring a case-by-case assessment of jurisdiction: 'In sum, "health" is not a matter which is subject to specific constitutional assignment but instead is an amorphous topic which can be addressed by valid federal or provincial legislation, depending in the circumstances of each case on the nature or scope of the health problem in question.'

In a nutshell, the issue is whether Aboriginal health governance is properly characterized as (1) an 'Indian' matter, and so within federal jurisdiction, (2) a 'health' matter, and so within provincial jurisdiction, or (3) a federal incursion into provincial jurisdiction which must be legitimated on a case-by-case basis.

In most situations where a question of jurisdiction arises, both levels of government claim authority and, thus, the right to assert a governance regime. Aboriginal matters are an exception to this rule. But as

Aboriginal law scholar Kent McNeil argues, it is not jurisdiction per se that the governments are trying to avoid, but rather responsibility.[28] Thus, it is hardly surprising that most provinces characterize Aboriginal health as an 'Indian' issue – and, as such, within federal jurisdiction and a matter to be addressed through federal funding and programming.[29]

Ottawa's position on the jurisdictional question is complex. Early federal activity suggests that Canada understood itself to be responsible for providing for Aboriginal health needs. The federal government began to formally provide medical services for Aboriginal people in the early 1900s.[30] The first federal official directly responsible for Aboriginal health was appointed in 1904,[31] and a general practice was to couple visits by Indian Agents to pay treaty annuities with visits by a physician.[32] The Department of Indian Affairs (DIA) continued to provide these services until 1945. By then the DIA had assumed responsibility for medical transportation, drugs, mental health, and communicable diseases. In 1945 this responsibility was transferred to the then 'Department of Health and Welfare.'

Currently, Health Canada provides distinctive health programming for Status Aboriginal people through its First Nations and Inuit Health Branch (FNIHB). Ottawa commits approximately $500 million per annum to six major health programs: Community Health Services, Non-insured Health Benefits, Environmental Health and Surveillance, National Native Alcohol and Drug Abuse Program, Hospital Services, and Capital Construction.[33] 'Non-Insured Health Benefits' provide insurance coverage for some services and products that are not included within provincial health plans, such as drugs, glasses, medical transportation, and dental work. The federal government also provides services that are typically considered a provincial responsibility, such as physician services, to Aboriginal communities 'where normal provincial services [are] not available.'[34]

Despite providing these services, the federal government has consistently claimed that it bears no statutory, constitutional, or treaty obligation to provide health services to Aboriginal people. Having disavowed any legal obligations, Ottawa explains that it accepts responsibility for Aboriginal health services 'for humanitarian reasons,'[35] or on the basis of 'custom and historic commitment.'[36] Obviously, such a position supports an arbitrary regime where Ottawa could theoretically withdraw its support at any moment.

Looking beyond the Constitution and Domestic Legislation

Many Aboriginal peoples argue that the constitutional division of powers is irrelevant for identifying state accountability as historically Aboriginal peoples entered into lawful relationships with the Dominion, not with the provinces. Under this theory, potential sources for Ottawa having special health obligations to Aboriginal peoples include treaties, the Rupert's Land Agreement, the Royal Proclamation of 1763, and the general fiduciary principles[37] that colour the relationship between the Crown and Aboriginal peoples.

The Treaty Theory Argument

Only the treaty theory has been tested in court proceedings. The Plains Cree cite a lawful health obligation in Treaty 6 – and its two promises of a 'medicine chest' which would be 'kept at the house of each Indian Agent for the use and benefit of the Indians at the direction of such agent' and that, in the event of a 'pestilence' or 'general famine,' the Queen would provide 'sufficient' assistance 'to relieve the Indians from the calamity.'[38]

The first action was brought in 1935. In *Dreaver v. The King*,[39] Chief Dreaver claimed, among other things, that expenses for medicines had been wrongfully debited against band funds. Chief Dreaver argued that 'drugs, under the treaty, were to be provided free.'[40] Justice Angers found that Treaty 6 did not grant the federal Crown the 'privilege of deciding which medicines, drugs, and medical supplies were to be furnished to the Indians gratuitously and which were to be charged to the funds of the band.'[41] Rather, he found that the Treaty guaranteed a right of general access to health products such that 'the Indians were to be provided with all the medicines, drugs or medical supplies which they might need entirely free of charge.'[42]

This interpretation of Treaty 6's access obligations was rejected by the Saskatchewan Court of Appeal in 1966 in *R v. Johnston*.[43] Here a status Indian, Walter Johnston, who had failed to pay a provincial hospital tax, had relied upon Treaty 6's medicine chest clause to guarantee him a right to access free medical care. At first instance, the judge of the Magistrate's Court followed *Dreaver*, and expanded upon it, finding that the Treaty granted a right of access, not only to gratuitous medicines, but also to medical services such as hospital care.[44] On appeal, Chief Justice Culliton, however, interpreted the Treaty more narrowly and concluded that a 'plain reading' did not support Mr Johnston's claims. Rather, 'medicine chest' rights were subject to the discretion of the Indian Agent and the term 'medicine chest' did not, in any case, extend to access to medical services such as hospital care.[45]

Chief Justice Culliton reaffirmed his position four years later, when he wrote the decision for *R. v Swimmer*.[46] Once again, the Aboriginal litigant had been successful at first instance. Mr Swimmer had argued that Treaty 6 precluded the state from having the authority to require treaty members to pay provincial health care taxes. The Chief Justice allowed the appeal, finding that the trial judge ought to have followed *Johnston*, and interpreted 'medicine chest' rights as limited and discretionary.

Subsequent jurisprudence on treaty interpretation suggests that Justice Culliton's decisions were wrong. The Supreme Court of Canada determined in *Nowegijick v. The Queen* that treaties relating to Indians 'should be liberally construed and doubtful expressions resolved in favour of the Indians.'[47] In its most recent pronouncement on treaty interpretation, *R. v. Marshall*,[48] the Supreme Court affirmed that the historic and cultural context in which the treaty was signed *must* be taken into account, even if there is no ambiguity on the face of the treaty. As well, the court is to 'choose from among the various possible interpretations of the common intention [of the parties] the one which best reconciles' the interests of the Crown and the Aboriginal parties to the treaty.[49] In searching for this 'common intention,' the integrity and honour of the Crown is presumed.[50] A final key principle of interpretation is that treaty rights are not to be interpreted in a static fashion. Rather they are to be updated to provide for their modern exercise by determining what modern practices are reasonably incidental to the core treaty right in its modern context.[51] As a consequence, similar litigation today may result in a finding that Treaty 6 Aboriginal peoples have a treaty right of gratuitous access to a broad range of health services and products.

This conclusion is supported by the recent findings of Prothonotary Hargrave in *Wuskwi Siphk Cree Nation v. Canada*, where the Prothonotary observed that *Johnson*'s dicta, that Treaty 6 did not require Canada to provide medical services, 'is now in all probability wrong.'[52] He wrote, 'Justice Angers took a proper approach in his 1935 decision on *Dreaver* ... reading the Treaty No. 6 medicine chest clause in a contemporary manner to mean a supply of all medicine, drugs, and medical supplies. Certainly, it is clear that the Saskatchewan Court of Appeal took what is now a wrong approach in its literal and restrictive readings of the medicine chest clause in the 1966 decision in *Johnson* ... In a current context the clause may well require a full range of contemporary medical services.'[53]

There is some evidence that Canada, or at least its agents, understood Canada to have health obligations under the treaties generally. One example involves the first federal official directly responsible for Aboriginal health, Dr Peter Bryce. Shortly after his appointment in 1904, he began to investigate the status of Aboriginal health. He found that, over a 15-year period, between 25 to 35 per cent of all Aboriginal children attending residential schools had died, primarily of tuberculosis or measles.[54] Bryce informed his superiors that this situation violated Canada's treaty obligations. Specifically, he accused the state of having 'criminal disregard for the treaty pledges to guard the welfare of the Indian wards' and that the degree and extent of this disregard could be gauged from the facts of the widespread devastation caused by tuberculosis.[55] Bryce contended that the Dominion's health obligations would only be adequately addressed if 'Indian health' was moved from the envelope of Indian Affairs to the new Department of Health. Many of Bryce's recommendations were eventually adopted. Thus, there is some evidence that health services were contemplated to be an aspect of the Crown's general obligations to Treaty 6 signatories.

The Rupert's Land Agreement Argument

Prior to Confederation, Charles II purported to grant Rupert's Land to the Hudson's Bay Company in 1670.[56] The grant included the hydrographic basin of Hudson's Bay, what are today northern Quebec and northern Ontario, the entire province of Manitoba, most of Saskatchewan, and part of southern Alberta. Although this area was not part of Canada in 1867, Canada successfully made pleadings to Great Britain shortly after Confederation to admit the territory.[57]

Kent McNeil canvassed the interactions leading up to the admission of Rupert's Land. In pleading its case, Canada committed to undertakings in an 1869 Address, which included making 'adequate provisions for the protection of the Indian tribes whose interests and well-being are involved in the transfer.'[58] McNeil presents a detailed analysis of the undertakings, and especially of the term 'well-being.' He concludes that 'the duty the Canadian government undertook includes an obligation either to ensure that the Indian tribes have the resources to provide health services and social and economic assistance to tribal members who need it, or to provide those services and that assistance itself.'[59]

McNeil's assessment of the term 'well-being' is certainly broad. However, it does align with a definition adopted by the Government of Canada. Following the publication of the Royal Commission's *Report on Aboriginal Peoples*, the Department of Indian Affairs and Northern Development (DIAND)[60] drafted a response and gave it the title *Gathering Strength: Canada's Aboriginal Action Plan.* In this document, Ottawa defines 'well-being' as including 'access to the health, social and cultural supports needed to ensure that people can remain healthy.'[61]

One difficulty with this argument is that the undertaking to provide for the 'well-being' of Indian tribes was not reiterated in the actual order that admitted Rupert's Land into Canada. McNeil argues that this omission is not relevant, as the undertaking was incorporated by reference through the Preamble to the Order. In particular, the Preamble stated that the terms in the 1869 Address had been approved and that the Address was attached as an Annex to the Order.[62]

The Royal Proclamation Argument

Like the Treaty 6 argument, a case based on the Rupert's Land Agreement would only extend to those specific Aboriginal populations who are connected to the relevant geographic area. A more general obligation can be traced to the Royal Proclamation of 1763. As John Borrows has documented, although the Royal Proclamation was merely an order when it was first issued, it became a treaty at Niagara in 1764 because it was at that time both presented by the colonists for affirmation and also accepted by the Aboriginal peoples.[63]

Borrows argues that insight into the Aboriginal understanding of the Royal Proclamation – as a treaty – can be gleaned through an assessment of the parties' subsequent conduct[64] and that this understanding must inform the interpretation of the treaty's terms. Borrows presents evidence that Aboriginal participants had understood the agreements to have created general obligations to sustain the welfare of First Nations and to protect their interests.[65] In particular, Borrows relies upon a transcribed exchange between Anishnabe people and representatives of the Crown in 1818. This transcript indicates that an Anishnabe speaker presented the Crown representative with a wampum belt that had been made in 1764, and in doing so stated, among other things: 'On giving us the Belt of Peace [i.e., the wampum belt], you said – 'If you should ever require my assistance, send this Belt, and my hand will be immediately stretched forth to assist you.'[66]

This general pledge of assistance could extend to health matters, given the generous interpretation applied to the scope of treaty promises. The Supreme Court of Canada considered whether the Royal Proclamation's obligations could extend to First Nations located in British Columbia in the case of *Calder v. AGBC*.[67] The Court split on this question. Three judges concluded that only those Aboriginal peoples who were 'under British protection' in 1763 were within the scope of the Proclamation. As the northern limit on British territory on the west coast was not determined until 1825, and sovereignty was not asserted until some years later, these judges concluded that bands within British Columbia were excluded. But three judges found otherwise. They characterized the Proclamation as 'a law which followed the flag as England assumed jurisdiction over newly-discovered or acquired lands or territories.'[68] They found that the United Kingdom was well aware of the existence of western territories and peoples in 1763 and that the Proclamation, on its face, was expressly intended to include the lands west of the Rocky Mountains.[69] Although the Royal Proclamation could certainly not be construed as a treaty for these western peoples, as it was never presented to them for affirmation, it still stands as a Royal Order to which the Crown is bound.

The Fiduciary Duty Argument

Claims have been made, but not litigated, based upon the fiduciary relationship between the Crown and Aboriginal peoples.[70] Recent Supreme Court of Canada jurisprudence suggests that this line of argument would have difficulty standing on its own. In *Wewaykum Indian Band v. Canada*,[71] Justice Binnie, writing for the Court, stated that the fiduciary relationship 'is called into existence to facilitate supervision of the high degree of discretionary control gradually assumed by the Crown over the lives of [A]boriginal peoples.'[72] Where the Crown does not exercise a degree of control over an Indian interest, fiduciary obligations would not arise. That is, the fiduciary relationship rides upon existing or proposed legal interests and cannot create a new and independent legal right (such as a free-standing right to health services). However, if such a right already exists – whether through statute, treaty, or some other mechanism – then the Crown's fiduciary obligations may well be invoked, as long as the legal framework entertains Crown exercise of discretionary power. Given that the *Indian Act* expressly permits the federal government to make regulations regarding the provision of medical treatment and health services for Indians, a determinative question is whether this statutory provision, through the operation of the fiduciary relationship, ought to be read as imposing proactive responsibilities upon Ottawa to pass such regulations and ensure that they serve the best interests of Aboriginal peoples.

Of the various avenues addressed above regarding whether Canada has a lawful obligation to provide Aboriginal peoples with access to health care services above and beyond that of other Canadians, the strongest claim is that based upon Treaty 6. As noted earlier, however, even if successful it would provide relief to only a small percentage of Canada's Aboriginal people. An argument based upon fiduciary obligations, while more difficult to make, would result in benefits for many more Aboriginal people.

Provincial and Federal Practice

Legal theory aside, what does the ongoing jurisdictional uncertainty lead to in governance practices? An example can be drawn from HIV/AIDS programming, which reveals a countrywide patchwork of health initiatives. Interjurisdictional HIV/AIDS coordinating committees have been established in a few provinces, notably, Alberta, British Columbia, and Manitoba, but not in others.[73] Some provinces, such as Ontario, specifically fund a provincial Aboriginal HIV/AIDS strategy. Other provinces, such as Nova Scotia and New Brunswick, take the position that they are not responsible for supporting such targeted programs because Aboriginal people fall within federal jurisdiction and so should be served through federal funding and programming.[74]

Nova Scotia's stance resonates with that of some Aboriginal communities. Although Ontario sought the participation of on-reserve Aboriginal communities in its HIV/AIDS strategy, these communities refused to join.[75] Presumably, the communities took this position out of concern that participation in a provincial, as opposed to federal, initiative could compromise their ability to pursue health-based treaty and Aboriginal rights claims against Canada.

There are also general AIDS/HIV funding sources, but these programs are also undercut by jurisdictional divisions. Community groups in Canada, including Aboriginal communities, can apply for funding from the AIDS Community Action Program (ACAP); this funding is not available, however, for on-reserve Aboriginal communities.[76] Likewise, the First Nations and Inuit Health Branch within Health Canada funds AIDS/HIV programs, but only for on-reserve communities.[77] The reserve boundary thus forms a barrier for AIDS/HIV programming purposes, resulting in fragmented initiatives and irregular access situations because of Aboriginal mobility between on-reserve and off-reserve residences.[78] It is clear, in short, that HIV/AIDS programming for Aboriginal peoples is fragmented and nationally inconsistent.

Some federal initiatives to improve Aboriginal access to health have been directly impeded by jurisdictional confusion. For example, Canada has been trying for over twenty-five years to provide equitable programs and services for Aboriginal peoples with disabilities. In 1981 a special House of Commons committee urged all levels of government to work together to develop programs to address the needs of disabled Aboriginal people. The major problem areas that the committee identified were housing, employment and economic security, education, emotional support, and service delivery.[79] This proposal languished for a decade. Then, in 1991, Ottawa announced a national strategy intended to assist all persons with disabilities: this included the then Department of Indian Affairs spending $5 million 'to improve co-ordination and accessibility and to promote sensitive design and delivery of existing programs and services to people with disabilities living on-reserve.'[80]

In 1993 a House of Commons Standing Committee released another report on Aboriginal people with disabilities and in it pointed out that no comprehensive plan of action covering all Aboriginal peoples with disabilities had been developed and no single agency had been charged with developing one.[81] The Committee concluded that 'the government has taken a strikingly fragmented approach to Aboriginal issues – let alone disability issues – within the federal system. Areas of responsibility for various groupings of Aboriginal people are scattered amongst different departments and there is certainly no concentrated focus on disability.'[82] In 1993 this Standing Committee recommended that immediate action be taken to coordinate federal programs and activities and that a tripartite federal / provincial-territorial / band governmental action plan be formed by late 1993. However, ten years later, in 2003, another House of Commons Standing Committee observed that the problems caused by jurisdictional incongruence and lack of coordination remained: 'The challenges facing Aboriginal children with disabilities have been identified in the past yet continue to exist. The 1996 Federal Task Force on Disability noted that the lack of disability-related services available on reserve often forces Aboriginal people to abandon their communities in search of supports. Once off-reserve, Aboriginal persons with a disability face jurisdictional barriers in accessing these supports and services.[83]

Legislated Divisions

In addition to the constitutional uncertainty as to whether Aboriginal health is an 'Indian' matter or a 'health' matter or whether the constitutional division of powers is actually irrelevant, given that First Nations' relationships are with Canada, there are also legislative divides that further complicate and hinder the deployment of effective governance structures to improve Aboriginal people's access to health care.

For example, while many bands have control over band membership, the federal government determines who may qualify for registration as a status Indian under the *Indian Act*, and there is no necessary correlation between Ottawa's legislated criteria for status and any given band's criteria for membership. To present a simplified explanation of the legislative system, only an individual who has at least two status grandparents qualifies for registered status.[84] So, in the event where a woman who is considered 50 per cent status – that is, she has one status and one non-status parent – has a child with a non-status man, that child will not have status. Band membership, however, quite often only requires that the individual to prove 'native ancestry' in the First Nation. Thus, one can be recognized as a member of an Indian band, live on reserve, speak an Aboriginal language, and live in an Aboriginal household, yet not qualify for registration as an Indian. Genetics and externally imposed kinship presumptions, not cultural or pragmatic factors, inform this federally imposed statutory division.

In terms of access to basic health care and services, as long as the non-status Indian lives on a reserve (that is, as long as she has band membership *and* housing is available for her), she will receive the same level of public and community health service as any other resident of that community.[85] However, federal policy is such that only status Indians have access to comprehensive benefits under the Non-Insured Health Benefits Program, which covers medication, dental work, medical transportation, and devices such as eyeglasses.[86] As a consequence, children living in the same extended family on a reserve may experience quite different levels of access based upon how Canada's health policy framework has been wedded to its existing legislative regime. The arbitrariness of this situation is illustrated by an exception to it, which provides that children of a status parent, regardless of whether or not they qualify for status themselves, receive full service coverage on a par with status children up until they are one year old. When that first birthday arrives, differentiation in access to health services begins.

The Health Transfer Program

Current initiatives to improve Aboriginal health have inherited these jurisdictional and legislative complications and so must navigate complex governmental relations from the 'outside.' One flagship initiative to improve Aboriginal health is the Health Transfer Program (HTP) which reassigns administrative responsibility for some elements of health services from Health Canada to Aboriginal communities, together with a negotiated funding envelope. The Program is intended to allow First Nations communities to develop health programs that will address their particular needs and empower them to draw up their own solutions.[87]

The Cree community of Pukatawagan, Manitoba, found that drawing up one's own solution can be an exercise in abandonment disguised as empowerment. In November 1993 the environmental health officer for the Cree Nation Tribal Health Centre issued a 'boil water' order because of high coliform counts. Provincial authorities characterized the problem as an environmental one, that is, contaminated water. Since the water was located on a reserve, which is federal land, Manitoba concluded that Canada was responsible for addressing the situation. Federal authorities, however, characterized the problem differently. Instead of viewing the problem as the environmental contamination of federal land (and thus within federal jurisdiction), they described the situation as a public health problem. Further, federal spokespeople concluded that because the Band had taken responsibility for public health programming through the Health Transfer Program, the Band was responsible for solving the problem. The Band argued that federal authorities were responsible, as the federal government had constructed the faulty water and sanitation systems. The Band also noted that the HTP envelope had no budget for such expenses, so repairs would require the Band to pull funding from its primary health care purse. The roulette game was in motion.

Critics of the Health Transfer Policy had anticipated such problems, having described HTP as a mechanism for the federal government to abdicate lawful responsibilities for the delivery of health care services to Aboriginal peoples.[88] Although it is arguably necessary to transfer responsibility into the hands of Aboriginal communities while Aboriginal health is still in crisis (or the crisis may never end), it is highly problematic that the transfers are occurring before Aboriginal communities have developed sufficient infrastructure and capacity to be successful on their own.

Nine months after the boil water order was issued, the Minister of Indian Affairs agreed to provide some assistance. In 1995 the sewage discharge pipe was moved downstream from the drinking water source, but jurisdictional arguments regarding responsibility persisted. Interestingly, Canada published a policy paper in 1995 with regard to Aboriginal self-determination that included the statement: 'There is no justifiable basis for the Government to retain fiduciary obligations in relation to subject matters over which it has relinquished its control and over which an Aboriginal government or institution has, correspondingly, assumed control.'[89] This position is in tension with the fundamental principle of the Royal Commission on Aboriginal Peoples for moving forward – that an on-going fiduciary relationship is essential for developing a renewed relationship between the Aboriginal and the non-Aboriginal people of Canada.

The Royal Commission characterized this fiduciary relationship in terms of a political and constitutional partnership that involves shared responsibilities between the parties. The Royal Commission's ideal is that this partnership be based on respect and recognition of the mutual vulnerability of the parties, which give rise to mutual obligations.[90] Canada's position statement does not reflect this conceptualization. Rather, it resonates with an 'interpretation of the fiduciary relationship as based on notions of guardian and ward.'[91] This latter position seems to have been reflected in the Pukatawagan debacle, where the federal government attempted to sever the relationship when the 'ward' stepped forward into an 'adult' role.

The struggle to define the characteristics of the underlying relationship between Ottawa and Aboriginal peoples points to a larger political and legal question. This question is whether Aboriginal peoples are subsumed within the Dominion and its divisions of power and jurisdiction, or whether, instead, they are outside of that union but forever deeply intertwined with it because of unique legal and historical factors.

In the end, Indian and Northern Affairs did provide the $21 million that was required to construct a new water and sewage treatment plant, sewage lagoon, sewage lift station, and sewage collection lines in 2000.[92]

It took seven years, extensive negative media coverage and community mobilization, and many turns of the roulette wheel, for the Cree community of Pukatawagan to have safe drinking water and a proper sanitation infrastructure.

Aboriginal communities participating in the Health Transfer Program are further hampered by their inheritance of a funding formula that reflects the *Indian Act* definition of 'Indian' and takes it one step further. When health care funds are transferred, only status Indians – *who also happen to live on reserve* – are included in the head count: no money is allotted to the Band's coffers in recognition of non-status band members who live on reserve or for status band members who choose, or are forced, to live off reserve. Legislated definitions of Indianness that ignore social reality impede progress towards universal standards of good health for Aboriginal peoples.

Meanwhile, health problems arising from deficient housing, general community conditions, and limited economic development and jurisdictional scope cannot be addressed through the HTP negotiations.[93] These matters are outside of Health Canada's scope. Many fall under the jurisdiction of Indian and Northern Affairs or other federal departments that are not connected with the Health Transfer Program. The Royal Commission on Aboriginal Peoples cites one chief who described the HTP process as an attempt to 'have Indian people administer their own misery.'[94] Indeed, it is difficult to conceive of how local administrative control can significantly alter community health, especially where this control involves inadequate existing health services.[95] Despite such comments, Aboriginal participation in the Health Transfer Program is high, and as of December 2003 over 49 per cent of First Nations communities had entered into, or completed, the transfer process.[96] The offer of administering some health services is extremely attractive to people who have 'long been treated as if they are incapable of running their own affairs' and who are claiming a right to govern themselves.[97] However, such an offer, when made without the institution-building, human resources, and financial wherewithal needed to do the job is likely to continue to create situations of 'abandonment in the guise of empowerment.'[98]

Bridging Divides: Existing Proposals

What Aboriginal peoples often lack in accessing health care is a route for effectively bridging existing jurisdictional, departmental, and legislative divisions. Although the question of how to bridge these is beyond the scope of this chapter, it is worth noting that this matter is discussed in the *Report on Aboriginal Peoples*, in the *Kirby Report*, and in the *Romanow Report*. The Royal Commission's key recommendation is that levels of government reach agreements as to their respective jurisdiction pending the realization of Aboriginal self-government.[99] Having a list of which entity has agreed to be held responsible for which issue would certainly be helpful, but ultimately this recommendation fails to address the resolution of health issues that *legitimately straddle* multiple jurisdictions. It also conceptually dismisses the argument that Aboriginal health qua health is solely within federal jurisdiction – a position that is likely to meet resistance within some Aboriginal communities. The concerns that Aboriginal communities may have in working with both Ottawa and the provinces must be openly addressed. Given factors such as population density, the relative remoteness of areas where many Aboriginal communities are located, and the cost of providing health care services, pragmatic concerns dictate that Aboriginal communities and the provinces both need to move towards a cooperative health governance relationship.[100]

Where the Royal Commission's proposal would result in an itemized list, Romanow proposes abandoning the whole issue of jurisdictional assignment. As described by Janesca Kydd (chapter 9, this volume), Romanow suggests breaking down jurisdictional silos by pooling all existing federal and provincial Aboriginal health funding in each province into one envelope. That envelope would then be administered through Aboriginal Health Partnerships.[101] This proposal seems to be more promising and could be effective on many fronts. Where Kydd's concerns about this proposal are largely administrative in nature (for example, what form would the bureaucracy take or who holds the purse strings), a more pragmatic concern is that Romanow's provincial silos would reproduce the inconsistent level of funding directed to Aboriginal health by various provinces. The envelope would be considerably larger in Ontario where the province already supports Aboriginal health initiatives, but quite small in provinces that do not fund Aboriginal health. As well, this approach fails to encompass broader health determinants. It does not, for example, propose a way to bridge the gap created by reserve land being within federal jurisdiction while environmental regulation is a largely provincial concern.

Kirby's proposal of a population health strategy requiring 'extensive and on-going interdepartmental collaboration' seems at once the most promising and yet the most vague. Merging Kirby's recommendations with those of Romanow may well result in a viable plan.

Each of these proposals depends upon voluntarily assumed responsibilities and skirts issues of legal responsibility. Although such an approach may effectively bypass some of the jurisdictional confusion, it leaves unanswered the question of to whom Aboriginal peoples can ultimately turn if they hit a wall – whether Canada's obligations are lawful or merely moral.

All of these proposals seek resolution of jurisdictional difficulties. Given the number of parties involved – all of the provinces and territories and the federal government, as well as Aboriginal communities and their political organizations – one should expect that negotiations would take some time. As an interim measure, Ottawa certainly has the power to consolidate unilaterally its responsibilities, programs, and initiatives that touch on Aboriginal health.[102] This could bring matters such as housing within the same envelope as community health, resulting in a more unified and effective approach to improving Aboriginal access.

I close with another example that illustrates the awkwardness of the current situation. Eskasoni, a Mi'kmaq Band located in Cape Breton, Nova Scotia, has managed its own community-based health services under the Health Transfer Program since 1997. The parties had negotiated that the transfer would include creating a new health care complex, drawing upon both federal and provincial funding. Each level of government was committed to the project. However, difficulties arose over how to ensure that provincial money was directed into facilities for provincial staff and programs, and federal money into facilities for federal staff and programs. In the end, the parties built two separate buildings, with one connecting door.[103] This two-building complex is a physical manifestation of the jurisdictional fragmentation that forms one of the unique barriers to Aboriginal health. A connecting door is a considerable improvement over a roulette wheel, but nevertheless falls far short of the goal of ensuring that everyone sits in the same room and at the same table.

NOTES

I thank Karen McEwan, Bill Lahey, and Brian Noble for their critical intellectual feedback and uncritical emotional support in the drafting of this chapter.

1 Stefan Matiation, 'Aboriginal People and HIV/AIDS' (1999) 4 2:3 Canadian HIV/AIDS Policy and Law Newsletter 31 at 32 [Matiation 1].
2 Canada, Royal Commission on Aboriginal Peoples, *Report of the Royal Commission on Aboriginal Peoples*, vol. 3, *Gathering Strength* (Ottawa: Minister of Supply and Services, 1996) [*Report on Aboriginal Peoples*] at 192.
3 *Ibid.* at 191.
4 *Ibid.*
5 *Ibid.* at 199.
6 *Ibid.* at 199.
7 *Ibid.* at 119.
8 Canada, Senate Standing Committee on Social Affairs, Science and Technology, *The Health of Canadians: The Federal Role – Interim Report*, vol. 4, *Issues and Options* (Ottawa: Senate of Canada, 2002) at 130 (Chair: Michael J.L Kirby) [*Kirby Report*].
9 Canada, Commission on the Future of Health Care in Canada, *Building on Values: The Future of Health Care in Canada* (Saskatoon: author, 2002) at 211 (Chair: Roy Romanow) [*Romanow Report*]. Recent data published by the First Nations and Inuit Health Branch (FNIHB) of Health Canada also support these characterizations. See Health Canada, FNIHB, *A Statistical Profile on the Health of First Nations in Canada* (Ottawa: author, 2002) [*Statistical Profile*].
10 *Romanow Report, supra* note 9 at 211. For a more detailed description of Romanow's proposals, see Janesca Kydd (in this volume).
11 For example, the FNIHB drew up emergency plans to contain SARS should it be detected on reserves because 'overcrowding and disease make reserves breeding grounds for outbreaks.' Brian Laghi, 'Epidemic Feared if SARS Spreads to Native Reserves,' *Globe and Mail*, 16 June 2003, A1.
12 *Statistical Profile, supra* note 9 at 44.
13 *Ibid.* at 7.
14 Stefan Matiation, *HIV/AIDS and Aboriginal People: Problems of Jurisdiction and Funding*, 2nd ed. (Montreal: Canadian HIV-AIDS Legal Network, 1999) [Matiation 2] at 2.
15 Anne McLellan, Minister of Health, 'Minister's Message – National Aboriginal Day in Canada,' http://www.hc-sc.gc.ca/english/media/minister/message_Aboriginal.html (accessed 18 June 2003).
16 (U.K.), 30 & 31 Vict., c. 3, reprinted in R.S.C. 1995, App. II, No. 5.
17 *Ibid.* s. 91(24).
18 Provinces bring this claim pursuant to ss. 92(7), (13), and (16) of the *Constitution Act, 1867, ibid.* See also Matiation 2, *supra* note 14 at 16.

19 *Indian Act*, R.S.C. 1985, c. I-5.
20 For further discussion of s. 88, see Martha Jackman, 'Constitutional Juris-diction over Health in Canada' (2000) 8 Health L. J. 95 at paras. 21-23.
21 [1997] B.C.J. No. 2410 (S.C.) (Q.L.).
22 *Ibid.* at para. 54.
23 [2000] B.C.J. No. 501 (C.A.) (Q.L.).
24 *Ibid.* at para. 3.
25 [1994] 3 F.C. 449 (T.D.).
26 *Ibid.* at para. 13.
27 [1982] 2 S.C.R. 112.
28 Kent McNeil, *Emerging Justice? Essays on Indigenous Rights in Canada and Australia* (Saskatoon, University of Saskatchewan, Native Law Centre, 2001).
29 See, e.g., the discussion in Canada, House of Commons Standing Commit-tee on Human Rights and the Status of Disabled Persons, *Completing the Circle: A Report on Aboriginal People with Disabilities* (Ottawa: Supply and Services Canada, 1993) (Chair: Bruce Halliday) [*Halliday Report*].
30 James Waldram, D. Ann Herring, and T. Kue Young, *Aboriginal Health in Canada: Historical, Cultural, and Epidemiological Perspectives* (Toronto: Uni-versity of Toronto Press, 1995) at 141.
31 *Ibid.* at 156.
32 *Ibid.* at 149.
33 James Frideres and Rene Gadacz, *Aboriginal Peoples in Canada: Contempo-rary Conflicts,* 6th ed. (Toronto: Prentice-Hall, 2003) at 68–9.
34 See Minister of National Health and Welfare, 'Policy of the Federal Gov-ernment Concerning Indian Health Services,' which was tabled in 1974 and is cited in FNIHB, 'History of Providing Health Services to First Nations and Inuit People,' http://www.hc-sc.gc.ca/fnihb-dgspni/fnihb/history.htm. For funding trends leading to current levels of transfer, see www.hc-sc.gc.ca/fnihb-dgspni/fnihb/bpm/hfa/ten_years_health_transfer/index.htm (accessed 23 Aug. 2005).
35 See discussion in Waldram et al., *supra* note 30 at 146 regarding statements made by representatives of the federal government between 1945 and 1970.
36 Frideres and Gadacz, *supra* note 33 at 69.
37 For example, see Union of B.C. Indian Chiefs, 'Aboriginal Health Rights Position.' This paper, last updated in 2003, is available at http://www.ubcic.bc.ca/health.htm (accessed 13 Nov. 2004).
38 *Treaty 6, Between Her Majesty the Queen and the Plain and Wood Cree Indians and Other Tribes of Indians At Fort Carlton, Fort Pitt and Battle River With*

Adhesions, 1876, 1889. A copy of this treaty is reproduced by Indian and Northern Affairs Canada as IAND publication no. QS-0574-000-EE-A-1, cat. no. R33-0664.

39 (1935), 5 C.N.L.R. 92 (Ex. Ct.).

40 *Ibid.* at 95.

41 *Ibid.* at 115.

42 *Ibid.*

43 (1966), 56 D.L.R. (2d) 749 (Sask. C.A.).

44 *Ibid.* at 751. Here the Court of Appeal cites directly from the decision at first instance.

45 *Ibid.* at 753.

46 *R. v. Swimmer* (1970), 17 D.L.R. (3d) 476 (Sask. C.A.).

47 *Nowegijick v. The Queen*, [1983] 1 S.C.R. 29 at 36.

48 [1999] 3 S.C.R. 456 at para. 11.

49 *Ibid.* at para. 14.

50 *R. v. Badger*, [1996] 1 S.C.R. 771 at para. 41.

51 *R. v. Sundown*, [1999] 1 S.C.R. 393 at para. 32; *Simon v. The Queen*, [1985] 2 S.C.R. 387 at 402.

52 [1999] 4 C.N.L.R. 393 (Fed.Ct.T.D.) at para. 12.

53 *Ibid.* at para. 14.

54 Peter Bryce, 'The History of American Indians in Relation to Health' (1914) 12 Ontario Historical Society 128–41 as cited in Waldram et al., *supra* note 30 at 156.

55 Peter Bryce, *The Story of a National Crime: An Appeal for Justice to the Indians of Canada* (Ottawa: James Hope, 1922) at 8, as cited in Waldram *et al.*, *supra* note 30 at 157.

56 McNeil, *supra* note 28 at 326.

57 *Ibid.* at 326–7.

58 *Ibid.* at 328–9.

59 *Ibid.* at 340.

60 Canada, Minister of Indian Affairs and Northern Development, *Gathering Strength: Canada's Aboriginal Action Plan* (Ottawa: IAND, 1997), available at http:www.ainc-inac.gc.ca/gs/chg_e.html (accessed 23 Aug. 2005).

61 *Ibid.* at 18. When accessing document on the internet, see s. IV.

62 McNeil, *supra* note 28 at 331.

63 John Borrows, 'Wampum at Niagara: The Royal Proclamation, Canadian Legal History, and Self-Government,' in Michael Asch, ed., *Aboriginal and Treaty Rights in Canada: Essays on Law, Equality and Respect for Difference* (Vancouver: UBC Press, 1997) at 161.

64 *Ibid.* at 165.

65 *Ibid.* at 166–8.
66 Capt. Thomas G. Anderson, 'Report on the Affairs of the Indians of Canada, Section III' App. No. 95 in App. T of the *Journals of the Legislative Assembly of Canada*, vol. 6 (1818) cited in Borrows, *supra* note 63 at 166.
67 (1973), 34 D.L.R. (3d) 145 (S.C.C.).
68 *Ibid.* at 203.
69 *Ibid.* at 206.
70 See, e.g., the Assembly of First Nations, 'First Nations Health Priorities,' http://www.afn.ca/Programs/Health/First%20Nations%20Health% 20Priorities.htm. (accessed 2 December 2003).
71 [2002] 4 S.C.R. 245.
72 *Ibid.* at para. 79.
73 Matiation 2, *supra* note 14 at 35.
74 *Ibid.* at 27–9.
75 *Ibid.* at 37.
76 *Ibid.* at 19.
77 *Ibid.* at 30.
78 Political, economic, and legal factors that have historically forced Aboriginal people to live off-reserve, to leave their communities, or travel between on-reserve and off-reserve residences are discussed at length in *Corbiere v. Canada*, [1999] 2 S.C.R. 203. See paras. 19, 32, 62, 71, and 84.
79 *Report on Aboriginal Peoples, supra* note 2 at 152.
80 *Ibid.* at 151.
81 *Ibid.* at 13.
82 *Ibid.*
83 Report of the Standing Committee on Human Resources Development and the Status of Persons with Disabilities, *Building a Brighter Future for Urban Aboriginal Children* (Ottawa: House of Commons, June 2003) at 20–1.
84 The system for determining eligibility for status is considerably more complex. See *Indian Act, supra* note 19, at c. 6, ss. 6, 7.
85 The FNIHB does not discriminate on the basis of status when it comes to these health services. See *Statistical Profile, supra* note 9 at 18.
86 *Ibid.* at 18–19.
87 See, e.g., FNIHB, 'Transfer Issues,' http://www.hc-sc.gc.ca/fnihb-dgspni/ fnihb/bpm/hfa/transfer_issues.htm (accessed 25 November 2003).
88 Assembly of First Nations *Special Report: The National Indian Health Transfer Conference* (Ottawa: author, 1988) at 4.
89 *Aboriginal Self-Government: The Government of Canada's Approach to Implementation of the Inherent Right and the Negotiation of Aboriginal Self-*

Government (Ottawa: Minister of Public Works and Government Services, 1995) at 14.

90 See discussion in Matiation 2, *supra* note 14 at 14.

91 *Ibid.*

92 INAC, *News Release*, 2-00141 'Mathias Colomb Cree Nation Celebrates Several Improvements to Its Community Infrastructure' (2 June 2000), http://www.ainc-inac.gc.ca/nr/prs/m-a2000/2-00141_e.html (accessed 23 Aug. 2005).

93 David Gregory et al., 'Canada's Indian Health Transfer Policy: The Gull Bay Band Experience' (1992) 51:3 Human Organization 214–22 at 217. Gregory cites this point to John O'Neil, 'The Politics of Health in the Fourth World: A Northern Canadian Example' (1986) 45 Human Organization 119–28.

94 *Report on Aboriginal Peoples, supra* note 2 at 117.

95 See discussion of this matter in Gregory, *supra* note 93 at 221.

96 The FNIHB posts data on participation in the Health Transfer Program on its website. The information is updated periodically. See Health Canada, 'Status of First Nations Control Activity,' http:www.hc-sc.gc.ca/fnihb-dgspni/fnihb/bpm/hfa/transfer_status/control_activity.htm (accessed 23 Aug. 2005).

97 *Report on Aboriginal Peoples, supra* note 2 at 165.

98 Here I paraphrase language that the Royal Commission used to describe a situation where Canada told a community it must solve its own problems when it requested assistance in dealing with two pedophiles. *Ibid.*

99 Ibid. at 234 (recommendation 3.3.3).

100 I am grateful to William Lahey for this observation.

101 *Romanow Report, supra* note 9 at 224.

102 I thank William Lahey for this observation.

103 Nicki Sims-Jones, 'The Eskasoni Primary Care Project' (2003) 5 Health Pol. Research Bulletin 14 at 16.

9 The Rural Aboriginal Health Gap: The Romanow Solutions?

JANESCA KYDD

Despite its obvious merits, the Canadian health care system continues to suffer from disparities both in the health status of Canadian citizens and in their ability to access health care.[1] One source of these disparities is geographic.[2] The problems created by geography are particularly acute for rural Canadians. Moreover, given that more than 50 per cent of Canada's Aboriginal peoples[3] live in rural areas,[4] rural health concerns directly affect the well-being of Canada's Aboriginal population as a whole.

In this chapter, I will analyse the problem faced by rural Aboriginals in accessing health care services and improving their health status. I refer to this problem as the 'rural Aboriginal health gap.' My primary focus in this chapter is on one of the latest and most comprehensive attempts at addressing this plight, *Building on Values: The Future of Health Care in Canada*[5] (the *Romanow Report*). My argument is that, while Romanow's recommendations on rural health may appear to close the rural Aboriginal health gap, more is required if the specific needs of Canada's Aboriginal population are to be met.

The Plight of Aboriginal Canadians in Rural Areas

Rural Canada is varied and diverse.[6] So, too, is the health of its residents. Health indicators developed by Statistics Canada and the Canadian Institute for Health Information have shown that 'the health status of people living in rural communities, especially people in northern communities, is not as good as the rest of the Canadian population.'[7] Access to health care services remains a problem in rural areas. In 1999, the Centre for Health Services and Policy Research at the University of

British Columbia issued a report surveying the initiatives in place across Canada that have the primary objective of improving access to medical care in areas that were considered underserved.[8] Its authors wrote that 'the number of policies and practices one finds as one canvasses the provinces and territories is astonishing,' adding that 'it is obvious Canada continues to suffer from relative policy impotence in this arena.'[9] This policy impotence, as I will argue below, is further exacerbated when longer-term determinants of health are at issue.

While long-term solutions aimed at addressing the determinants of health have been pursued by both provincial and federal governments, quick solutions remain elusive. It has been recognized that in order for initiatives aimed at addressing the determinants of health to be success-ful, the '"silos" that currently exist between health policy and other social policy areas such as education, housing or social services' must be broken down.[10] Partnerships between Aboriginal communities and various levels of government are required.[11] But such partnerships, while individually worthy, are collectively insufficient to meet the needs of rural Aboriginals. In what follows, I examine whether the *Romanow Report* has succeeded in articulating the solutions that have long eluded others.

Overview of the *Romanow Report*

Introduction

Romanow presents his solutions to the rural Aboriginal health gap in two separate chapters of his report: one on rural health (chapter 7) and another one that is specifically about Aboriginal health (chapter 10). Romanow takes this approach because, although Aboriginals comprise a large part of the rural demographic, they also have issues specific to themselves as Aboriginal peoples. I propose to merge the two chapters in my review, however, as everything Romanow writes with regard to rural areas has relevance to Aboriginal health access and status.

Romanow begins by identifying the particular problems that must be addressed before his vision – one in which 'Canadians residing in rural and remote regions and communities are as healthy as people living in metropolitan and other urban centers'[12] – can be realized. In regard to rural communities in general, Romanow points out that there is no coherent approach to addressing health concerns. Among other things, he points out that there is a lack of consensus on what adequate access should include; that there is a need for more effective linkages with larger centres, especially when challenged with serving the smallest and most remote of communities; and that there is a need to reorient the focus from symptoms to causes. That is, strategies appear to focus more on health care delivery rather than on addressing the fundamental causes of the rural health deficit.[13]

Romanow identifies four issues – in addition to those mentioned above – that in his opinion contribute to the *Aboriginal* aspect of the rural Aboriginal health gap. These issues are: (1) competing constitutional assumptions; (2) fragmented funding for health services; (3) poorer health outcomes; and (4) different cultural and political influences.[14] Addressing these problems, Romanow argues, requires a national response that cuts across administrative and jurisdictional barriers: 'only by designing programs which respect the cultures of the nations' people and communities and by celebrating Canada's diversity, can health professionals help improve the health of vulnerable populations and reduce the demands on the health system as a whole.'[15]

Romanow's Rural and Aboriginal Recommendations

Rural Recommendations
Romanow recommends an infusion of $1.5 billion of federal government funding to address the access needs of rural Canadians. He calls this infusion '[t]he Remote and Rural Access Fund' (RRAF). Romanow's first two recommendations are aimed at improving access to health care providers. Money from the RRAF would be used to 'attract and retain health care providers' and 'support innovative ways of expanding rural experiences for physicians, nurses and other health care providers as part of their education and training.'[16] The third recommendation seeks to improve current health care services by expanding telehealth approaches.[17] These solutions would constitute little more than a recommendation for more resources for established policy initiatives.

Romanow's fourth recommendation for rural communities is aimed specifically at improving health status. He submits that a portion of the RRAF 'should be used to support innovative ways of delivering health care services to smaller communities and to improve the health of people in those communities.'[18] 'The objective is to find the best approaches to strengthen community resiliency, social capital and local capacity, improve healthy behaviours and lifestyles, and improve the overall health status of people in rural and remote communities.'[19] Romanow states that the provinces and territories would still have discretion regarding which approaches are most appropriate for their communities.[20] However, he also states that a process must be put in place to monitor, evaluate, and disseminate the results of these projects.[21] These responsibilities would likely be allocated to the National Health Council, a new bureaucratic entity recommended earlier in the report. A Council has been established 'to monitor and make annual public reports on the implementation of the Accord, particularly its account- ability and transparency provisions,'[22] but it has not been given any responsibility to administer an RRAF fund as envisaged by Romanow.

Aboriginal Recommendations: Consolidation of Funding and Aboriginal Health Partnerships

In addressing the specific concerns on Aboriginal health, Romanow is quite clear that a new approach is needed to cut across policy silos and jurisdictional barriers. He makes two recommendations towards achiev- ing this goal. First, with regard to the problem of fragmented sources of funding he states: 'Current funding for Aboriginal health services pro- vided by the federal, provincial and territorial governments and Ab- original organizations should be pooled into single consolidated budgets in each province and territory to be used to integrate Aboriginal health services, improve access, and provide adequate, stable and predictable funding.'[23]

The consolidation of funds would be the first step to establishing the goal of creating Aboriginal Health Partnerships (AHPs) that 'would be responsible for developing policies, providing services and improving the health of Aboriginal peoples.'[24] The funds would provide a stable financial base to support the AHPs, and distributions would be made on a per capita basis according to the number of Aboriginals who sign up to be served by an AHP as well as interested non-Aboriginals who may choose to be served by an AHP.[25]

AHPs could take many forms in order to 'reflect the needs, character- istics and circumstances of the population served.'[26] Romanow expects that, in general, they would take a holistic approach to health, consider- ing 'broader conditions that help build capacity and good health in individuals and communities, such as nutrition, housing, education, employment and so on.'[27] The programs would thus be adapted to the 'cultural, social, economic and political circumstances unique to Aboriginal groups' and would 'give Aboriginal peoples a direct voice in how health care services are designed and delivered.'[28]

In terms of structure, the AHPs would be organized 'as a "not-for-profit" community corporation with a board of directors comprised of representatives of the funders (primarily Aboriginal organizations with direct control over funds designated for the provision of health services, together with federal, provincial, and territorial governments) and other individuals involved in establishing the Partnership (for example, key organizers, users, and health care providers).'[29]

The responsibilities of an AHP board would include 'organizing, purchasing and delivering health care services that could range from establishing primary health care networks to more integrated organizations responsible for managing a larger range of services.'[30]

Finally, in terms of accountability, each AHP should be responsible and accountable for the funds it receives and how they are used.[31] Romanow states that clear conditions must be in place to address and clarify responsibility and accountability.[32] This should include an explicit mandate, up-to-date information on performance indicators, and the capacity to make decisions based on the best available evidence.[33] Furthermore, 'structures would have to be in place to allow the Partnership to discuss options, exchange ideas, and also to produce financial accounts that are public and open to all those involved.'[34]

Analysis of the Romanow Recommendations

Many Canadians responded positively to the Romanow recommendations in the areas of rural and aboriginal health.[35] But I see a number of significant obstacles to the successful implementation of these recommendations, particularly those relating to Aboriginal health.

Rural Concerns

Romanow's recommendations for rural health care largely build on pre-existing initiatives. His suggested $1.5 billion infusion of funding for the creation of the RRAF was generally well received,[36] although, as previously mentioned, these funds have not yet materialized. However, it is important to note that although it would be earmarked by the federal government for certain initiatives, the money would still be subject to the discretionary use of the provincial governments. Romanow recommended that the Health Council be charged with monitoring the use of the funds on behalf of the public.[37] The two major areas of concern with Romanow's rural recommendations also apply to many of the other areas of his report: dissatisfaction over the level of funding proposed and scepticism about the proposed Health Council.

First, with respect to funding, concerns have been raised over whether an infusion of new money would do anything to change the system in any significant way. One commentator wrote that Romanow's proposed increases in spending would not even scratch the surface in a system that currently spends $100 billion a year.[38]

Other, however, others have commented that Romanow's suggested monetary infusions are too high.[39] Some might also find that the RRAF is unnecessary, as it simply builds on pre-existing initiatives that will likely continue to exist even without the new funds. The response to this argument, however, is that since these initiatives are a necessary component of our health care system, we should provide funding for their improvement. Given that the relative success of rural health initiatives is not entirely known, to adequately determine the necessity or feasibility of additional rural health care funding, one would need more information about the relation between expenditures and outcomes. Funding concerns, therefore, directly shade into concerns over accountability for health care funding and, more specifically, into concerns about Romanow's proposal for a National Health Council.

Romanow recommended that a National Health Council monitor health care funding to ensure accountability. That is, the Health Council should track the effectiveness of the funds spent by the provinces and territories on health care delivery. Critics of the Council have pointed out that ensuring accountability is something that Health Canada, the provincial ministries of health, and all of their related agencies, have been unable to do to date.[40] Canada's *Constitution* has been interpreted to make health a provincial responsibility.[41] Romanow's suggestion for a Health Council, then, has been said to be an attempt to federalize health care. Some have also complained that it amounts to unnecessary bureaucratic overkill.[42]

These objections are answerable. Romanow responded to the worries about increased bureaucracy by noting that the federal government had already tried allocating new funds to the provinces without agreement as to what those funds would be spent on (in 2000, for example, $23.4 billion in new federal money was allotted for health care)[43] – and that it did not work. The Canadian Medical Association has also responded to those who balk at the notion of federal funding with strings attached:

'It's difficult to see how the ungainly marionette of Canadian health care can be managed *without* strings. A worse idea would be to let anti-federalist wrangling trammel any chance of meaningful change.'[44] The notion of a Health Council therefore would appear to be a step in the right direction in dealing with health care difficulties grounded in lack of accountability.[45]

Aboriginal Concerns

Romanow's recommendations on Aboriginal health seek to achieve all that is aimed for with his rural health recommendations and then some. As I will argue below, these suggestions, while laudable, are fraught with difficulty.

Consolidation Framework Agreement

As mentioned above, the first step to achieving Romanow's goals for Aboriginal health is consolidating all of the existing funds for Aboriginal health into one base to support Aboriginal health care programs and services through the AHPs. Romanow recommends that the consolidation of funding agreements be done generally on a provincial and territorial basis. He then moves on to discuss how the AHPs would work before fully addressing the critical topic of the framework agreement.

Who, however, would ultimately hold the purse strings? Would some new entity be created to take charge of distributing the pooled funds to the AHPs? Romanow does not address this point other than to note that the framework agreements should address who will contribute what and on what terms. Some form of mediating bureaucratic structure supervising distribution of the consolidated funds to the AHPs would likely be required. Acknowledging the need for such a structure to manage and allocate pooled resources raises the following questions: First, what would be its composition? Second, on what terms would it operate? Third, what would be the processes for appointment of its members? The *Romanow Report* speaks to none of these issues, perhaps hoping that the contributing parties would find their own solutions. Still, Romanow should have made some suggestions in order to create a dialogue. For example, a committee could be struck by representatives of all contributing parties to manage the consolidated pool, or the federal government could take on that role. The National Health Council might be an entity which could oversee the management of the funds and deal with any sort of disputes that might arise.

Funding Considerations

Romanow appears to believe that the existing funds are sufficient to achieving the ends that he has in mind, but he does not depart from the traditional notion of per capita funding. Unfortunately, standard per capita funding does not work in areas where the population is sparse and residents must travel great distances to access health care.[46] On average, rural residents are ten kilometres away from a physician, compared with less than two kilometres for residents of urban areas.[47] In remote and northern areas that ten-kilometre average jumps to 100 kilometres for two-thirds of the population; and in the Arctic, many have to travel for up to six hours by airplane for hospital-based services.[48] A fair funding formula demands that account be taken of the increased cost of travel in various rural communities.

Per capita funding was a contentious issue during the First Ministers Conference on Health Care in February 2003. The three territorial leaders urged Ottawa 'to alter its per capita health-care funding formula for the territories because it overlooks the high costs of caring for small populations spread across remote regions.'[49] The territories wanted a special base fund of $20 to $25 million to be set up to help meet their special needs. Because the Prime Minister refused to agree to such a proposal, the territorial leaders walked out of the meetings, 'stating that there was nothing there for them and that they had again been left behind by a government that does not understand the needs of their mostly Aboriginal populations.'[50] A tentative resolution, however, was later reached on this matter.[51]

Presumably, given Romanow's vision, funds would only be distributed to an AHP once a viable plan was presented and approved. But who would approve the AHP proposals? Would it be the same entity that holds the purse strings to the consolidated funds? Surely a decision-making process with 'approval criteria' against which to judge the AHP proposals would need to be established. Therefore, the individuals of the 'consolidated fund structure' would need not only an understanding of budgets and finance but also of evaluating health care proposals.

Finally, while Romanow states that an individual must sign up to be served by an AHP, there is no discussion of what financial consequences flow should that individual change his or her mind and decide to opt back into the current system of health care delivery. For example, the *Romanow Report* is silent on whether the monies allotted to an individual under the AHP would be returned back to its sources or whether there would be restrictions placed on switching between AHPs and the status quo system.

Information Sharing and Accountability

Romanow suggests that the AHPs develop a system to share information and learn from one another, but he glosses over the logistics of carrying out this task. Romanow further suggests that each order of government that contributes funds should be accountable to its own legislative body. However, this is a much more problematic notion of accountability than is the case, for example, between provincial governments and regional health authorities, given the various pipes of funding potentially flowing to AHPs. Many masters could make operational life very difficult for the AHPs. Perhaps it would make more sense if the AHPs were held accountable by the 'consolidated fund structure,' but, as stated above, it is unclear to whom the 'consolidated fund structure' would, in turn, be accountable.

Economic and Administrative Considerations over New Bureaucracy

Romanow's recommendations are innovative. But they create the need for several bureaucratic structures and thus give rise to many hidden costs, for example, computers, office space, and administrative support. At first blush, the only new bureaucratic entities that arise from Romanow's rural Aboriginal recommendations are the AHPs and the National Health Council. However, my analysis thus far has revealed at least four additional structures: the consolidated budget structure, an information-sharing structure, and accountability structures for both the consolidated fund structure and the various AHPs (unless this responsibility is undertaken by the National Health Council). The generality of the recommendations made and their unprecedented nature suggest that the benefits of these reforms could be outweighed by the additional costs of maintaining this additional bureaucracy. Romanow should address these issues in order to strengthen his recommendations.

Manpower and Knowledge

In addition to the administrative costs identified above, each and every AHP would require a board of directors. While each AHP would have representatives from the community serve on the board, Romanow does not address whether the government representatives on the board of one AHP could sit on another. Even if government representatives *could* sit on more than one board, they would run the risk of overextending themselves if they were to sit on several AHP boards.

Another problem with the concept of AHPs is that it presupposes the availability of a certain degree of knowledge to set up the board of directors, create the necessary infrastructure, contract with outside health care providers, utilize resources to best suit the community's needs, and so on. A prerequisite to AHP implementation therefore appears to be educational and training of the community members involved. Funding for recruitment and training is therefore another hidden cost of this regime.

Community Conflict
Even if the barriers mentioned above could be overcome, there is no requirement that all the individuals of a particular community would have to be covered by the same AHP. Although generally an AHP would cover several communities of small sizes and similar regional character, it is also possible for one larger community to be served by two or more AHPs. In the latter case, an AHP would have an incentive to compete for more individuals to join it over another AHP in order to qualify for more funding. The pros and cons of joining a particular AHP would have to be weighed by community members. However, because of the tightly knit character of many rural Aboriginal communities, disagreement over an issue as important as health care has the potential for leading to community conflict.

Conclusion

The disparities in access experienced by Aboriginal people and rural Canadians mocks Canada's portrayal of its health care system as one of the best in the world. The sorry statistics for Aboriginal health also underscore how a health care system designed for the majority of the population does not serve the needs of smaller, more vulnerable portions of the population.

The Romanow Commission is the latest in a line of task forces and commissions empowered to address these key issues. But, although Romanow's recommendations for Aboriginal health are laudable, they remain fraught with difficulty. It is tempting to conclude that his recommendations with respect to Aboriginal health could be subsumed within his recommendations for rural health where there are far fewer concerns regarding implementation.

Nonetheless, the fact remains that the health status of rural Aboriginal Canadians is worse than that of rural Canadians, and this suggests that there is a missing ingredient in Romanow's rural recommendations. My analysis of Romanow's Aboriginal recommendations has revealed several problems that are largely related to hidden bureaucratic entities and their related costs. Because Romanow's Aboriginal recommendations are novel, their contingencies need to be addressed. A cost-benefit analysis of these additional layers of bureaucracy would need to be undertaken. In addition, a funding system based on something other than a per capita scale would need to be developed. The potential for community conflict would also need to be addressed, and the additional costs of manpower and knowledge must be taken into account. Romanow's recommendations have potential, but with so many important questions left unanswered they risk being ignored. A more specific plan, in my opinion, would have had a greater hope of implementation.

Romanow's recommendations were considered at the First Ministers Conference on Health Care in February 2003. Although $34.8 billion in federal funding over the next five years was promised,[52] none of Romanow's recommendations for alleviating the rural Aboriginal health gap were implemented. There was no RRAF. Instead, funding for rural health seems to come from several different areas of the Accord.[53]

My conclusions to this point have been largely negative, so let me end with the following, more positive, observation. Although disappointing, the failure of the First Ministers to effectively deal with the rural Aboriginal health gap does not mean that nothing is being done about it. There is hope, with the implementation of the National Health Council, that we will be better equipped to assess the effectiveness of new rural Aboriginal health expenditures and to suggest alternatives for reform in the future. Moreover, the failure of the First Ministers to address the difficulties inherent in Romanow's rural Aboriginal recommendations at the 2003 conference on health care does not mean that these recommendations cannot be explored in the future. It is abundantly clear that cooperation between the federal and provincial governments is required if the health concerns of rural Aboriginal people are to be adequately addressed and resolved. Without that cooperation, government leadership, and willingness at both the federal and provincial levels, the best laid plans will come to naught.

NOTES

This chapter is based on a paper Ms Kydd produced in completing her JD at the Faculty of Law, University of Toronto.

1 The disparities of the Canadian health care system were recently addressed by the Commission on the Future of Health Care in Canada in *Building on Values: The Future of Health Care in Canada – Final Report* (Saskatoon: Commission on the Future of Heath Care in Canada, 2002) (Chair: Roy Romanow), http://www.hc-sc.gc.ca/english/pdf/romanow/pdfs/HCC_Final_Report.pdf (accessed 29 August 2005) [*Romanow Report*].
2 *Ibid.* at 159.
3 In this chapter, I define 'Aboriginal peoples' as including First Nations, Inuit, and Métis, while acknowledging that there is much diversity between these communities. 'There are more than 600 First Nations communities across the country, speaking over 50 languages,' according to Canada's Ministerial Advisory Council on Rural Health, *Rural Health in Rural Hands: Strategic Directions for Rural, Remote, Northern and Aboriginal Communities* (Ottawa: author, 2002) (Chair: Colin Kinsley), online: http://www.hc-sc.gc.ca/english/pdf/rural_health/rural_hands.pdf (accessed 29 August 2005) [*Rural Health Report*] at 48; *Romanow Report, supra* note 1 at 221.
4 *Rural Health Report, ibid.* at 48, based on Statistics Canada 1996 Population Census data.
5 *Ibid.*
6 *Rural Health Report, supra* note 3 at 1 and 9; *Romanow Report, supra* note 1 at 160.
7 *Romanow Report, supra* note 1 at 161.
8 Morris L. Barer *et al.,* 'Toward Improved Access to Medical Services for Relatively Underserviced Populations: Canadian Approaches, Foreign Lessons' (May 1999) Centre for Health Services and Policy Research, University of British Columbia, http://www.hc-sc.gc.ca/english/media/releases/1999/pdf_docs/99picebk7.rtf (accessed 29 August 2005) [*Toward Improved Access*].
9 *Ibid.*
10 *Ibid.* at 221.
11 *Ibid.* at 220.
12 *Ibid.* at 165.
13 *Ibid.* at 163–5.

14 *Ibid.* at 212. For an excellent discussion of the constitutional problems facing health care reformers, see Constance MacIntosh's contribution to this volume.
15 *Ibid.,* referring to viewpoints expressed at the National Aboriginal Health Organizations forum, *Dialogue on Aboriginal Health: Sharing Our Challenges and Our Successes. Draft Proceedings,* held in partnership with the Romanow Commission, 26 June, Aylmer, Quebec, and during other public hearings, as well as in the written submission to the Romanow Commission by the Canadian Public Health Association, 'Creating Conditions for Health.' (2001).
16 *Romanow Report, supra* note 1 at 166.
17 *Ibid* at 162. Telehealth 'uses information technologies to link patients and health care providers to a spectrum of services that can be brought together to provide higher quality care. It offers tremendous possibilities for overcoming the obstacles of distance and improving access to health care in rural communities.' Canada, Medical Services Branch, Program Transfer and Policy Development, *The Context of Delivery of Health Services to Status Indians and Inuit by Medical Services Branch* (Ottawa: Medical Services Branch, 6 Sept. 1988) at 3. http:// www.cpha.ca/english/pstatem/creat/creating_e.pdf (accessed 29 August 2005).
18 *Romanow Report, supra* note 1 at 168.
19 *Ibid.* at 169.
20 *Ibid* at 166.
21 *Ibid* at 169.
22 See http://www.hc-sc.gc.ca/english/media/releases/2003/2003_97bk1.htm (accessed 8 June 2005). See also the first report of the Health Council available at http://hcc-ccs.com/docs/BkgrdHealthyCdnsENG.pdf (accessed 29 August 2005).
23 *Romanow Report, supra* note 1 at 223.
24 *Ibid.* at 223.
25 *Ibid.* at 226 and 227.
26 *Ibid.* at 223.
27 *Ibid.*
28 *Ibid.* at 212.
29 *Ibid.* at 228.
30 *Ibid.* at 227.
31 *Ibid.* at 228.
32 *Ibid.*
33 *Ibid.*
34 *Ibid.*

35 For example, see '$1.5 Billion for Rural Health' *Rural News*, 29 November 2002, http://www.srpc.ca/News/issue430.html; Jim Bell, 'Romanow Inspires Hope for Better Health Care in Nunavut,' *Nunatsiaq News*, 6 December 2002, http://www.nunatsiaq.com/archives/nunavut021206/news/nunavut/21206_01.html (accessed 29 August 2005); Assembly of First Nations, Press Release, 'National Chief Welcomes Focus on Health, But More Details Needed' (28 November 2002), http://www.afn.ca (accessed 8 June 2005); Registered Nurses Association of Ontario, 'RNAO Response to the Romanow Commission Report' (December 2002) at 21, http://www.rnao.org/html/PDF/Final_Romanow_response.pdf (accessed 29 August 2005).

36 '1.5 Billion for Rural Health,' *ibid.*; 'Romanow Inspires Hope,' *ibid.*

37 Dennis Buekert, 'Reforms Wouldn't Trample Provincial Jurisdiction, Romanow Says,' *Canadian Press* (3 December 2002), http://www.canada.com/national/features/healthcare/story.html?id=3D7F7A3A-C817-42C8-A1E2-1C8CCFD1CB0A (accessed 8 June 2005).

38 Robert Daniel, 'Considering Romanow: A look at the Romanow Commission's Report on the State of Health Care in Canada' (2002) 45 *CSA News*, http://www.snowbirds.org/csanews/issues/45/22.html.

39 For example, see Drew Hasselback, 'Ideas Would Eat Surplus and More – Funding Triage: Economists Wary About the Impact of Spending Billions' *Financial Post*, 29 November 2002, http://www.canada.com/national/features/healthcare/story.html?id=BA3468A1-0DF2-4FA8-9F15-45B6DCD07D9A (accessed 29 August 2005).

40 *CSA News, supra* note 38.

41 *Ibid.*

42 *Ibid.*

43 André Picard, 'Where the Health Dollars Go Depends on Who You Believe,' *Globe and Mail*, 7 February 2003. '[A]n estimated 70 per cent of that money went to wages for health-care workers, not for any change whatsoever.'

44 'Perchance to Dream: Mr. Romanow's Final Report,' Editorial (2003), 168:1 *Canadian Medical Association Journal*, http://www.cmaj.ca/cgi/content/full/168/1/5 (accessed 29 August 2005).

45 See also the first report of the Health Council available at http://hcc-ccs.com/.

46 *Ibid.*

47 *Rural Health Report, supra* note 3 at 13.

48 *Ibid.* at 2 and 13.

49 Kim Lunman, 'PM Draws Fire for Shunning Territories' *Globe and Mail*,

7 February 2003, AI, http://www.globeandmail.com (accessed 29 August 2005).

50 Brian Laghi and Shawn McCarthy, 'Premiers Grumble, but PM Gets Deal on Health' *Globe and Mail*, 6 February 2003.

51 After the Accord was released, Prime Minister Chrétien acknowledged that the territories could not be treated like other provinces and that the per capita funding model was not viable for the North. He agreed to adjust the territories' funding on a bilateral basis ('Health Deal Ignores North,' *ibid.*). He then met with the territorial leaders and Health Minister Anne McLellan. An agreement was reached to provide a $60-million 'floor' to the three territories for health care, over and above the per capita funding stipulated by the Accord. Although further details were required to 'hammer out the details,' it was expected that the territorial leaders would begin to participate in the Accord. Jeff Gray, 'PM, Territorial Leaders Resolve Health Spat,' *Globe and Mail*, 20 February 2003, http://www.globeandmail.com ; '60M for Northern Premiers' *Rural News*, 21 February 2003, http://www.srpc.ca (accessed 29 August 2005).

52 Canada, 2003 First Ministers' Accord on Health Care Renewal, *Health Care Renewal Accord 2003: Federal Health Investments,* http://www.hc-sc.gc.ca/english/hca2003/factsheets2.html (accessed 29 August 2005).

53 For example, $16 billion was dedicated to establishing a five-year Health Reform Fund targeted to primary health care, home care and catastrophic drug coverage. The First Ministers agreed that 'the ultimate goal of primary health care reform is to provide all Canadians, wherever they live, with access to an appropriate health care provider, 24 hours a day, 7 days a week.' However, this was qualified to mean at least 50 per cent of Canadians would have this access, as soon as possible, and that this target would be met within eight years. The Accord also provided that $600 million would be invested 'in health information technology for electronic health records, telehealth and information infrastructure,' as it was agreed that these systems are critical to improving accessibility and quality care, patient safety and sustainability for Canadians who live in rural and remote areas (*ibid.* and the 2003 Accord, *supra* note 52).

10 Access to Treatment of Serious Mental Illness: Enabling Choice or Enabling Treatment?

SHEILA WILDEMAN

Canadian mental health policy over the past few decades has centred upon the dual objectives of ensuring that persons with serious mental illness[1] receive effective, timely treatment in instances of acute crisis and ongoing health maintenance in the community.[2] These objectives have roundly been deemed to have been obstructed by a lack of governmental commitment and funding at both the provincial and federal levels, a problem that shows up most starkly when the importance of non-medical supports such as basic income and secure housing are contemplated under the rubric of the social determinants of health.[3] The resulting situation for persons with serious mental illness may be regarded as broadly comparable to that of the Aboriginal communities discussed in the two preceding chapters by Constance MacIntosh and Janesca Kydd, in that the principle of respect for autonomy or agency (individual or in the case of Aboriginal peoples, also communal) tends to manifest itself in these settings as abandonment to conditions of extreme material hardship. Moreover, although the 'vulnerability' linking Aboriginal peoples and persons with serious mental illness is a contentious one at best, a common complexity is apparent in the ways the health needs of these constituencies have historically been conceived by government under a totalizing model of beneficence and guardianship, with few conceptual resources for acknowledging the diverse values and interests (let alone the agency) of those cast as wards.

That said, aspirationally at least, much contemporary mental health policy persists in pressing the conceptual and systemic implications of recognizing persons with serious mental illness as citizens or full community members. This accords with the logic of deinstitutionalization which, along with a deep background commitment to economic efficiency, claims as its objective the dismantling of the total psychiatric institution while increasing persons' freedom and well-being in the context of community life.[4]

My purpose in this chapter is to raise some concerns about whether the orientation of mental health policy towards *improving access* to treatment of serious mental illness ultimately translates to a project of enabling and supporting treatment choices or simply enabling treatment – within and beyond the walls of the psychiatric hospital. These concerns are directed in part towards the implications of the discursive shift in position of the subject of mental health policy from inmate to citizen, calling into question just how deep is the commitment to promoting equal rights of citizenship among persons diagnosed with mental illness.[5] I suggest that mental health policies and laws directed at affirming citizenship or community membership – in particular, those focused upon enabling access to treatment – tend in the case of serious mental illness to amount to an imperative of compliance with medication at all costs. As such, a strict dualist alternative is constructed between involuntary maintenance in hospital and involuntary (or significantly coerced) compliance with treatment in the community. What is apparently closed off is the project of enabling and respecting persons' ability to make treatment choices reflecting their wider projects of defining and pursuing personal well-being – or defining and pursuing lesser forms of personal suffering. That is, what is closed off is the project of enabling and respecting personal autonomy in this core area of the lives of persons who have been diagnosed with serious mental illness. I wish to show that much current mental health policy and law participates in the subversion of the liberal legal value of autonomy, specifically by refraining from meaningful engagement with the vital project of defining, assessing, and promoting capacity to make treatment decisions on the part of persons diagnosed with serious mental illness.

Reorienting mental health policy from the objective of compliance with treatment to the complexities of defining and enabling decisional capacity will require renewed attention to the values in play in individual treatment choices and in wider policy choices about mental health treatment. In this chapter, rather than attempting to address in any detail the criteria by which capacity for treatment choice should be defined, I offer a preliminary critique of the occlusion of capable treatment choice in much contemporary law and policy oriented to the treatment of serious mental illness.

I begin with a brief discussion of the fundamental commitment in Canadian law to autonomy as this plays out in the arena of medical treatment choice, here introducing the Supreme Court of Canada's recent statement on capacity to make treatment choices under Ontario law in *Starson v. Swayze*.[6] I then examine some key documents from the domain of national mental health policy formation that may be understood to deploy the discourse of access in order to advance the project of enabling treatment, while diminishing the importance of enabling and respecting capable treatment choices. Next I identify three areas of mental health law and policy that demand renewed attention in light of the need to rethink the nature and importance of treatment choice in the psychiatric context: provincial laws providing for involuntary treatment of persons subject to involuntary psychiatric hospitalization, laws providing for mandated community treatment (community treatment orders), and policies and practices of assertive community treatment. In closing I raise a set of possible legal and policy responses to what I suggest is the continuing discriminatory disregard of the capable treatment choices of persons deemed seriously mentally ill and the accompanying disregard for the conditions required to enable such choices.

A final introductory note: I employ the term 'serious mental illness' with the understanding that its use in mental health policy is not precisely fixed. The term is generally associated with severity and duration of symptoms, their interference with social functioning, and specific diagnoses (for example, schizophrenia, bipolar disorder, and major depression).[7] By adopting this descriptor I am able to map my critique onto the arena of contemporary mental health policy; however, I am aware that I risk thereby obscuring the importance of the social and institutional structures that condition the phenomena that the descriptor tracks (symptoms, social functioning, and diagnosis). In addition, I acknowledge a particularly troubling tension in my use of the term given that I seek to draw specifically on the perspectives of persons who reject the very category of illness into which their diagnoses would place them.

Autonomy and Capacity in the Psychiatric Context

The Right to Make Treatment Decisions

The right to make treatment decisions is a basic tenet of health law in Canada and internationally. Some Canadian provinces have recognized this right in health legislation.[8] But the right is in any case well established at common law, where it is articulated under the general principle of respect for autonomy (grounding claims in battery and/or negligence),[9] and is further encompassed in the right to liberty and security of the person under section 7 of the *Charter of Rights and Freedoms*.[10] Moreover, unconsented-to physical interference may constitute the criminal offence of assault.

The importance of the right to make treatment decisions in accordance with one's unique values underpinned the Ontario Court of Appeal's decision in *Malette v. Shulman*.[11] There, a physician was held liable in battery for giving a blood transfusion to a Jehovah's Witness in defiance of a directive on her person indicating that she did not wish to receive such transfusions. The court stated that for the freedom to make choices about medical treatment to be meaningful, 'people must have the right to make choices that accord with their own values regardless of how unwise or foolish those choices may appear to others.'[12]

The 1991 decision of the Ontario Court of Appeal in *Fleming v. Reid* held that the right to make treatment decisions is protected under section 7 of the *Charter*.[13] In so doing, *Fleming* struck down a law that allowed the Ontario Consent and Capacity Board to authorize physicians' best-interest–based treatment plans for involuntary psychiatric patients deemed incapable of making treatment decisions, without consideration of those patients' prior capable wishes. Leaving open the potential that provisions could be made to guide the ascertainment of prior capable wishes or their applicability to changed circumstances, the court held that mere disregard of such wishes was indefensible, stating: '[A]s a general proposition, psychiatric patients are entitled to make competent decisions and exercise their right to self-determination in accordance with their own standards and values and not necessarily in the manner others may believe to be in the patients' best interests.'[14]

Recently, the Supreme Court in *Starson* positioned the right to refuse treatment as 'fundamental' to dignity and autonomy.[15] This, too, was a decision arising out of the context of involuntary psychiatric hospitalization. The majority adopted from *Fleming* the notion that the prospect of involuntary treatment with antipsychotic medications suggests a heightened engagement of the autonomy interest, quoting the latter decision on this point: 'Few medical procedures can be more intrusive than the forcible injection of powerful mind-altering drugs which are often accompanied by severe and sometimes irreversible adverse side effects.'[16]

Starson *and Capacity*

Starson involved the interpretation and application of the test for capacity to make treatment decisions under Ontario's *Health Care Consent Act*.[17] Starson was involuntarily hospitalized following a finding that he was not criminally responsible on account of mental disorder on charges of uttering death threats. His diagnosis was schizoaffective disorder or, alternatively, bipolar disorder. The commentary of the courts and media centred upon Starson's unique intelligence, particularly his accomplishments in the field of theoretical physics despite his lack of formal training in the area. Upon his involuntary placement in hospital, Starson refused treatment with antipsychotic medications, whereupon his doctor declared him incapable of making this treatment decision.

The test under which the Ontario Consent and Capacity Board affirmed the declaration of incapacity was the following: 'A person is capable with respect to a treatment ... if the person is able to *understand* the information that is relevant to making a decision about the treatment ... and able to *appreciate* the reasonably foreseeable consequences of a decision or lack of decision'[18] (emphasis added). This test has two prongs: the ability to understand in the sense of comprehending the relevant information and the ability to appreciate that information in the sense of grasping its relevance to one's own circumstances (for example, weighing risks and benefits).[19]

Rather than go into the detailed factual and interpretative disputes that marked the Board's and courts' approaches in *Starson*, I will simply highlight the central elements of the Supreme Court's decision. First, the Court emphasized that mental disorder is not equivalent to incapacity to make treatment decisions, noting that vigilance is required to counter the discriminatory assumption that a diagnosis of mental illness justifies abrogation of all or any autonomy-based rights.[20] Second, the majority endorsed the idea that a patient need not agree with his or her diagnosis to be deemed capable,[21] grounding this tenet of capacity assessment in a conception of legitimate differences of opinion on either or both the facts and/or the values underpinning diagnoses. Justice Major stated: '[A] patient is not required to describe his mental condition as an "illness," or to otherwise characterize the condition in negative terms. Nor is a patient required to agree with the attending physician's opinion regarding the cause of that condition.'[22] However, these reasons continue, to be deemed capable of making a given treatment decision the person must be able to recognize that he or she 'is affected by [the condition's] manifestations.'[23]

The *Starson* majority's articulation of the principle that one's mental condition may be subject to radically different yet equally legitimate value-laden interpretations registers as a strong commitment to value pluralism.[24] That is, the majority acknowledges that persons may value their mental (or, one might add, physical) differences in ways that depart markedly from prevailing medical or social norms, and against this background advances the view that persons should not be forced to adhere to dominant conceptions of a valuable or good life. The emphasis on identifying and respecting persons' value-laden reasons for refusing medication is borne out in the majority's approach to Starson's testimony. Justice Major cited Starson's express resistance to the prospect of antipsychotic medications 'slowing down' his thoughts so that he would think like other people, quoting his statement that this 'would be worse than death for me, because I have always considered normal to be a term so boring it would be like death.'[25]

Ultimately, the majority of the court understood Starson to positively value his unusual thought processes despite their sometimes negative personal and social consequences. His experience of medication as leaving him slow of thought and slurred in speech – like 'a struggling-to-think "drunk"'[26] – was further cited by the Court in support of his decisively valuing his unmedicated over his medicated state.

Underlying the *Starson* decision are a set of highly charged questions about how, in the determination of capacity, beliefs and values properly grounding choice may be distinguished from factual and evaluative delusions and/or lack of insight into illness. Yet at the decision's core is the imperative of liberal legalism that the diverse experiences and potentially incommensurable values informing the choices that persons make be respected. Applied to the domain of capacity determination, this requires that space be made for appreciation of individuals' value-laden reasons for refusing (or choosing) treatment,[27] and where applicable, for refusing to acknowledge illness.[28]

Although the decision in *Starson* places respect for value pluralism at the centre of the analysis of decisional capacity, there is in addition an important source of empirical support for the proposition that many persons with serious mental illness, including those subject to involuntary hospitalization, are well equipped (or as well equipped as other persons) to make treatment decisions. The MacArthur Treatment Competence Study[29] drew upon multiple sources in U.S. law for criteria[30] with which to assess the 'treatment competence' of selected involuntary psychiatric patients (diagnosed with schizophrenia or major depression) as well as medical patients and other community members. The study found that, while the patients hospitalized with mental illness 'more often manifested deficits in [decision-making] performance,'[31] the majority of those hospitalized with major depression and almost half of those hospitalized with schizophrenia performed well on all the measures of capacity that were assessed.[32] This study ultimately suggests that '[m]ost patients hospitalized with serious mental illness have abilities similar to persons without mental illness for making treatment decisions.'[33] Thus, the researchers conclude that 'the justification for a blanket denial of the right to consent to or refuse treatment for persons hospitalized because of mental illness cannot be based on the assumption that they uniformly lack decision-making capacity.'[34]

Access

Numerous policy documents and consultation processes over the past few decades have sought to identify ways of meeting the medical, psychological, and social needs of persons with serious mental illness.[35] Among the barriers to well-being commonly invoked – and traced to deinstitutionalization policies in place since the 1960s – are poverty, homelessness or substandard housing, trans-institutionalization (for example, imprisonment), and recurring ('revolving-door') hospital admissions.[36] Yet systemic problems such as low rates of disability assistance[37] and disincentives to seeking part-time or contract employment[38] have typically been overshadowed by policy objectives targeting nonadherence to medication.

Policy Formation and Adherence to Treatment

The lack of community supports for individuals with serious mental illness and their families received new attention in 2002 with the release of the *Romanow Report*.[39] In a phrase much quoted by the media, that report positioned mental health care as the 'orphan child' of Canadian health policy.[40] Its two main critiques in this regard were the unavailability (or inconsistent availability across provinces) of home care services for the seriously mentally ill and (contained within a broader critique of the lack of universal prescription drug coverage) the lack of coverage outside hospital for the high cost of psychiatric drugs.[41]

On home care, the report recommended that funds be earmarked out of federal transfer payments to the provinces 'to support expansion of the *Canada Health Act* to include medically necessary home care services.'[42] Among the services to fall immediately under this rubric were '[h]ome mental health case management and [crisis] intervention services.'[43] Yet the Report's elaboration upon these services invites concern about its commitment to enabling and respecting capable treatment choices. That is, the importance of providing mental health home care quickly fuses with assumptions about the central mandate in mental health policy to ensure that persons take and continue to take their medications: 'Treating people effectively in the community rather than in institutions or hospitals requires home care, particularly in order to ensure that people with mental illnesses continue to take their medications appropriately and do not need repeated re-admissions.'[44] Here, ensuring medication compliance is cast as central to the overarching objective of promoting a cost-effective and less restrictive alternative to involuntary inpatient care. However, beyond questions about whether these objectives are indeed served through regimes focused on medication compliance, this vision of the mandate of mental health home care places the imperative of respect for capable treatment choice in jeopardy.

Similar concerns may be raised about the discourse employed in the *Romanow Report* on access to prescription drugs, specifically its proposed medication management program: 'If people refuse to take necessary drugs because of the costs, it affects not only the individuals involved but also their families, their communities, and the overall health of the population. It can also increase costs in the longer term.'[45] This observation is made in the context of the laudable project of enabling access to expensive medications, and further, it is not limited to persons with mental illness; nevertheless, it communicates the wider message that refusal (this word is chosen over the language of inability to access) of necessary drugs ('necessary' suggesting an absence of value-ladenness) is unacceptable because of the attendant 'costs.'

Another policy formation document of note in this regard is *A Report on Mental Illnesses in Canada*, released in 2002 under the joint sponsorship of Health Canada and the leading mental health advocacy, research, and professional organizations in the country.[46] Again, a strong association between community-based case management and ensuring compliance with medication is expressed. Case management is described as follows: 'Case management programs ... generally consist of multidisciplinary teams that share the clinical responsibility for each individual receiving care in the community. A team aims to help individuals with mental illness to achieve the highest level of functioning possible in the least restrictive setting. *To this end the team works to ensure compliance with treatment (particularly for those with schizophrenia and other psychotic illnesses)* and, consequently, improve functioning in order to reduce the need for hospital readmission' (emphasis added).[47]

There is no reference in the document to the issue of capacity or incapacity to make treatment decisions or explicit limitation of this approach to persons formally under community treatment orders or on leave during a period of involuntary committal. The emphasis in the above passage on ensuring medication adherence may be viewed in conjunction with this statement in the opening chapter: 'The active involvement of the individual in the choice of therapy and his/her adherence to the chosen therapy are critical to successful treatment.'[48] 'Involvement' and 'adherence' here stand in for the right to make autonomous choices based on full disclosure of information. Similarly, in discussing the role of the primary care provider in caring for persons with mood disorders, the report states: 'Educating family and primary care providers is essential not only to ensure the recognition of early warning signs of depression, mania and suicide and to implement appropriate treatment, but also to ensure adherence to treatment in order to minimize future relapses.'[49]

The Right-to-Treatment Lobby

Discussion of the erasure of treatment choice in recent mental health policy formation documents would not be complete without reference to the discourse of the 'right to treatment,' which has a peculiar history of deployment by certain elements in the mental health policy lobby in the attempt to vitiate express treatment refusals. This has particularly been the case in the United States, where the approach is rooted in case law recognizing a right on the part of involuntarily committed psychiatric patients to some form of appropriate treatment rather than simple incarceration.[50] This line of cases extends to decisions recognizing a right to a least restrictive form of treatment, including community-based treatment where available and deemed medically appropriate.[51] Yet U.S. lobby organizations such as the Treatment Advocacy Center (TAC) draw upon these principles by pitting the right to treatment against the 'right to be sick' or the 'right to rot,' with the objective of expanding the scope of committal criteria and restricting the right to refuse treatment.[52] The current approach of this lobby consists in great part in attempts to forge a strong connection between refusal of psychiatric treatment and decisional incapacity. This connection turns upon the concept of lack of insight, naturalized as 'the medical condition of anosognosia,' so giving little if any scope to the reasons or values that may underlie specific treatment refusals or denials of illness.[53]

In the Canadian context, the Schizophrenia Society of Canada (SSC) has adopted an orientation to treatment laws and policies that reflects the right-to-treatment approach. In its intervenor factum in the *Starson* case at the Supreme Court, the SSC stated its interest in the appeal as follows: 'The Society's mission is to alleviate the suffering caused by schizophrenia … [It] has a significant interest in the Court's interpretation and application of the law as it relates to involuntary detention and, particularly, to the availability and timeliness of appropriate treatment for serious mental illness. *The Society supports the right to freedom for psychiatric patients that only treatment can bring*' (emphasis added).[54] In a press release following the decision in *Starson*, the Society's president stated: 'We are disappointed by the Supreme Court of Canada's decision in the *Starson* case. It appears that in Ontario, it will continue to be difficult to provide involuntary patients with severe mental illnesses, including schizophrenia, with the treatment they need to alleviate their suffering on a timely basis and to facilitate their release from hospital.'[55]

Finally, the right-to-treatment discourse is evident in a recent major text on Canadian mental health law and policy by John Gray, Margaret Shone, and Peter Liddle.[56] These authors appeal to the right to treatment as trumping the right to refuse treatment in an extended response to the Ontario Court of Appeal's judgment in *Fleming*.[57] In challenging the *Fleming* Court's situating refusals of psychiatric treatment at the core of the autonomy interest, the authors revisit the *Charter* to argue that the fundamental interests it protects are best advanced by treatment aimed at liberating persons from psychiatric incarceration. Thus, they invoke section 7 in stating that 'deprivation of the security of a person which restores liberty, as is possible with non-consensual psychiatric treatment, is in accordance with the *Charter* as long as the treatment is carried out in accordance with the principles of fundamental justice';[58] section 2(b) with their position that involuntary treatment advances the interest in freedom of thought, as disordered thought processes are the antithesis of freedom 'in the sense of being rational, analytical and showing proper judgment';[59] section 12 in support of the argument that involuntary treatment frees persons from such cruel and unusual security practices as seclusion, restraints, and prolonged detention;[60] and section 15 in holding that the equality rights of persons involuntarily hospitalized in jurisdictions prohibiting involuntary treatment may be infringed through impeded access to the benefits of treatment.[61] Gray, Shone, and Liddle further argue that any infringement of *Charter* rights may be justified under section 1 in light of the clinical, institutional, and economic costs of respecting capable refusals in the context of involuntary hospitalization.[62]

These arguments, like the policy formation documents examined above, are rooted in a 'human needs' approach to mental health interventions,[63] reflecting a concern for the well-being of persons with serious mental illness, while at the same time attending to the interests of those who work and live in proximity to such persons. This approach may be regarded as advancing a fundamental conceptual shift in mental health law and policy, away from a focus on autonomy as negative liberty (emphasizing the right to refuse) and towards promoting a form of liberty situated within the community and defined with reference to shared values – a liberty more robust and meaningful to the individual even as it is offset by the interests of others. On my analysis, however, the form that this attempted shift takes in the arguments noted above is misguided. To prioritize (specifically for the population of psychiatric patients) the freedom to live in the community and to think rationally – freedoms which arguably amount to thinking and acting in accordance with community norms – over the interest in having one's capable treatment choices respected imports a best interests standard for this group that unduly compromises the core interests protected by section 7 and by section 15. At the very least, it is important to resist the tendency of such arguments to obscure the distinction between involuntary treatment (overriding capable wishes) and non-voluntary treatment (where capable wishes cannot be ascertained) – and the associated tendency to suggest that treating in the face of capable refusal may be justified with reference to the individual's interest in receiving treatment rather than, for example, the state's interest in treating.[64]

Laws and Policies: Enabling Treatment or Enabling (Capable) Choices?

My concern with the orientation towards treatment compliance and disregard for decisional capacity in the discourse of mental health policy formation extends to certain existent laws and policies. Three key areas in which the conflict between enabling treatment and enabling choice is engaged are laws on involuntary treatment of persons subject to involuntary psychiatric committal, community treatment orders (CTOs), and policies and practices of assertive community treatment (ACT).

Involuntary Committal and Treatment

Despite the reasoning in *Fleming*[65] and in the background to *Starson*[66] on the importance of the right to make treatment decisions in the context of involuntary psychiatric hospitalization, many provincial and territorial jurisdictions provide that persons subject to involuntary hospitalization may be treated involuntarily, without regard for their capacity to make treatment decisions. These may be divided into a first category of legislation that simply does not contemplate the relevance of capacity to make treatment decisions in circumstances of involuntary hospitalization (this is the case in British Columbia and in Newfoundland and Labrador),[67] and a second category which provides for assessment of capacity but invests a tribunal with the power to override capable refusals[68] expressed by involuntary patients (Alberta, the Yukon, and New Brunswick).[69] These aspects of provincial mental health law have not been put to the test of the *Charter* (sections 7 or 15). A Section 15 challenge, for instance, might press the implications of the differential treatment to which persons with psychiatric disorders are subject in this context, in disregard of individual capacities.[70]

The Saskatchewan model deserves separate discussion. That province's *Mental Health Services Act* premises involuntary psychiatric committal in part on a finding of incapacity (or the person's inability 'to fully understand and to make an informed decision regarding his need for treatment or care and supervision').[71] Following committal, treatment is a matter of physician discretion.[72] It may be argued that this accords with respect for at least contemporaneous capable choices (but not prior capable wishes), as individuals who are capable of making treatment choices are apparently not committed in the first place.[73] However, two key concerns may be raised.

First, the requirement of 'full' understanding of one's 'need' for treatment (*or* care and supervision) strongly suggests a 'best-interests' standard is incorporated into the test for decisional capacity in the specified areas.[74] A second and related concern is that in the circumstances of psychiatric assessment with a view to committal there may be great pressure placed on this determination of capacity.[75] That is, objectives such as stabilizing the patient or containing a potentially explosive familial or social situation may motivate doctors, on protective or beneficent grounds, to commit – and so to make the requisite finding of incapacity. Given the lack of precise scientific measures for determining decisional capacity and the unspecific nature of the type of decision contemplated by the provision in question, the Saskatchewan regime is unlikely to give significant protection to the right to make treatment decisions.

Community Treatment Orders

Saskatchewan adopted a regime of community treatment orders under its *Mental Health Services Act* in 1995;[76] Ontario introduced a similar regime under its *Mental Health Act* in 2000.[77] In both provinces, CTOs are doctors' orders that a person adhere to a program of treatment, supervision, or care in the community for a (renewable) period of time.[78] These regimes are directed at persons with a history of psychiatric hospitalization who meet at least the committal criterion of a likelihood of substantial mental or physical deterioration if not treated and who are deemed appropriate candidates for community rather than hospital-based treatment.[79] In Ontario, consent to the order must be given by the person or his or her substitute.[80] In both provinces, if the person does not comply with the treatment plan, she or he can be taken by force to the issuing physician for examination to determine whether to order a psychiatric assessment in hospital with a view to a longer period of involuntary committal.[81]

I will not here rehearse the arguments for and against community treatment orders.[82] My point is that this type of regime reproduces and exacerbates the tensions in mental health policy between ensuring compliance and enabling choice. As such I would question the claim that CTOs constitute a least restrictive form of treatment of those who meet committal criteria. For, in the first place, introduction of the CTO option risks encouraging doctors to exercise their discretion in favour of finding that committal criteria are met. Second, and more broadly, the danger of CTOs is that coercive relationships oriented towards treatment enforcement may be further entrenched in the community, thereby displacing the project of enabling self-determination through the fostering of relationships of trust and practices of reflection within a context of meaningful social and therapeutic options.[83]

Assertive Community Treatment Teams

Assertive community treatment (ACT) is a leading model of community care and supervision of individuals with serious mental illness. Developed in Wisconsin in the 1970s, the model was more recently introduced into Canada; most of Ontario's sixty-one ACT teams were established with that government's major commitment to the model in 1998–9.[84] ACT is characterized by multidisciplinary support teams (for example, psychiatrists, occupational therapists, nurses, social workers, and sometimes peer support workers) dedicated to reducing symptoms and maintaining the community residence of persons with serious mental illness. Teams are available to clients twenty-four hours a day, and they make regular ('assertive') attempts to seek them out at home or elsewhere.[85]

The incidence and quality of consent in ACT interventions demands more study. Some commentators have noted the potential for this 'hospital without walls' model to introduce or exacerbate coercive practices,[86] a concern informed in part by the lack of the sort of procedural protections that are afforded in the hospital setting. Some research, however, including preliminary results of a recent study sponsored by the Canadian Mental Health Association,[87] suggests a significant level of client satisfaction with ACT teams.[88] Ongoing empirical work specifically attentive to the experiences of persons subject to ACT interventions may serve as an important indicator of whether ACT can move beyond the pervasive focus on enforcing medication compliance to more flexible modes of supporting self-determination: for example, helping persons access housing and other community supports while encouraging considered treatment choices and remaining respectful of capable refusals.[89]

Conclusions: Building Capacity in and beyond Law

The discussion above identifies significant tensions between contemporary mental health laws and policies oriented towards the treatment of serious mental illness, on the one hand, and the liberal legal commitment to individual autonomy and to respecting diverse conceptions of value, on the other. Resistance to viewing decisional capacity through the lens of value pluralism may be linked not only to a human-needs orientation that posits need and not choice as the ground of legal and social obligations towards persons diagnosed with serious mental illness (the orphan children of the health care system's 'orphan child'), but also to strong public apprehensions associating serious mental illness with dangerousness. Such apprehensions have inspired quick political solutions (on the model of community treatment orders) promising increased public security through medication enforcement. I have suggested that classifying all persons deemed seriously mentally ill as lacking the capacity to make treatment decisions is deeply problematic. Here I would add that apart from the flawed empirical basis for the further perception of dangerousness,[90] such matters of public security (real or imagined) must be kept separate from the determination of persons' capacity to decide about proposed treatments. If involuntary treatment is to be justified on the basis of public security, let this argument stand or fall on its own rather than drawing upon the false assumption that serious mental illness, or for that matter involuntary hospitalization, necessarily implies the inability to make treatment decisions.

So we return to the pressing question of how capacity to make treatment decisions is (justly) to be gauged among persons deemed to have serious mental illness. There is not space here to explore the diverse legal and clinical models of capacity assessment in place in different jurisdictions,[91] and the attentiveness or non-attentiveness of these models to the mixed cognitive, emotional, and social dimensions of decision-making practices. The empirical work of Appelbaum and Grisso referred to above[92] (along with continuing critical appraisals of that work more oriented to the normative issues underlying definitions of capacity) is just one example of ongoing research in psychiatry and law that addresses the challenges of capacity assessment. Mental health policy, too, must address these challenges. This means, beyond becoming apprised of the current debates on the cognitive and emotional bases of decision,[93] also giving close attention to the effects of poverty, of accessibility of therapeutic and social-vocational options, and of coercive institutional contexts in conditioning persons' presentation as decisionally capable or incapable. Finally, in accordance with the core commitment of a liberal constitutional order to value pluralism, mental health policy must attend to the adequacy of practices of capacity determination to identifying and respecting the values of those assessed[94] – most notably by drawing upon the experiences and perspectives of persons who have undergone assessment.

Legal and policy reform might begin with internal governmental review of and/or *Charter* challenges to involuntary treatment regimes applicable to persons subject to involuntary psychiatric committal and such suspect elements of law as Saskatchewan's elevated standard of capacity under its *Mental Health Services Act*.[95] In addition, efforts to bring capacity assessment into accord with the imperatives of value pluralism might include articulation of prohibited inferences in provincial health care consent legislation: for example, rules against inferring incapacity solely from non-compliance with treatment, or denial of illness (at least not without investigating the subject's awareness of concrete symptoms), or denial of potential adverse consequences of refusal (at least not without investigating the nature and circumstances of disclosure and the basis for denial). More positively, increased efforts should be made to educate physicians on engaging with patients in reflective discussions about diagnoses and possible treatments. Educational efforts may further include fostering processes of self-education and peer or advocate support of considered treatment decisions.[96] Finally, to increase the diversity of perspectives applied in the assessment of capacity, policy-makers might provide that administrative panels adjudicating the issue include persons with a history of psychiatric diagnosis or hospitalization and/or members of the mental health bar. All this presumes a background commitment to enabling and justly assessing decisional capacity through provision of human and other resources directed to this end.

I want to suggest, however, that such changes are unlikely without significant transformation in the prevailing assumptions conditioning what is and is not entertained in the formation of policy on the treatment of serious mental illness. Arguably, policy deliberations in this area have a tendency to descend into a form of stylized debate, pitting a thin conception of autonomy as negative liberty against a strong, value-laden paternalism. While the one side risks ignoring the social or relational foundations of self-determination and, in the tradition of libertarian antipsychiatry[97] may reject incremental reforms as masking the fundamental nature of psychiatry as a tool of social conformism, the other side threatens to entrench dominant conceptions of normalcy or 'the good life' within the very concept of what it is to be autonomous or decisionally capable. Each of these approaches culminates in imputations of false consciousness onto an entire class of persons: those who accept treatment are the dupes of psychiatric power; those who refuse treatment are the victims of failed insight. The standoff I describe was evident in the public reception of *Starson*, which consisted less in deliberation on the implications of value pluralism for capacity assessment than careening attempts to portray the case either as a romantic story of misunderstood genius or a story of misplaced romanticism, behind which the 'true' story of the dangerousness and inherent incapacity of the seriously mentally ill lurked.[98]

Given this environment, the prospects for significant transformation in mental health policy and practice may seem dim. Yet beyond the polarized positions I have described are forms of cultural production and critique that attend both to the hard-won nature of self-determination on the part of individuals diagnosed with serious mental illness and the systemic reforms necessary for it.[99] Most notable is a growing literature aimed at exploring the nature and conditions of self-determination from the perspectives of persons diagnosed with mental illness who are intimately familiar with the coercive as well as enabling aspects of the mental health system.[100] Here I would cite the popular works of Canadian journalists Pat Capponi[101] and Scott Simmie,[102] who combine autobiography and intimate accounts of others' experiences with critical analyses of the institutional settings that have shaped their stories. Both acknowledge the benefits that many persons derive from psychiatric medications, but regard such benefits as contingent upon each person's unique experience and values.[103] Thus, they place central emphasis on pursuing and attaining such knowledge of oneself and of proposed and alternative treatments (including the alternative of no treatment) as may enable one to make informed choices.[104] At the same time, they draw attention to the social and institutional reforms necessary to support self-determination among those caught in self-perpetuating cycles of poverty and mental distress.[105]

Such efforts do not in themselves resolve the continuing complexities of capacity assessment, for instance, the need to negotiate competing domains of knowledge in distinguishing unconventional values from evaluative delusions or from an inability to appreciate salient facts. However, these interventions in the cultural arena open new spaces for articulating or rendering visible the diverse ways that persons' experiences and values may inform their choices about psychiatric treatment. As such, these accounts disrupt the abstract standoff between autonomy and beneficence that can render mental health policy debates an exercise in mutual incomprehension.

In closing, I return to the theme of access to health care that has inspired this collection of essays. In much health policy the objective of enabling access may be assumed to advance both the values of beneficence and autonomy; what is more, access to treatments deemed medically necessary is increasingly regarded as a right of citizenship. Yet we are reminded in this brief survey of contemporary laws and policies on the treatment of serious mental illness that not all treatment is experienced as a benefit and that the discourse of access may at least in this context mask a deeper orientation towards ensuring compliance as opposed to enabling choice. My critique of laws and policies on the treatment of serious mental illness is by no means an argument 'against access.' It is, rather, a warning that in the drive towards access we disregard the imperative of respect for choice at our peril – or at least, at the peril of those of us classified under the historically despised and feared title of serious mental illness. Unmasking the discourse of access to reveal its troubling illiberal premises in this setting is not enough, however. The work ahead consists in carefully revisiting the theory and practice of assessing capacity to make treatment decisions, with an eye to determining whether the prevailing means of discerning such capacity in persons deemed seriously mentally ill may be more a matter of enforcing conformity with dominant values and assuaging public fears than of protecting the autonomy-based interests of those under scrutiny.

NOTES

Thanks to David Dyzenhaus, Colleen Flood, and Vaughan Black for helpful comments, and the Social Sciences and Humanities Research Council for a fellowship in support of my ongoing research on capacity to make treatment decisions.

1 See, e.g., Ontario Ministry of Health Long-Term Care, *Making It Happen* (Implementation Plan for Mental Health Reform) (Toronto: Ministry of Health and Long-Term Care, 1999) at 13–14. 'The priority population for mental health reform is people with serious mental illness,' defined with reference to 'disability, anticipated duration and/or current duration, and diagnoses.'
2 See, e.g., Health Systems Research Unit, Clarke Institute of Psychiatry, *Review of Best Practices in Mental Health Reform* (Ottawa: Minister of Government Works and Public Services Canada, 1998) [*Review of Best Practices*], Section I.
3 See, e.g., the Canadian Mental Health Association (CMHA), *Access to Mental Health Services: Issues, Barriers, and Recommendations for Federal Action* (submission to the Standing Senate Committee on Social Affairs,

Science and Technology) (Toronto: CMHA, 2003), http://www.cmha.ca/ english/research/index.html (accessed 6 March 2004) at 1, 3–5, 13 [*Access to Mental Health Services*].

4 Canada, Commission on the Future of Health Care in Canada, *Building on Values: The Future of Health Care in Canada – Final Report'* (Saskatoon: Commission on the Future of Heath Care in Canada, 2002) (Chair: Roy Romanow) at 178–9 [*Romanow Report*]; S. Goodwin, *Comparative Mental Health Policy: From Institutional to Community Care* (London, Sage, 1997); Andrew T. Scull, *Decarceration: Community Treatment and the Deviant – A Radical View* (Cambridge: Polity, 1984).

5 For a critical assessment of recent efforts to engage persons diagnosed with mental illness in mental health policy formation, see Barbara Everett, *A Fragile Revolution: Consumers and Psychiatric Survivors Confront the Power of the Mental Health System* (Waterloo: Wilfred Laurier University Press, 2000). For a wide-ranging critique of the curtailment of citizenship rights among persons with disabilities, see Dianne Pothier and Richard Devlin, 'Introduction: Toward a Critical Theory of Disitizenship,' in Dianne Pothier and Richard Devlin, eds., *Critical Disability Theory: Essays in Philosophy, Politics, Policy and Law* (Vancouver: UBC Press, 2005).

6 [2003] 1 S.C.R. 722 [*Starson*].

7 See *supra* note 1.

8 See, e.g,. *Health Care Consent Act, 1996*, S.O. 1996, c. 2, Sch. A [*Health Care Consent Act*]; *Hospitals Act*, R.S.N.S. 1989, c. 208; *Health Care (Consent) and Care Facility (Admission) Act*, S.B.C. 1993, c. 48; *Health Act*, S.Y.T. 1989–90, c. 36; Art. 11 C.C.Q.; *Health Care Directives Act*, S.M. 1992, c. 33.

9 *Reibl v. Hughes*, [1980] 2 S.C.R. 880; *Ciarlariello v. Schacter*, [1993] 2 S.C.R. 119.

10 *Canadian Charter of Rights and Freedoms*, Part I of the *Constitution Act, 1982*, being Schedule B to the *Canada Act 1982* (U.K.), 1982, c.11 [*Charter*]. See *R. v. Morgentaler*, [1988] 1 S.C.R. 30 (s. 7 encompasses the right to make decisions concerning one's own body) [*Morgentaler*]; *Fleming v. Reid* (1991), 4 O.R. (3d) 74 (C.A.) (s. 7 encompasses the right to refuse treatment) [*Fleming*].

11 (1990), 72 O.R. (2d) 417.

12 *Ibid.* at 424.

13 *Charter, supra* note 10.

14 *Fleming, supra* note 10 at 94.

15 *Starson, supra* note 6 at 759.

16 *Fleming, supra* note 10 at 88; *Starson, supra* note 6 at 759.

17 *Health Care Consent Act, supra* note 8, s. 4(1).

18 *Ibid.*

19 *Starson, supra* note 6 at 760–1.

20 *Ibid.* at 760.

21 *Ibid.* at 762, citing David N. Weisstub, *Enquiry on Mental Competency: Final Report* (Toronto: Queen's Printer for Ontario, 1990) at 229, 250n443.

22 *Ibid.*

23 *Ibid.*

24 Value pluralism is the thesis, developed, e.g., in the work of Isaiah Berlin and explored more recently by liberal pluralists such as William Galston, that human values are multiple and irreducible to a single overarching value. The thesis also tends to posit conflict among as well as the incommensurability of (at least some) values, and so their non-amenability to ranking according to a common metric. Value pluralism on some conceptions is taken to ground arguments for state tolerance of or even positive support for a multiplicity of valuable ways of life or conceptions of the good. See, e.g., William Galston, *Liberal Pluralism: The Implications of Value Pluralism for Political Theory and Practice* (Cambridge: Cambridge University Press, 2002).

25 *Starson, supra* note 6 at 770.

26 *Ibid.* at 771.

27 The great majority of assessments of capacity to make treatment decisions occur where medication is refused. See Bruce Winick, *The Right to Refuse Mental Health Treatment* (Washington, DC: American Psychological Association, 1997) at 350–4.

28 The majority also directed that adjudicators of capacity inquire into the reasons behind a failure to appreciate the consequences of a decision, suggesting that a failure to inform meaningfully may sometimes be the root problem. *Starson, supra* note 6 at 762–3.

29 Paul Appelbaum and Thomas Grisso, 'The MacArthur Treatment Competence Study I' (1995) 19:2 Law and Human Behavior 105 ['Competence study I']; Thomas Grisso *et al.*, 'The MacArthur Treatment Competence Study II' (1995) 19:2 Law and Human Behavior 126; Thomas Grisso and Paul Appelbaum, 'The MacArthur Treatment Competence Study III' (1995) 19:2 Law and Human Behavior 149 ['Competence Study III'].

30 See 'Competence Study I', *ibid.* at 108–11. These criteria were the ability to 'communicate a choice,' 'understand relevant information,' 'appreciate the nature of the situation and its consequences,' and 'manipulate information rationally.' Standardized measures were then used to assess 498 participants from three sites.

31 'Competence Study III,' *supra* note 29 at 169.
32 'Nearly one half of the schizophrenia group and 76% of the depression group performed in the "adequate" range (according to ad hoc definitions of adequacy used in this study) across all decision-making measures, and a significant portion performed at or above the mean for persons without mental illness' (*ibid.* at 171).
33 This statement is taken from 'The MacArthur Treatment Competence Study: Executive Summary' (Feb. 2001), http://www.macarthur .virginia.edu/treatment.html (accessed 26 July 2003).
34 'Competence Study III,' *supra* note 29 at 171.
35 Ontario's numerous initiatives are briefly surveyed in the Ontario Ministry of Health and Long-Term Care, *The Time Is Now: Themes and Recommendations for Mental Health Reform in Ontario* (Report of the Mental Health Implementation Task Force Chairs) (Ontario: Ministry of Health and Long-Term Care, 2002) [*The Time Is Now*] at 22–4.
36 See *Access to Mental Health Services, supra* note 3 at 13; the *Romanow Report, supra* note 4 at 178; Barbara Everett *et al., Recovery Rediscovered: Implications for Mental Health Policy in Canada* (CMHA, 2003), http://www.cmha.ca/ english/research/index.html (accessed 7 March 2004) at 14–18 [*Recovery Rediscovered*].
37 See John Fraser, Cynthia Wilkey, and Joanne Frenschkowksi, *Denial by Design: The Ontario Disability Support Program* (Report on the Ontario Disability Support Legislation) (Toronto: Income Security Advocacy Centre, 2003).
38 *Access to Mental Health Services, supra* note 3 at 14; *The Time Is Now, supra* note 35 at 52.
39 *Romanow Report, supra* note 4.
40 *Ibid.* at xxxi and 178.
41 *Ibid.,* chaps. 8 and 9.
42 *Ibid.* at 176.
43 *Ibid.*
44 *Ibid.* at 179.
45 *Ibid.* at 207.
46 Health Canada, *A Report on Mental Illness in Canada* (Ottawa: Health Canada, 2002).
47 *Ibid.* at 26.
48 *Ibid.* at 24.
49 *Ibid.* at 39. The failure to address the issue of treatment choice in the current mental health policy climate is further evidenced in Donald Wasylenki et al., 'Tertiary Mental Health Services: I. Key Concepts' (2000)

45 Can. J. Psychiatry 179. This article describes primary and secondary care services for treating serious mental illness as 'characterized by accountability, a heavy reliance on case management, appropriate housing, and *medication compliance*' (at 179, emphasis added). The paper describes, in addition, a more aggressive form of tertiary care.

50 *E.g.*, *Rouse v. Cameron*, 373 F.2d 451 (D.C. Cir. 1966); *O'Connor v. Donaldson*, 422 U.S. 563 (1975); *Youngberg v. Romeo*, 457 U.S. 307 (1982).

51 See A.B. Klapper, 'Finding a Right in State Constitutions for Community Treatment of the Mentally Ill' (1993) 142 U. of Penn. L.R. 739.

52 See the Treatment Advocacy Center (TAC) website, http://www.psychlaws .org, e.g., E.F. Torrey and M. Zdanowicz, 'A Right to Mental Illness?' editorial, *New York Post*, 28 May 1999, http://www.psychlaws.org/ GeneralResources/article14.htm (accessed 7 March 2004).

53 See Xavier Amador, *I Am Not Sick: I Don't Need Help! Helping the Seriously Mentally Ill Accept Treatment* (New York: Vida, 2000); and TAC, *Impaired Awareness of Illness (Anosognosia): A Major Problem for Individuals with Schizophrenia and Bipolar Disorder* (Briefing Paper), http://www.psychlaws .org/BriefingPapers/BP14.htm (accessed 7 March 2004).

54 *Starson, supra* note 6 in: Factum of the Intervener Schizophrenia Society of Canada, at 1.

55 'Schizophrenia Society Disappointed with Supreme Court Decision' *Schizophrenia Society of Canada News Release* (6 June 2003), http://www .schizophrenia.ca/releases/starsonrelease.pdf (accessed 7 March 2004).

56 *Canadian Mental Health Law and Policy* (Markham, ON: Butterworths, 2000) [*Canadian Mental Health Law and Policy*].

57 *Ibid.* at 193–212.

58 *Ibid.* at 197.

59 *Ibid.* at 197–8.

60 *Ibid.* at 198–200.

61 *Ibid.* at 200.

62 *Ibid.* at 200–12.

63 *Ibid.* at 10–12; John E. Gray and Richard O'Reilly, 'Clinically Significant Differences among Canadian Mental Health Acts' (May 2001) 46 Can. J. Psychiatry 315.

64 At a later point in their analysis (*Canadian Mental Health Law and Policy, supra* note 56 at 360), the authors propose a model statute that would sanction involuntary committal only where incapacity to make treatment decisions is established. As I note below in connection with the regime in Saskatchewan, while this may appear to demonstrate respect for capable treatment decisions, the high threshold of capacity suggested in the

provision (which demands that persons 'fully understand' and 'fully appreciate the consequences of making an informed decision regarding the person's need for admission to a psychiatric facility and for treatment') renders the move suspect.

65 *Fleming, supra* note 10.

66 *Starson, supra* note 6.

67 Under B.C.'s *Mental Health Act*, R.S.B.C. 1996, c. 288, ss. 8(a) and 31(1), treatment of involuntary patients may be authorized by the director of the institution; under the Newfoundland and Labrador *Mental Health Act*, R.S.N. 1990, c. M-9, s. 6(3), the administrator or medical director may 'detain and treat' patients under a confirmed certificate of admission. In neither province do the criteria for committal require a finding of incapacity to make treatment decisions.

68 For reasons of space, I leave aside the important issue of how the regimes in question structure the identification and import of prior capable wishes.

69 See the Alberta *Mental Health Act*, R.S.A. 2000, c. M-13, s. 29; Yukon *Mental Health Act*, S.Y.T. 1989–90, c. 28, ss. 21(2)(c) and 23(2)(a); and New Brunswick *Mental Health Act*, R.S.N.B. 1973, c. M-10 s. 8.11(3).

70 *Law v. Canada (Minister of Employment and Immigration*, [1999] 1 S.C.R. 497 at paras. 53 and 69. There is not space here to explore the particulars of how such a challenge might be constructed.

71 *Mental Health Services Act*, S.S. 1984–85–86, c. M-13.1, s. 24(2)(a)(ii).

72 *Ibid.*, s. 25(1).

73 Note that the *Mental Health Services Act* does not explicitly provide the power to involuntarily treat persons involuntarily hospitalized under Part XX.1 of the *Criminal Code*, R.S.C. 1985, c. C-46.

74 This is particularly notable from an equality perspective when compared with the definition of capacity to make treatment decisions in Saskatchewan's *Health Care Directives and Substitute Decision Makers Act*, S.S. 1997, C. H-0.001, s. 2(1)(b), as the ability '"(i) to understand information relevant to a health care decision respecting a proposed treatment; (ii) to appreciate the reasonably foreseeable consequences of making or not making a health care decision respecting a proposed treatment; and (iii) to communicate a health care decision on a proposed treatment."'

The authority of advance health care directives is curtailed under this statute where persons are subject to involuntary hospitalization or a community treatment order under the *Mental Health Services Act*; such persons' directives relating to treatment of a mental disorder are 'to be used for guidance as to the wishes of the person making the directive' only (s. 5(4)(a)).

75 This concern applies also to the alternative committal standard introduced in Ontario in 2000 which, along with the relaxed criterion of a likelihood of 'substantial mental or physical deterioration,' requires that the person has been found incapable of consenting 'to his or her treatment in a psychiatric facility' and that substitute consent has been obtained (*Mental Health Act*, R.S.O. 1990, c. M.7, s. 20 (1.1)).

76 *Supra* note 75, ss. 24.2–24.7.

77 *Supra* note 79, ss. 33.1–33.8.

78 In Saskatchewan, up to three months (*Mental Health Services Act*, s. 24.5); in Ontario, six months (*Mental Health Act*, s. 33.1 (11) and (12)). Note that CTOs do not apply to persons detained in psychiatric hospitals following a finding of unfitness to stand trial or not criminally responsible on account of mental disorder, who come under the authority of the provincial review boards established under the *Criminal Code*, R.S. 1985, c. C-46, s. 672.38. On the relationship between CTOs and provisions for leave from hospital during a period of civil committal, see Archie Kaiser, 'Mental Disability Law,' in Jocelyn Downie, Timothy Caulfield, and Colleen Flood (eds.), *Canadian Health Law and Policy*, 2nd ed. (Toronto: Butterworths, 2002) 251 [*Mental Disability Law*] at 304–5.

79 The CTO criteria are set out in the Saskatchewan Act at s. 24.3(1)(a) and in the Ontario Act at s. 33.1(4). In Saskatchewan, the committal criterion requiring that the person be unable 'to fully understand and to make an informed decision regarding his or her need for treatment or care and supervision' is restated as a criterion for imposing a CTO (s. 24.3(1)(a)(v)).

80 Ontario *Mental Health Act*, s. 33.1(4)(f).

81 Ibid., s. 33.3; Saskatchewan *Mental Health Services Act*, s. 24.6.

82 In the Canadian context, arguments against are posed by Kaiser in *Mental Disability Law, supra* note 78 at 303–6; arguments for are posed by Richard O'Reilly et al., 'Mandatory Outpatient Treatment' *Canadian Psychiatric Association Press Release* (Jan. 2003), http://www.cpaapc.org/Publications / Position_Papers/mandatory.asp (accessed 8 March 2004). A nuanced discussion of the empirical research on CTOs that emphasizes the normative issues driving these debates is found in John Dawson *et al.*, 'Ambivalence about Community Treatment Orders' (2003) 26 Int'l J. Law and Psychiatry 243. Similarly, see Virginia Hiday, 'Outpatient Commitment: The State of Empirical Research on its Outcomes' (2003) 9 Psychol. Pub. Pol. and L. 8 ['Outpatient Commitment'].

83 Kaiser makes this point, *supra* note 78 at 303, 305. A further concern about the Saskatchewan model is that it extends into the community the problems noted above on the high (arguably discriminatory) threshold inscribed in that Act's definition of capacity.

84 See Ontario Ministry of Health and Long-Term Care, *Recommended Standards for Assertive Community Treatment Teams* (Toronto: Ministry of Health and Long-Term Care, 1998); Forensic Mental Health Services Expert Advisory Panel for the Ontario Ministry of Health and Long-Term Care, *Assessment, Treatment, and Community Integration of the Mentally Disordered Offender* (Ontario: Ministry of Health and Long-Term Care, 2002) at 60 [*The Mentally Disordered Offender*].

85 *Review of Best Practices in Mental Health Reform, supra* note 2, Section I, Chapter 1.

86 Ontario opponents of coercive psychiatry protested the introduction of ACT teams in that province, deeming them 'mental health police' with a mandate to enforce treatment. See, e.g., the statement of G. Bacque in the archives of the Homeless People's Network (5 June 1998), http://aspin .asu.edu/hpn/ archives/Jun98/0041.html (accessed 11 March 2003). Also see Joanna Watts and Stefan Priebe, 'A Phenomenological Account of Users' Experience of Assertive Community Treatment' (2002) 16 Bioethics 439.

87 Cristina Redko et al., 'Participant Perspectives on Satisfaction with Assertive Community Treatment' (Winter 2004) 27 Psychiatric Rehabilitation Journal 283. While this research reveals considerable satisfaction with some aspects of the ACT program, interviewees expressed particular dissatisfaction about not 'having enough say' in ACT interventions.

88 A summary of research on ACT to 1997 is found in *Review of Best Practices in Mental Health Reform, supra* note 2, Section I, Chapter 1.

89 See the recommendations on 'assertive case outreach management' in *The Mentally Disordered Offender, supra* note 84 at 61, emphasizing respect for clients' medication choices and promoting a model of psychosocial rehabilitation.

90 Research indicates that the prevalence of violence among persons with mental illness who do not engage in substance abuse is no higher than among other community members. See Henry Steadman *et al.*, 'Violence by People Discharged from Acute Psychiatric Inpatient Facilities and by Others in the Same Neighbourhoods' (1998) 55 Arch. of Gen. Psychiatry 393; Health Canada, *Mental Illness and Violence: Proof or Stereotype?* (Study of Mental Illness and Dangerousness) by J. Arboleda-Flórez *et al.* (Ottawa: Health Canada, 1996); 'Outpatient Commitment,' *supra* note 82 at 32n4.

91 See, e.g., Kathleen C. Glass, 'Revising Definitions and Devising Instruments: Two Decades of Assessing Mental Competence' (1997) 20 Int'l J. Law and Psychiatry 5 ['Revising Definitions']; J.W. Berg *et al.*, 'Constructing Competence: Formulating Standards of Legal Competence to Make Treatment Decisions' (1996) 48 Rutgers L.R. 345.

92 *Supra* note 29.

93 See, e.g., Louis C. Charland, 'Appreciation and Emotion: Theoretical Reflections on the MacArthur Treatment Competence Study' (1999) 8 Kennedy Inst. of Ethics J. 359; Paul Appelbaum, 'Ought We to Require Emotional Capacity as Part of Decisional Competence?' (1998) 8 Kennedy Inst. of Ethics J. 377.

94 An emphasis on value pluralism is found in a number of commentators on decisional capacity. See, e.g., Benjamin Freedman, 'Competence, Marginal and Otherwise: Concepts and Ethics' (1981) 4 Int'l J. Law and Psychiatry 53; Robert Pepper-Smith and William Harvey, 'Competency and Practical Judgment' 17 Theor. Med. 135; 'Revising Definitions,' *supra* note 91; Barbara Secker, 'Labelling Patient (In)Competence: A Feminist Analysis of Medico-Legal Discourse' (1999) 30 J. of Soc. Philosophy 295.

95 *Supra* note 71. The more complicated question of subjecting Ontario's and/or Saskatchewan's community treatment order regimes to *Charter* challenge is beyond the scope of this chapter.

96 See 'Revising Definitions,' *supra* note 91 at 30–2.

97 I refer to the libertarian antipsychiatry exemplified in the work of Thomas Szasz, *The Myth of Mental Illness* (New York: Hoeber-Harper, 1961)). However, as a complex social movement opposing coercive psychiatric practices, antipsychiatry cannot be confined to the libertarian model.

98 For instance, sentimental reference to the popular film *A Beautiful Mind* is made in Kirk Makin, 'Brilliant Man in an Asylum Fights Doctors to Top Court,' *Globe and Mail*, 5 May 2003, A3, and Juliet O'Neill, 'The Patient Who Won't Take His Medicine,' *Ottawa Citizen*, 6 June 2003, A1–A2. Sceptical responses to the Supreme Court's decision included Kirk Makin, 'High Court Supports Mentally-Ill Physicist,' *Globe and Mail*, 7 June 2003, A7, and Margaret Wente, 'The Case of the Crazy Professor,' *Globe and Mail*, 10 June 2003, A17.

99 Exceptions to my depiction of the policy formation climate include the report *The Time Is Now, supra* note 35, in which 'recovery' is 'defined by the individual, not by service providers' (at 21), and the recent CMFA report 'Recovery Rediscovered,' *supra* note 37.

100 For background, see Judith Cook and Jessica Jonkins, 'Self-Determination among Mental Health Consumers/Survivors: Using Lessons from the Past to Guide the Future' (2002) 13 J. Disability Policy Studies 87. See also the diverse approaches to self-determination in the papers collected for the National Leadership Summit on Self-Determination and Consumer-Direction and Control, Bethesda, MD, 21–3 Oct. 1999 http://cdrc.ohsu .edu/selfdetermination/leadership/alliance/papers.html (accessed

8 March 2004). Also see the historical research of Geoffrey Reaume, which illuminates diverse forms of agency experienced by persons committed to psychiatric hospital in the nineteenth and twentieth centuries. Geoffrey Reaume, *Remembrance of Patients Past: Patient Life at the Toronto Hospital for the Insane, 1870–1940* (Oxford: Oxford University Press, 2000).

101 Pat Capponi, *Upstairs at the Crazy House: The Life of a Psychiatric Survivor* (Toronto: Viking, 1992); Pat Capponi, *Beyond the Crazy House: Changing the Future of Madness* (Toronto: Penguin, 2003) [*Beyond the Crazy House*].

102 Scott Simmie and Julia Nunes, *The Last Taboo: A Survival Guide to Mental Health Care in Canada* (Toronto: McClelland and Stewart, 2001) [*The Last Taboo*]; Scott Simmie and Julia Nunes, *Beyond Crazy: Journeys Through Mental Illness* (Toronto: McClelland and Stewart, 2002).

103 *Beyond the Crazy House, supra* note 101 at 111–12; *The Last Taboo, supra* note 102 at 214–39.

104 *Beyond the Crazy House, ibid.,* at 151–7; *The Last Taboo, ibid.* at 36, 229. Also see J. Chamberlin, 'Confessions of a Noncompliant Patient' (1998) 36 J. Psychosocial Nursing 49 at 50.

105 *Beyond the Crazy House, ibid.,* at 172, 224–8.

PART FOUR

Rationing Access: The Role of the
Physician Gatekeeper

11 The Legal Regulation of Referral Incentives: Physician Kickbacks and Physician Self-Referral

SUJIT CHOUDHRY, NITEESH K. CHOUDHRY,
AND ADALSTEINN D. BROWN

Introduction: Referral Incentives and the Law

The regulation of private health care has become a central issue in Canadian health policy. The specific issue that has attracted the most attention is whether physicians and patients may opt out of the single payer system for physician services and set up a parallel private system. Although the prohibition of opting out is not a condition for federal-provincial transfer payments under the *Canada Health Act*,[1] a recent paper notes that all provinces have enacted prohibitions and disincentives to curtail opting out by physicians and patients.[2] In addition, the Supreme Court of Canada has recently found unconstitutional under the *Canadian Charter of Rights and Freedoms*[3] the prohibition on private health insurance in circumstances under which individuals cannot access care within a reasonable time frame within the public system.[4]

By contrast, there has been relatively little discussion of the regulation of independent health facilities (IHFs), even though they are, for the most part, privately owned, for-profit entities, and are assuming increasing prominence in the landscape of health care institutions. IHFs provide a range of diagnostic and therapeutic services, such as physiotherapy and laboratory testing. IHFs provide services on a fee-for-service basis to individuals, who may pay out of pocket or may have coverage from private health insurance companies or provincial health insurance plans. Because of the multiple sources of payment, IHFs, unlike many other health care providers, operate simultaneously within the public and private health care systems. There may be as many as 1,000 IHFs in Ontario alone.[5]

As with other health care facilities, IHFs depend on physician referrals for patients. Because IHFs bill on a fee-for-service basis, physician referrals ultimately determine revenues and profitability. This raises two important issues for public policy. First, as experience in the United States has shown, institutional providers such as hospitals and IHFs have often compensated physicians for patient referrals. If physicians are compensated for making referrals, they may be placed in a financial conflict of interest, because referral incentives may overwhelm their clinical judgment. This may threaten cost-containment efforts and quality of care, as patients may receive unnecessary testing and treatment or as patients are referred to a provider who is not necessarily selected on the basis of the quality of care that he or she provide. Moreover, inducing a larger volume of referrals to particular providers may compromise access for those patients who actually need it, particularly in areas with limited physician and other resource availability. Second, experience in the United States has also shown that similar incentives can exist when physicians refer to IHFs in which they have an investment interest, giving rise to similar problems. Indeed, both kickbacks and self-referral were regarded as serious enough to prompt federal regulatory intervention in the United States.[6] Despite the worrisome American evidence and the spread of IHFs in Canada, kickbacks and self-referral were not mentioned either by the report of the Senate Standing Committee on Social Affairs, Science and Technology (*Kirby Report*)[7] or by the final report of the Royal Commission on the Future of Health Care in Canada (*Romanow Report*).[8] Moreover, the topic has generated limited scholarly commentary in Canada.[9]

The potential for both kickbacks and self-referral to give rise to financial conflicts of interest raises the question of what the existing regulatory framework is, if any. To be sure, financial conflicts of interest that involve physicians are regulated by the common law.[10] But in this chapter, we review provincial laws and regulations to determine whether they adequately protect patients against conflicts of interest arising from referral incentives. These rules take the form of rules of professional conduct for physicians. Our conclusion is mixed; in some respects these rules adequately protect patients, but in others they do not.

This lack of adequate regulation of referral incentives is of concern as provincial governments increasingly look to IHFs as a means to achieve greater efficiencies in delivering publicly insured health care services and to create the incentives for greater private capital investment in the health care infrastructure. Moreover, physician investment in IHFs is likely to grow as well. Physician investment may be motivated by a mixture of objectives, such as enhancing access to care, increasing physician income by circumventing billing caps and other limits on physician revenues, and providing better control over quality. The growth of alternate payment mechanisms that cover the range of currently insured services may also encourage physicians to seek other revenue streams. In short, IHFs are likely to become a more important part of the landscape of health care institutions, underlining the need for adequate regulation. Following our review of existing regulation, in this chapter we propose regulatory models to be implemented before the further proliferation of IHFs. Indeed, given that conflict of interest guidelines are currently under review in Ontario,[11] this is an opportune time to explore the issue across Canada.

Defining Kickbacks and Self-Referral

An IHF and a referring physician may have two kinds of financial relationships. The first is a *kickback*, whereby a physician receives financial compensation for referring patients to a particular IHF for health-related services. In many markets, client referrals are compensated since they are of economic value to the party receiving the referral. Accordingly, we should not be surprised to see similar forms of compensation emerge in markets for health care, as has happened for many years in the United States.

Compensation can flow from IHFs to referring physicians or from specialists to primary care physicians, where the payment of kickbacks is often referred to as *fee-splitting*. Moreover, compensation can take many forms. In some cases, it may consist of a simple cash payment for each patient referred, or a percentage of the billings resulting from the referred patient. Complicated arrangements may consist of more favourable terms for office space, leases for medical equipment, or business loans, if the referring physician is a tenant or landlord, an equipment lessee or lessor, or a borrower or lender.

In many markets, compensation for referrals is unobjectionable. However, in health care this is ethically problematic because it creates a potential conflict of interest between physicians' financial self-interest and their duty to advise patients solely on the basis the patients' health needs. That is, the best interests of patients, not the financial interests of physicians, should guide decisions to refer. If the opposite is true, physicians may make unnecessary referrals, which could mean that patients will be subjected to medically unnecessary care. Moreover, even if a referral is necessary, a kickback could lead physicians to direct referrals to particular providers for reasons other than the quality or accessibility of care. Finally, the incentives to increase referral volume and to direct referral stream to particular providers may create inefficiencies, increase waiting times, decrease access, and potentially increase costs.

Similar considerations of cost and quality arise in cases of *self-referral*, where the IHFs to which physicians refer their patients are partly or completely owned by those physicians, or in which referring physicians hold some other kind of investment interest. Physicians benefit from self-referral not by receiving kickbacks, but through the revenues generated by the IHF. Self-referral has generated more controversy in the medical community than have kickbacks.[12] Some physicians have argued that physician-owned IHFs are merely extensions of physician practices, even if they are situated in a different location and even if the referring physicians do not personally provide services at those facilities themselves. For this reason, self-referral is fundamentally different from referral to other providers. Defenders of self-referral have also argued that ownership by referring physicians does not represent a financial conflict of interest because it is a warrant of quality. Indeed, because of their expertise, physicians are more likely to apprehend the need for new IHFs and to design innovative ways for delivering high quality care. In addition, physician-owners, because of their ethical obligation to promote patient well-being, would be less profit-oriented than non-physician owners; this would provide a guarantee of the quality of care that patients receive. These physicians might even be able to provide better continuity of care by referring to their own facilities. Therefore, far from jeopardizing the quality of care, some would argue that self-referrals further patient well-being and that restricting self-referrals hurts patients.[13]

The Relevance of the American Experience for Canada

In deciding how to address these concerns, Canadian regulators have much to learn from the experience of the United States. American lawmakers have taken it to be self-evident that kickbacks negatively affect quality and costs by altering physician behaviour. By contrast, probably driven by the ethical controversy over self-referral, a large body of empirical literature has attempted to assess the effects on quality and cost, if any, of physician self-referral to IHFs.

Taken as a whole, this research suggests that self-referral increases referral volume and health care costs. Mitchell and Scott[14] studied the effects of physician ownership of physical therapy and rehabilitation facilities in Florida. They found that patients who received care in facilities jointly owned by physicians (joint-venture clinics) had 40 per cent more visits per year on average than patients treated in non–joint-venture centres. In addition, gross and net revenues per patient were 30 to 40 per cent higher in joint-venture facilities and their percentage mark-up (that is, net profit before taxes expressed as a percentage of total operating expenses) was almost two times higher (44.8 per cent versus 23 per cent). Similar results were found by Hillman et al., who compared the use of radiological tests (including chest x-ray, spine x-ray, and ultrasound) by physicians who had imaging equipment in their offices (self-referring physicians) with physicians who always referred their patients to radiologists for testing (radiologist-referring physicians). They found that self-referring physicians were 4 to 4.5 times more likely to obtain radiological investigations than radiologist-referring physicians, and they charged significantly more for tests of the same complexity.[15]

The impact of self-referrals on health care quality is less clear. Overall, although the evidence is limited, it would appear that facilities jointly owned by physicians provide care that is, at best, of equivalent quality to that provided by other facilities. Mitchell and Scott's study found that joint-venture physiotherapy facilities employ proportionately fewer licensed therapists, and these licensed individuals spend about 60 per cent less time per patient per visit treating patients than do licensed therapists in non–joint-venture facilities.[16] Similarly, a study of radiation therapy clinics demonstrated that radiation therapists, who are the principal personnel involved in quality control for patients undergoing radiation therapy other than physicians, spent 18 per cent less time per patient in joint-venture clinics.[17] While these results suggest that the use of unlicensed physiotherapists or less frequent use of radiation therapists is a marker of poor quality in joint-venture facilities, empirically it is unclear whether these factors have any appreciable consequences for more concrete patient outcomes such as satisfaction, morbidity, or mortality. In contrast, it is possible that the joint-venture physiotherapy clinics that schedule frequent patient visits, or the physicians with diagnostic equipment in their own offices who order tests more readily, may be doing so appropriately and therefore may be benefiting patients. This seems unlikely; nevertheless, there is an absence of evidence to support or refute these assertions.

These findings raise interesting questions for Richard Saver's position (chapter 12, this volume) in which he advocates physician gainsharing. Saver argues that financial incentives analogous to those created by kickbacks and self-referral relationships may allow for the achievement of efficiencies in health care delivery that may not jeopardize quality and that may, in fact, enhance it. In support, he cites the experience of the Medicare Participating Heart Bypass Center Demonstration Project in the United States. The data on self-referral demonstrate, however, that physician investment interests are likely to increase costs. The question for Saver is whether it is possible to design a regulatory regime that avoids or minimizes these difficulties while harnessing their potential benefits.

The substantial differences in the financing and organization of the American and Canadian health care systems counsel caution in drawing lessons from the United States, both with respect to observed behaviours of providers and of patients. However, the need for caution should not prevent Canadian regulators from identifying particular aspects of the American health care system that seem to map onto existing or emerging features of the Canadian health care system. In the United States, referrals to IHFs generated a set of financial arrangements (kickbacks and self-referrals) prompted a set of provider behaviours that have been regarded as inappropriate. As similar structural features emerge in the Canadian health care system, we should be concerned that they may create similar behaviours in Canada. Given the potential for kickbacks and self-referral to generate inappropriate physician behaviour in Canada, it is important to assess the adequacy of the current regulatory framework.

Legal Rules on Kickbacks and Self-Referral

General

In Canada, kickbacks[18] and self-referrals[19] are regulated by the rules of professional misconduct. These rules are generally found in by-laws and regulations promulgated pursuant to provincial laws governing the practice of medicine. Some of these rules have been enacted by provincial governments; in other cases, they have been generated by provincial medical licensing authorities themselves. In one province (British Columbia), the rule regarding self-referral is located in a statute. It is worth noting that provincial laws governing the structure and financing of health insurance programs do not regulate referral incentives. By comparison, in the United States, kickbacks and self-referral are located in portions of the *United States Code* governing Medicare Medicaid, and other federal health insurance programs.[20]

The regulation of kickbacks and self-referral through rules governing professional misconduct has two important consequences. First, the responsibility for enforcing these rules falls to provincial medical licensing authorities and, therefore, provincial ministries of health are not involved in enforcement. That fact that provincial medical licensing authorities have traditionally been the line departments for enforcement may reflect how kickbacks and self-referral in Canada have historically been conceptualized as raising concerns regarding the quality of care and professional ethics as opposed to health system design and financing. By contrast, in the United States, both the Department of Health and Human Services and the Department of Justice are vested with primary responsibility for the enforcement of federal laws on kickbacks and self-referral, clearly reflecting concerns over cost. Therefore, in Canada, lack of regulation of kickbacks and self-referral by provincial ministries of health may be a case where the legal and institutional framework for regulation has not kept pace with the unintended evolution of the health care system (for example, the proliferation of IHFs) or its intended evolution (for example, an integrated health system that try to align incentives across providers).

The role of provincial medical licensing authorities as the bodies responsible for enforcement of the rules around kickbacks and self-referrals may also reflect an historical situation where there were relatively few incentives for physicians to engage in self-referral and relatively few pressures or incentives for the development of IHFs. Consequently, the licensing authorities have relatively little experience in detecting and determining conflicts of interest in relationship to kickbacks and self-referrals. This lack of experience raises questions about the capacity of provincial licensing authorities to effectively investigate and police these situations. Further, as the number of IHFs grows and the potential opportunities for conflicts of interest also grow, provincial licensing authorities may have insufficient resources to police these conflicts of interest. Finally, provincial medical licensing authorities may encounter practical difficulties in regulating referrals across provincial and international borders. For example, physicians could refer patients to IHFs in another province in which they have a financial interest.

A second and related point is that the sanctions that can be imposed by provincial medical licensing authorities are severe but limited in scope. For example, if it finds that a physician has committed an act of professional misconduct, the College of Physicians and Surgeons of Ontario (CPSO) may reprimand the physician; revoke or suspend the physician's licence to practice; or attach terms, conditions, and limitations to the physician's certificate of registration. The CPSO has a limited power to impose fines (up to $35,000). By contrast, in the United States, violation of the anti-kickback provisions of the federal Social Security Act is a criminal offence, punishable by a fine of up to $25,000 and/or imprisonment of up to five years.[21] Physicians who violate the federal Stark Laws (which prohibit physician self-referral for Medicare and Medicaid patients) may be denied payment for insured services and may be required to refund payments already made.[22] Moreover, physicians who violate the anti-kickback statute and the Stark Laws may face heavy fines for each individual violation (for example, each self-referral that contravenes the Stark Laws) or exclusion from federal health care programs.[23] The CPSO lacks these powers.

Kickbacks

Table 11.1 summarizes the rules of physician professional misconduct governing kickbacks. Eight provinces (Alberta, British Columbia, Manitoba, New Brunswick, Newfoundland, Ontario, Quebec, and Saskatchewan) explicitly regulate kickbacks. The remaining two provinces (Nova Scotia and Prince Edward Island) do not explicitly prohibit kickbacks, although it is legally possible that the general prohibition on professional misconduct in those provinces could be interpreted to prohibit kickbacks. Furthermore, although the College of Physicians and Surgeons Nova Scotia has issued non-binding guidelines, these do not have legal force.

Anti-kickback provisions vary somewhat in the scope of the conduct they regulate. All eight provinces that regulate kickbacks regulate the *receipt* of compensation by physicians for referrals. Seven of these provinces categorically prohibit receiving any kickback. For example, Ontario prohibits 'receiving fees from any person to whom a member has referred a patient or requesting or accepting a rebate or commission for the referral of a patient.'[24]

The Alberta provision is similar, but in addition to prohibiting the receipt of kickbacks, it also prohibits the solicitation of kickbacks: 'A registered practitioner shall not *seek* or accept any payment or benefit,

Table 11.1 Rules of Professional Misconduct and Physician Kickbacks

	Kickback Arrangement				What Is Regulated				How Kickbacks Are Regulated		Exceptions
	Physician as Payor of Kickback	Physician as Recipient of Kickback	Any Person as Payor of Kickback	Drug/Device Supplier as Payor of Kickback	Referrals to Physicians	Referrals to IHFs	Referrals to Pharmaceutical Suppliers	Referrals to Medical Device Suppliers	Disclosure	Prohibition	Market Value Rentals & No Volume Incentive[a]
Alberta	X	X	X		X	X	X	X		X	
British Columbia		X		X			X	X		X	
Manitoba[b]		X	X	X	X	X	X	X		X	X
New Brunswick	X	X	X		X	X	X	X		X	
Newfoundland		X		X	X	X	X	X		X	X
Nova Scotia[c]											
Ontario	X	X	X	X	X	X	X	X		X	X
Prince Edward Island											
Quebec[d]	X	X	X		X	X	X	X	X	X	
Saskatchewan	X	X	X	X	X	X	X	X		X	X

Sources: CPSA By-laws, ss. 48 and 51.1; B.C. *Medical Practitioners Act*; CPSM By-Law 1, CPSM 'General Ethical Statement 124'; Regulation 9, Nfld. *Medical Board Regulations (MBR)*; Nfld. s. 35; *MBR*, ss. 16 and 17; *Ontario Professional Misconduct Regulation*, s. 11; *Ontario General Regulation: Medicine Act*, ss. 15 and 16; and Quebec *Code of Ethics of Physicians*, ss. 73 and 79. (Full references in note 18 of the text.)
[a] These exceptions allow for rental agreements at market value between physicians and parties (i.e., physicians, IHFs, pharmacies, medical device suppliers) to whom those physicians may make referrals.
[b] Manitoba, Ontario, and Saskatchewan each have two provisions governing kickbacks. One provision prohibits kickbacks in general language whereas the second provision is also a wide-ranging provision, but has more specific rules. See text for more discussion.
[c] Nova Scotia has issued guidelines that are not legally binding and are therefore not included in this table.
[d] Quebec has two provisions governing kickbacks. One prohibits the receipt of kickbacks, but only if the kickback 'would jeopardize ... [the] professional independence' of a physician (no further definition of the amount or nature of such a kickback is provided). The other provision permits the physician to receive royalties for prescribing 'products having a benefit to health,' if those royalties are disclosed to patients. See text for more discussion.

directly or indirectly, for any service rendered to a patient by any other practitioner or person.'[25]

Quebec's provision, by contrast, only prohibits physicians from receiving 'any commission, rebate or material benefit that would jeopardize … [the] professional independence' of a physician.[26] Unfortunately, the Quebec provision does not provide any guidance on what kickbacks would impair a physician's professional independence.

Rules in only five provinces (Alberta, New Brunswick, Ontario, Quebec, and Saskatchewan) expressly prohibit physicians from *paying* kickbacks for referrals to other individuals, including other physicians. For example, the Saskatchewan provision makes '[s]haring fees with any person who has referred a patient'[27] professional misconduct. By implication, in the remaining five provinces (British Columbia, Manitoba, Newfoundland, Nova Scotia, and Prince Edward Island), it is not professional misconduct for physicians to compensate persons for referrals or to offer compensation for referrals. The caveat here is that referring physicians would be prohibited from receiving such fees in three of these five provinces (British Columbia, and Manitoba, Newfoundland), providing for some kind of regulation.

Provincial rules vary with respect to the detail in which they specify the entity that pays the kickback to the physician for a patient referral. The rules of six provinces (Alberta, Manitoba, New Brunswick, Ontario, Quebec, and Saskatchewan) do not specify the entity that pays kickbacks. For example, the Manitoba provision states that physicians must 'not enter any agreement where a reward, direct or indirect, is associated with the volume of your work, your referrals, your orders, or your fees.'[28]

These rules are broad enough to cover not only kickbacks paid by physicians, but also kickbacks paid by other health professionals who receive patient referrals from physicians such as physiotherapists. Moreover, they are broad enough to capture payments made by corporations, such as IHFs and pharmaceutical companies, as well as by individuals associated with those corporations (for example, directors, shareholders, and marketing representatives). Note, though, that these rules do not and cannot prohibit the making of such payments by non-physicians, because they are found in rules of physician professional misconduct. The rules of four provinces (British Columbia, Ontario, Newfoundland, and Saskatchewan) specifically refer to the payments of kickbacks by suppliers of pharmaceuticals and suppliers of medical goods and services, both of which benefit from referral streams. British Columbia's provision, for example, states: 'A member of the college must not take or receive remuneration by way of commission, discount, refund or otherwise from a person who fills a prescription issued by the member or who makes or supplies appliances.'[29]

Since British Columbia does not have a provision identifying other persons as potential payors of kickbacks, it appears not to constitute professional misconduct in that province for physicians both to pay and to receive kickbacks for patient referrals (that is, to participate in fee-splitting). It also appears not to constitute professional misconduct for physicians to receive kickbacks from IHFs that do not supply appliances.

Four provinces (Manitoba, Newfoundland, Ontario, and Saskatchewan) have enacted identically worded exceptions to the prohibition on kickbacks, which allow for rental agreements between physicians and parties (for example, other physicians, IHFs, pharmacies, suppliers of medical devices) to whom those physicians may make patient referrals. The danger of rental arrangements is that they may be structured to disguise kickbacks, for example, by setting leases at below-market rates (where referring physicians are tenants) or above-market rates (where referring physicians are landlords), or by tying rental rates to the volume of patient referrals. Accordingly, in these four provinces, rental arrangements are permissible only if rent is set at market rates and contains no volume incentive for referrals.

Finally, Quebec permits physicians to receive royalties for prescribing 'products having a benefit to health,' if those royalties are disclosed to patients.[30] This provision is broad enough to cover pharmaceuticals and medical devices and could contradict Quebec's more general provision on kickbacks. Furthermore, it does not indicate on its face how it interacts with the general provision.

Physician Self-Referral

Table 11.2 summarizes rules of physician professional misconduct on self-referral. Seven provinces (Alberta, British Columbia, Manitoba, New Brunswick, Ontario, Quebec, and Saskatchewan) regulate self-referral to IHFs. Self-referral to health facilities is not expressly regulated in the remaining three provinces (Newfoundland, Nova Scotia, and Prince Edward Island), meaning that self-referral by physicians to facilities in which they or their family members have an investment interest does not constitute professional misconduct. However, there is considerably more variation in the regulation of self-referral than in the regulation of kickbacks.

The paradigmatic case of self-referral by physicians entails referrals

Table 11.2 Rules of Professional Misconduct and Physician Self-Referral

	Who Has Investment Interest			How Self-Referral Is Regulated				Exceptions		
	Physicians	Immediate Family[a]	Extended Family	Disclosure	Prohibition	Restrictions on Investment Interest[b]	Other	Otherwise Not Available/Community Need[c]	Medically Necessary[d]	Publicly Traded Corporation Not Closely Held
Alberta[e]	X				X	X		X	X	
British Columbia	X	X	X		X			X		
Manitoba[f]	X	X[g]		X		X	X			
New Brunswick	X				X					
Newfoundland										
Nova Scotia										
Ontario	X	X	X	X						X[h]
Prince Edward Island										
Quebec	X			X						
Saskatchewan	X	X	X		X				X	

Sources: SCPS By-laws, ss. 51(1)(f)(i) and 51(2)(n); CPSM By-laws, ss. 47 and 49; B.C. *Medical and Health Care Services Regulation,* ss. 38-40; B.C. *Medicare Protection Act,* s. 35(1); CPSM By-Law 1, s. 55; CPSM 'General Ethical Statement 124'; Regulation 9, Nfld. s. 36; *Ontario General Regulation: Medicine Act; Quebec Code of Ethics of Physicians,* s. 77; and SCPS By-laws, s. 51(1)(f)(v) (diagnostic facilities). (Full references in notes 18 and 19 of the text.)

[a] Defined as a spouse, child, or parent.

[b] The terms of investment cannot include a requirement that referrals be made or any volume incentive for referrals. Manitoba additionally requires that the investment be offered at fair market value, presumably to preclude the masking of volume incentives.

[c] These exceptions require prior approval by a regulatory authority in order to apply.

[d] Self-referral is permitted if it is medically necessary.

[e] Alberta has two provisions. One prohibits self-referral except in cases of 'demonstrable objective medical benefit.' The other prohibits self-referral to IHFs except in cases of community need or where the practitioner provides care directly.

[f] Manitoba has two provisions. One requires physicians to 'avoid inappropriate personal benefit' in self-referral, which may prohibit certain kinds of self-referrals. The other requires disclosure of a financial interest.

[g] Refers to 'indirect ownership' interests, which probably encompass familial investment interests (at least by an immediate family member).

[h] Ontario does not require disclosure if the physician does not have a controlling interest.

by physicians to facilities in which they hold a personal investment interest. Not surprisingly, all seven provinces that regulate self-referral to health facilities regulate physicians' investment interests. Since it would be easy to circumvent such rules by putting an investment interest in the name of a family member, three provinces (British Columbia, Ontario, and Saskatchewan) also regulate referrals to health facilities in which family have an ownership interest. In table 11.2, we define 'immediate family' as including a spouse, child, or parent and 'extended family' as including other family members.

These three provinces include both immediate and extended family within the scope of rules on self-referral. The definition of family in Saskatchewan's provision is representative: 'member of the physician's family' means anyone connected with her or him by blood relationship, marriage, or adoption. Here (1) connected by blood relationship means that one is the child or other descendent of the other or one the brother or sister of the other; (2) connected by marriage means that one is married to the other or to a person who is connected by blood relationship to the other; and (3) connected by adoption means that one has been adopted, either legally or in fact, as the child of the other or as the child or a person who is connected by blood relationship (otherwise than as a brother or sister) to the other.[31]

In addition, one of Manitoba's rules refers to 'indirect ownership' interests, which we interpret to encompass the investment interests of immediate family members. The remaining six provinces – the three with no regulations on self-referral at all (Newfoundland, Nova Scotia, and Prince Edward Island) and the three that limit the regulation of self-referrals to IHFs in which physicians are investors (Alberta, New Brunswick, and Quebec) – do not expressly prohibit physicians from referring patients to facilities owned by their family members.

Provinces regulate self-referral differently. Four provinces (Alberta, British Columbia, New Brunswick, and Saskatchewan) outright prohibit physician self-referral. This is the regulatory model in the United States under federal law.[32] By contrast, the remaining three provinces that regulate self-referral (Manitoba, Ontario, and Quebec) simply require that referring physicians disclose investment interests to patients. Quebec's provision is an illustrative example:[33] 'A physician must inform the patient of the fact that he has interests in the enterprise providing the diagnostic or therapeutic services he prescribes for him.'

Some provinces that regulate self-referral provide for exceptions. Alberta and British Columbia, which both presumptively prohibit self-referral, have a community need exception – that is, they permit self-referral in cases where an IHF that does not raise conflict of interest concerns is unavailable. This exception may be important in rural areas. Both provinces require prior approval by a regulatory authority for the community need exception to apply – in British Columbia this is the Medical Services Commission and in Alberta it is the Council of the College of Physicians and Surgeons of Alberta. Paradoxically, Alberta has another provision that permits self-referral in cases of 'demonstrable objective medical benefit,' which is difficult to reconcile with the strictly prohibitive nature of Alberta's other provision on self-referral.[34] Saskatchewan also permits self-referral in cases of medical necessity as an exception to the general rule of prohibition.[35] Ontario, which permits self-referral with disclosure, does not require disclosure in cases where the physician and family members do not have a controlling interest in the IHF: '[T]he facility is owned by a corporation the shares of which are publicly traded through a stock exchange and the corporation is not wholly, substantially or actually owned or controlled by the member, a member of his or her family or a combination of them.'[36]

Finally, Alberta and Manitoba regulate the terms of physicians' investment interests in IHFs, regardless of whether a physician engages in self-referral or not. Both provinces prohibit physician investment in IHFs from including a requirement that patient referrals be made to the IHF or volume incentives for patient referrals. Manitoba additionally requires that the investment be offered at fair market value, presumably to preclude the masking of volume incentives. By implication, Ontario and Quebec, which allow self-referral with disclosure to patients, permit such terms to be included in the terms of investment, as do the three provinces (Newfoundland, Nova Scotia, and Prince Edward Island) where self-referral is not regulated.

Discussion and Policy Recommendations

Although some provinces have rules of professional misconduct governing kickbacks and self-referrals, these rules are often inadequate. As we argue below, there are several areas in which provincial rules could be improved. In particular, we suggest that self-referrals should be more tightly regulated, although they may be unavoidable in limited circumstances. Given that conflict-of-interest guidelines are currently under review in Ontario, such proposals are timely. More generally, we recommend that provinces without legally binding rules enact such provisions, as opposed to relying on non-binding guidelines issued by provincial medical licensing authorities.

Lead Enforcement Institution

The approach in the United States to regulating kickbacks and self-referrals has been much more aggressive than that in Canada. In part, this aggressive approach may be a response to the presence of greater incentives for potential conflicts of interest in the United States, which in turn may be a result of the more entrepreneurial and market-driven approach to organizing and financing health care in that jurisdiction. However, contrasting the divergent regulatory approaches in the United States and in Canada identifies several weaknesses in the ability to police conflicts of interest in Canada under current arrangements. For example, provincial medical licensing authorities have limitations as the lead enforcement agency for referral incentives, including their limited experience and resources to deal with a potentially growing problem; their lack of power to administer strong disincentives such as exclusion from provincial health insurance programs; and their dependence on patient complaints to enforce rules of professional misconduct, which is problematic because kickbacks and self-referral are largely invisible to patients. In addition, issues of health care financing and system design fall outside the mandate of provincial medical licensing authorities, which more narrowly focus on professional misconduct. For these reasons, we suggest that the lead regulatory institution should be shifted from medical licensing authorities to provincial ministries of health.

Such a shift in responsibilities should strengthen the hand of provincial governments to combat kickbacks and self-referral. However, provincial medical licensing authorities should be involved in enforcement, because despite the limitations of self-regulation, patient complaints are a potentially useful source of information on kickbacks and self-referrals, and because provincial medical licensing authorities can revoke, suspend, or otherwise attach conditions to the licences of physicians. Thus, under our proposed arrangements, provincial licensing authorities would refer potential cases of kickbacks and self-referral to the ministries of health for investigation, and provincial ministries of health would refer cases where individuals have been found to be engaged in these practices for professional misconduct proceedings. Finally, it should be noted that shifting responsibility to provincial ministries of health does not eliminate the potential problems associated with cross-border instances of conflict of interest. Resolution of these problems will require interprovincial cooperation.

Kickbacks: Recommendations

Although eight provinces prohibit physicians from receiving kickbacks, only five prohibit physicians from paying or offering to pay kickbacks. But as a matter of professional misconduct, the payment of kickbacks represents as much of a conflict of interest as does the receipt of kickbacks, because these payments seek to induce referrals regardless of patient health status. Moreover, the growing role of non-physician health professionals (for example, physiotherapists) who may refer patients to physicians strengthens the case for prohibiting the payment of kickbacks by physicians. We recommend that all provinces prohibit physicians from paying or receiving kickbacks, not only to physicians, but to any other person. We also recommend that all provinces designate offering to pay kickbacks as professional misconduct.

Self-Referral to Independent Health Facilities: Recommendations

Three provinces do not expressly regulate self-referral to IHFs at all. Furthermore, six provinces permit self-referrals by physicians to IHFs owned by members of their immediate family. Given the cost and quality concerns raised by self-referral, and the ease of circumventing restrictions on self-referral through placing investments in the names of immediate family, provincial rules should be amended as necessary, both to regulate self-referral and to include referral to IHFs in which immediate and extended family members are investors within the ambit of regulation.

Three provinces that regulate self-referral to IHFs merely require referring physicians to disclose their investment interest to patients. In our view, disclosure may effectively police financial conflict-of-interest in cases where disclosure is made to someone with the requisite expertise to make an independent judgment. For example, disclosure works well in the context of medical research, where the audience consists of other physicians. But disclosure in clinical contexts to relatively inexpert patients does not work very well, particularly when those patients require treatment. Patients may also misinterpret disclosure, not as a warning to take care, but rather as a warranty of an IHF's quality.[37]

Finally, patients may not wish to refuse the referral in order not to strain the physician-patient relationship.

We recommend that self-referral be prohibited. However, there should be a community-need exception, as is currently in force in Alberta and British Columbia, in situations where self-referral is unavoidable. Prior approval by a regulatory authority is a necessary safeguard for ensuring that this exception is not abused, perhaps through techniques similar to those employed to define underserviced areas. A ban on self-referral would still permit physician investment in IHFs. Finally, a ban on self-referral, even with a community-need exception, would require reconsideration if governments encourage physicians to integrate financially with IHFs or hospitals (for example, through risk-adjusted capitation). The goal of financial integration is to align provider incentives and encourage providers to offer care as cost-effectively as possible. However, financial integration between physicians and IHFs would make self-referral difficult to avoid. In the United States, as a result of the tension between restrictions on self-referral and the financial integration of providers, a number of important exceptions have been created to the federal ban on self-referral.[38] Provincial governments would need to create similar exceptions in Canada.

If self-referral is permitted, the terms of physician investment must not create the incentive to either make referrals or to inflate the volume of referrals. Only two provinces impose such restrictions. When added to the four provinces where self-referral by physicians is prohibited, this means that at present these investment terms do not attract professional sanction in four provinces, where they should.

Conclusion

Physicians play a key role in Canada as gatekeepers to the health care system. Although some exceptions exist, patients are generally unable, without a doctor's prescription or referral, to access specialists, hospitals, x-rays, other diagnostic tests, and drugs. Patients, in general, rely on physicians not only to identify their health needs but also on what services they require to meet that need. Thus, the role of physicians in setting the boundaries of publicly funded Medicare – who gets what services and when – is critical. Unregulated kickbacks and self-referrals can potentially result in physicians sending patients for more tests and treatments than required by the standard of care.

Although provinces have enacted rules of professional misconduct on kickbacks and physician self-referral, the current regulatory framework is inadequate. As independent health facilities proliferate further, provincial governments should review current rules to 'get in front' of the important regulatory challenges that IHFs pose to cost and quality of patient care. As a number of policy advocates suggest changes to the way that health care is financed, it will be important to keep in mind how these changes affect the providers of care and their ability to organize themselves to oversee provision. A recent report, for example, recommends that governments move from annual, global budgets for hospitals to service-based funding, in part to stimulate the creation of 'specialized, stand-alone facilities.'[39] It will be critical to consider the consequences of such reform in smaller communities where there may be few physicians capable of integrating with other providers of care and, thus, avoiding self-referrals in such situations may be especially difficult.

NOTES

This is a revised and expanded version of Choudhry et al., 'Unregulated Private Markets for Health Care in Canada? Rules of Professional Misconduct, Physician Kickbacks and Physician Self-Referral' (2004) 170 Can. Med. Assoc. J. 115.

1 R.S.C. 1985, c. C-6.
2 Colleen M. Flood and Tom Archibald, 'The Illegality of Private Health Care in Canada' (2001) 164 Can. Med. Assoc. J. 825.
3 Part I of the *Constitution Act, 1982*, being Schedule B to the *Canada Act 1982* (U.K.), 1982, c. 11.
4 *Chaoulli v. Québec* (Attorney General), [2005] S.C.C. 35. See also Patrick J. Monahan and Stanley H. Hartt, 'The Charter and Health Care: Guaranteeing Timely Access to Health Care for Canadians,' C.D. Howe Institute Commentary 164 (May 2002), http://www.cdhowe.org (accessed 27 March 2004) and Colleen M. Flood, Kent Roach, and Lorne Sossin, eds., *Access to Care, Access to Justice: The Legal Debate on Private Health Insurance* (Toronto: University of Toronto Press, 2005).
5 Joan N. Gilmour, 'Regulation of Free-Standing Health Facilities: An Entrée for Privatization and For-Profit in Health Care' (2003) 11 Health L. J. 131.
6 *Social Security Act*, 42 U.S.C. s. 1320a-7b (1998); *Ethics in Patient Referral Act*, 42 U.S.C. s. 1395 (1998).

7 Canada, *The Health of Canadians – The Federal Role: Current Trends and Future Challenges*, vol. 2 (Ottawa: Standing Senate Committee on Social Affairs, Science and Technology, 2002) [*Kirby Report*].

8 Canada, *Building on Values: The Future of Health Care in Canada* (Saskatoon: Commission on the Future of Health Care in Canada, 2002) (Chair: Roy Romanow) [*Romanow Report*].

9 Moe Litman, 'Fiduciary Law and For-Profit and Non-For-Profit Health Care,' in Timothy A. Caulfield, ed., *Health Care Reform and the Law in Canada* (Edmonton: University of Alberta Press, 2002) 85.

10 Moe Litman, 'Self-referral and Kickbacks: Fiduciary Law and the Regulation of "Trafficking in Patients"' (2004) 170 Can. Med. Assoc. J. 1119.

11 College of Physicians and Surgeons of Ontario (CPSO) Policies, http://www.cpso.on.ca/Policies/policy.htm (accessed 25 November 2005).

12 Elizabeth H. Morreim, 'Conflicts of Interest: Profits and Problems in Physician Referrals' (1989) 262 J. Am. Med. Assoc. 390.

13 Council on Ethical and Judicial Affairs, American Medical Association (AMA), 'Conflicts of Interest: Physician Ownership of Medical Facilities' (1992) 267 JAMA 2366.

14 Jean M. Mitchell and Elton Scott, 'Physician Ownership of Physical Therapy Services: Effects on Charges, Utilization, Profits, and Service Characteristics' (1992) 268 J. Am. Med. Assoc. 2055.

15 Bruce J. Hillman *et al.*, 'Frequency and Costs of Diagnostic Imaging in Office Practice: A Comparison of Self-Referring and Radiologist-Referring Physicians' (1990) 323 New Eng. J. Med. 1604; Bruce J. Hillman *et al.*, 'Physicians' Utilization and Charges for Outpatient Diagnostic Imaging in a Medicare Population' (1992) 268) 2050.

16 Mitchell and Scott, *supra* note 14.

17 Jean M. Mitchell and Jonathan H. Sunshine, 'Consequences of Physicians Ownership of Health Care Facilities: Joint Ventures in Radiation Therapy' (1992) 327 New. Eng. J. Med. 1497.

18 By-Laws, College of Physicians and Surgeons of Alberta (CPSA), ss. 48 and 51.1; *Medical Practitioners Act*, R.S.B.C. 1996, c. 285, s. 90; By-Law 1, College of Physicians and Surgeons of Manitoba (CPSM), Schedule G, s. 53; 'General Ethical Statement 124 (Conflict of Interest),' CPSM; Regulation 9, College of Physicians and Surgeons of New Brunswick (CPSNB), s. 35; *Medical Board Regulations*, Nfld. Reg. 1113/96, ss. 16 and 17; *Professional Misconduct Regulation*, O. Reg. 856/93 as am., s. 11; *General Regulation: Medicine Act*, O. Reg. 114/94, ss. 15 and 16; *Code of Ethics of Physicians*, R.S.Q., c. M-9, r. 4.1, ss. 73 and 79; By-Laws, Saskatchewan College of Physicians and Surgeons (SCPS), ss. 51(1)(f)(i) and 51(2)(n).

19 CPSA By-laws, *ibid*. ss. 47 and 49; *Medical and Health Care Services Regulation*, B.C. Reg. 426/97, ss. 38–40; *Medicare Protection Act*, R.S.B.C. c. 286, s. 35(1); CPSM, By-Law 1, *ibid.*, s. 55; CPSM, 'General Ethical Statement 124,' *ibid.*; CPSNB, Regulation 9, *ibid.*, s. 36; *General Regulation: Medicine Act*, *ibid.*, s. 17; *Code of Ethics of Physicians, ibid.*, s. 77; SCPS By-laws, *ibid.*, s. 51(1)(f)(v) (diagnostic facilities).

20 See *supra* note 6 and accompanying text.

21 *Social Security Act*, 42 U.S.C. s. 1320a-7b (1998).

22 *Ethics in Patient Referral Act, supra* note 6.

23 Paul Kalb, 'Health Care Fraud and Abuse' (1999) 282 J. Am. Med. Assoc. 1163.

24 *Professional Misconduct Regulation, supra* note 18, s. 11.

25 CPSA, By-laws, *supra* note 18, s. 48 (emphasis added).

26 *Code of Ethics of Physicians, supra* note 18, s. 73.

27 SCPS, By-laws, *supra* note 18, s. 51(2)(n).

28 CPSM, General Ethical Statement 124, *supra* note 18.

29 *Medical Practitioners Act, supra* note 18.

30 *Code of Ethics of Physicians, supra* note 18, s. 79.

31 SCPS, By-laws, *supra* note 18, s. 51(1)(d).

32 *Ethics in Patient Referral Act, supra* note 6.

33 *Code of Ethics of Physicians, supra* note 18, s. 77.

34 CPSA, By-laws, *supra* note 18, s. 47.

35 SCPS, By-laws, *supra* note 18, ss. 51(1)(f)(iv) and (v).

36 *General Regulation: Medicine Act, supra* note 18, s. 17.

37 Morreim, *supra* note 12.

38 42 C.F.R. s. 411.355(c).

39 Michael J. Kirby and Wilbert Keon, 'Why Competition Is Essential in the Delivery of Publicly Funded Health Care Services' (2004) 5:8 Policy Matters 1 at 4.

12 The Costs of Avoiding Physician Conflicts of Interest: A Cautionary Tale of Gainsharing Regulation

RICHARD S. SAVER

There is little doubt that health care providers often face serious and troubling conflicts of interest in making health care allocation decisions. Because physicians, in particular, have the difficult role of gatekeeping, they frequently become the target of economic arrangements designed to influence their utilization patterns. Parties external to the doctor-patient relationship can, through financial incentives, exercise powerful, behind-the-scenes leverage over physician decision-making. Such financial incentives threaten to compromise physician judgment, bias clinical decisions, and promote objectives other than patient interests.[1]

Conflicts of interest should certainly concern Canadian health care policy-makers and scholars. All trends in Canadian health care seem to be leading towards an increasing array of conflicts of interest for physicians as gatekeepers (as comprehensively examined by Choudhry, Choudhry, and Brown in chapter 11). While perhaps slightly contrarian to their suggestions, and to the views of other commentators, I wish to sound a note of caution about how to deal with such conflicts. Finding conflicts of interest in health care allocation decisions is, in my view, the easy part of the analysis. The more difficult question for health law and policy is what to do about it?

In their thorough discussion of the potential problems posed by physician kickback and self-referral schemes, Choudhry et al. (this volume) note that the United States has had vastly more experience with legal attempts to manage such conflicts, and they suggest that Canadian regulators could benefit from paying attention to the U.S. experience. The general lesson they derive from looking to the United States is the need for Canadian regulators to adopt a more aggressive and more tightly regulated approach. I agree with their overall conclusion that the current lack of comprehensive, coordinated regulation of self-referral and kickback incentives poses problems for Canadian health care. However, I suggest that an additional important lesson can be learned from looking to the United States. Any move to develop a tighter regulatory scheme could easily result in the imposition of overly broad-based bans. Regulatory remedies may, despite the best of intentions, introduce new problems of their own. Thus, while there is a pressing need to proceed quickly and proactively to address conflict-of-interest problems, it is also important to remain circumspect, even-handed, and context-specific when confronting problems of conflict of interest that, at first blush, all seem equally troubling.

The U.S. experience shows that not all physician conflicts of interest are the same. Moreover, certain such conflicts may need to be tolerated, as a pragmatic matter, because they are a necessary means to accomplish broader, important health policy goals. Regulation in this area must be nuanced, well-tailored, and sufficiently flexible to proportionately accommodate the variety of situations that arise. Otherwise, unintended consequences can follow. Indeed, sometimes a zero-tolerance approach, with heavy-handed efforts to ban physician conflicts of interest in health care allocation decisions, can end up doing more harm than good.

As an example, and a cautionary tale, I will discuss the U.S. health care system's attempts to regulate the practice of hospital-physician gainsharing – a conflict-of-interest activity somewhat distinct from the kickback and self-referral schemes discussed by Choudhry et al. Under gainsharing arrangements, hospitals typically share a percentage of cost-savings with their medical staff physicians if the physicians succeed in implementing productivity improvements that result in lower costs for their institution. Gainsharing is subject to many restrictions under U.S. law, and few other countries actively encourage the practice as a matter of health policy. Gainsharing payments are generally viewed with much suspicion as rewards to physicians for stinting on care. Gainsharing also has been seen as a vehicle for disguised kickback-type payments used by hospitals to generate referrals of patients from participating physicians.[2] Thus, the beefed-up prohibitive approach to kickbacks that Choudhry et al. urge could, without sufficient exceptions or safe harbours, easily crowd out health care finance and delivery innovations such as gainsharing programs.

This would be an unfortunate outcome. The U.S. gainsharing experience serves as a warning about overregulation with regard to physician conflicts of interest. Legal restrictions on gainsharing may impede hospitals' ability to undertake important operational reforms, including the development of therapeutically important disease management programs (DMPs) for chronically ill patients.

What Is Gainsharing?

Gainsharing is a reward-and-participation system in which organizations and workers share the financial gains arising through improved productivity, quality enhancement, and cost reduction, as well as other reforms.[3] Most gainsharing programs involve at least the following three key features: (1) workers actively collaborate with management to generate ideas for improving productivity; (2) workers participate in actual decision-making regarding implementation of the reforms; and (3) workers as a group receive a direct financial bonus for any cost savings or productivity gains that the organization may experience.[4] Because of the bonus, workers are said to 'share' in the 'gain' that their reform efforts bring to the organization.

Applied to the hospital setting, a typical gainsharing program would work as follows. Suppose that a hospital wants to improve the productivity and quality of its cardiac surgery program. The hospital promises the cardiac surgeons on its medical staff a direct financial bonus, equal to 50 per cent of any institutional cost savings achieved, if they are able to develop and implement productivity reforms for treating the hospital's cardiac patients. As a result, imagine that the surgeons develop several new policies. They recommend opening surgical trays, cell saver units, and comparable supplies and equipment only as needed during a procedure, rather than in advance and discarding items if unused. They recommend standardizing the surgical equipment and supply orders, substituting less costly items when possible, and also creating savings opportunities for the institution from bulk-purchase orders. They suggest limiting the use of Aprotinin, an expensive antihemorrhaging medication, to a smaller number of patients based on specific criteria of clinical need. Finally, they recommend an aggressive schedule for starting patients on postsurgery rehabilitation therapy. The staff surgeons contend that the combination of these measures should lead to lower costs per patient case, shorter stays in the hospital, and a probable reduction in the number of patient readmissions that result from postsurgery complications.[5]

If total costs for the same volume of patients (adjusted for inflation) decline during the evaluation year compared with the baseline year, and other independent quality measures are satisfied, the physicians will earn 50 per cent of the cost savings that the hospital accrues.

Gainsharing has been a common practice in non–health care sectors of the economy for some time, particularly in the manufacturing sector. Of Fortune 1000 firms, 39 per cent had adopted some form of gainsharing, according to data from the early 1990s.[6] Other surveys suggest that 19 per cent of all U.S. businesses gainshare in some form.[7]

The Legal Background

In the United States, two large governmental health care programs operate alongside the private market. Medicare is the federal program for the elderly and disabled and Medicaid is the combined federal-state program for the poor. Both programs impose a near-ban on gainsharing. The federal Medicare/Medicaid statute[8] substantially restricts hospital gainsharing by imposing civil monetary penalties when a hospital 'knowingly makes a payment, directly or indirectly, to a physician as an inducement to reduce or limit services provided with respect to [Medicare or Medicaid] patients.'[9] To the extent that a gainsharing bonus induces physicians to achieve cost savings by reducing services to Medicare/Medicaid patients, it would run afoul of the statute. If the statute is violated, civil fines of up to $2,000 (U.S.) may be imposed *for each patient* affected. The fines can be imposed both on the hospital making the bonus payment and on the physician receiving it.[10]

In July 1999 the Office of Inspector General (OIG) of the U.S. Department of Health and Human Services (DHHS) issued a special advisory bulletin declaring that most hospital-physician gainsharing plans were illegal per se because of Medicare/Medicaid statutory restrictions.[11] But in January 2001 the OIG seemingly backtracked a bit, issuing an advisory opinion specifically approving a gainsharing program developed by St Joseph's Hospital in Atlanta to reduce that hospital's cardiac operating room costs.[12] The hospital and its staff surgeons developed many reform ideas akin to the hypothetical gainsharing program discussed in the previous section.[13] However, the 2001 OIG advisory opinion and subsequent opinions imposed rigorous requirements and relied upon mitigating factors that other hospitals interested in gainsharing will not easily be able to meet or replicate.[14] Thus, the OIG has created an extremely narrow exception to the gainsharing ban. Moreover, there are no regulatory safe harbours under the gainsharing law. As a result, the Medicare/Medicaid restriction has produced a considerable chilling effect. Gainsharing remains fraught with legal risk and currently there is a dearth of gainsharing by U.S. hospitals.[15]

Why Is Gainsharing Restricted?

The U.S. Congress added the statutory restriction on hospital-physician incentive programs such as gainsharing in the *Omnibus Budget Reconciliation Act* of 1986.[16] To appreciate why it did so, it is important to understand the basics of U.S. Medicare program reimbursement. In 1983 Congress established the Medicare Prospective Payment System (PPS) for reimbursing inpatient hospital services.[17] The PPS assign a patient to an elaborate set of diagnosis-related groups (DRGs) depending upon the patient's principal diagnosis. Medicare pays hospitals a pre-established flat payment for each patient depending upon that patient's DRG. The prospective payment rate is intended to reflect the costs that a typical hospital would incur in treating such a patient. The hospital generally receives the same fee for patients with the same DRG regardless of how much it actually costs to treat any one particular patient and regardless of the patient's actual length of stay in the hospital.[18] Further, Medicare still pays physicians on a fee-for-service basis,[19] which means that physicians can earn more money the more services they provide to the hospitalized patient. Thus, the PPS provides hospitals with clear incentives to provide more efficient care and to conserve resources to stay within a predetermined PPS payment, while at the same time physicians face opposite incentives through the Medicare reimbursement system.[20]

Congress was concerned that the payment system it designed could lead to overzealous cost-cutting measures by hospitals. Some hospitals might try to lower costs by rewarding physicians for discharging patients sooner than medically indicated.[21] Thus, along with introducing the new PPS, Congress statutorily banned hospitals from paying physicians to reduce services to hospitalized patients.

Lawmakers also believed that such incentive payments not only threatened the quality of care that patients would receive, but that the financial arrangements compromised physician decision-making.[22] Moreover, the Council on Judicial and Ethical Affairs of the American Medical Association (AMA) came out in opposition to hospital-physician gainsharing, warning that it put physicians in the difficult ethical position of placing hospital cost savings above their patients' welfare.[23]

Additional concerns raised include that gainsharing will lead to stinting on patient care and encourage hospitals and physicians to 'cherry pick' healthier patients to generate cost savings that would earn them bonuses. And, as previously noted, gainsharing payments have also been viewed with much suspicion as disguised kickback-type payments in order for hospitals to generate referrals of patients from participating physicians.[24]

The Gainsharing Experience in Non–Health Care Settings

Are these concerns justified? A brief review of the gainsharing experience in non–health care settings casts significant doubt on the basic patient protection premise of the opposition to gainsharing.

Health Care vs Other Markets

To start, it is acknowledged that evidence of the effects of gainsharing in non–health care settings may have only limited applicability to hospitals. Distinct conditions drive different markets. Health care operations are not easily broken down into repetitive, routine steps as are industrial processes, and serious information problems confronting patients make the health care market particularly vulnerable to failures.[25] All this suggests whether gainsharing works in other markets may not necessarily predict much about whether and how it would work with hospitals. Nonetheless, the only real available evidence on gainsharing at present comes from non-hospital industries, where the practice is much more common. Moreover, the success of gainsharing has been identified as the ability to collapse barriers between management and labour by motivating worker participation in organizational decision-making. Thus, there are obvious parallels to the hospital sector, where a very real divide exists between hospital management and hospital medical staff.

Productivity Impact and Service Sector Applications

Research estimates vary regarding the impact of gainsharing on productivity. Some studies find that almost two-thirds of organizations with gainsharing plans show productivity improvement,[26] while others note about half of firms with gainsharing yielding tangible productivity results.[27] A frequently cited U.S. General Accounting Office (GAO) survey finds that firms with gainsharing programs average cost savings of 16 to 17 per cent.[28] One must be wary about drawing broad conclusions from such data, as some gainsharing surveys suffer from a lack of generalizability and potential design flaws.[29] Still, in the non–health care sector, gainsharing has been at least moderately associated with increased productivity, higher profits, improved quality, less waste, fewer accidents, lower worker turnover, fewer employee grievances, and increased job satisfaction.[30]

Gainsharing may be more challenging to introduce in service sector organizations such as hospitals because of the lack of clear and uniform output measures by which to evaluate performance. For hospitals, developing accurate output measures can be a challenge as hospital services are characterized by heterogeneous output. Quality measurements, too, can be quite subjective, hard to quantify, and inconsistently applied.[31] Yet the evidence available to date suggests that gainsharing has achieved productivity results and other improvements in its more limited application to service industries such as banks, utilities, and restaurants.[32] Further, the few U.S. hospitals that instituted gainsharing often achieved cost savings.[33]

Quality and Other Benefits

Perhaps counter-intuitively, gainsharing programs have been associated not only with cost savings, but also with quality improvement. An in-depth field survey of the gainsharing experience of six manufacturing firms reveals that all of the participating organizations experienced improved quality of their products and services, with several of their facilities winning customer satisfaction awards.[34] Similarly, the Whirlpool Corporation's experiment with gainsharing at one of its plants in Michigan led to productivity increases of about 19 per cent annually and improved product quality: number of parts rejected at that plant dropped from 837 per million to 4 per million.[35]

Why might gainsharing lead to improved quality? First, many firms make payment of the gainsharing bonus contingent on achieving not only cost savings but also other independent quality measures. Thus, under well-designed gainsharing programs, workers have an economic incentive to achieve quality gains for the organization. Indeed, sometimes gainsharing can convince organizations to invest more in better equipment or to contribute other long-term capital to improve quality, in addition to reducing overall production inefficiencies.[36]

Second, many quality-related problems can drive cost. Poor quality imposes its own costs on an organization because of the need to address problems such as customer dissatisfaction, product defects, and other quality-related issues. Gainsharing's focus on improving efficiency should, therefore, induce institutions to look for opportunities to improve productivity by reducing quality-related costs. Third, quality improvement depends upon worker participation and the generation of credible information with which to confront quality problems. Gainsharing's ability to generate worker collaboration and increase communication flows should, therefore, help bolster independent attempts at quality improvement within the organization.[37]

The Appeal of Gainsharing to Hospitals

Many U.S. hospitals want to experiment with gainsharing as a way of introducing significant operational reform to control both cost and quality.

Limitations to Hospital-Physician Collaboration for Cost Control

As in Canada, most hospital medical staff physicians in the United States serve as independent contractors, and not as hospital employees.[38] Hospitals cannot exercise the degree of control inherent in most employment relationships, and therefore their authority over medical staff physicians remains constrained. Typically the organizational structure at a U.S. hospital is very complex, featuring multiple lines of authority, with hospital executives, the medical staff, and the hospital's Board of Directors all having parallel and, at times, conflicting lines of authority.[39]

As a result, medical staff physicians often do not view the hospital's operational objectives as a 'physician' issue. Indeed, physicians may perceive themselves to be practising at odds with the hospital and feel detached from the medical centre's institutional mission. This can lead to passive resistance or even open defiance of the hospital's efforts at productivity reform. As a result, hospital–medical staff relations can become quite strained.

Financial incentives, such as gainsharing bonuses, may thus be needed to stimulate physician participation in reforming a hospital's productivity. Largely because of the current lack of aligned incentives, other efforts by U.S. hospitals to encourage more cost-efficient physician

practice patterns have met with but limited success. Performing extensive utilization review of the services and items that staff physicians
provide has proven to be a weak and problematic cost-control strategy.[40] Meanwhile, dissemination of best-practice guidelines to physicians has proven to be less effective at motivating physician behaviour
than financial incentives as physicians often fail to follow the guidelines.[41] Their professional training makes physicians less responsive
than perhaps others to hierarchical mandates. They are more likely
influenced by appeals to consensus, collegiality, clinical experience, and
the application of professional judgment in resolving allocation issues.[42]
Because of its participative and collaborative nature, gainsharing may
be a more physician-friendly manner for engaging physicians to strive
for productivity reform.

A Needed Boost to Hospital Quality Reform?

The quality improvement activities of a hospital depend for their success upon established workplace cultures of physician participation
and their collaboration with hospital management.[43] Gainsharing,
through its emphasis on teamwork, joint decision-making, participative governance, and the linkage of performance results with rewards
may offer a better background environment for hospital quality reform.
   Gainsharing may be the right vehicle for introducing quality improvement because regular participation in gainsharing can help to
displace the current norms of detachment and non-alignment among
many medical staff physicians. Gainsharing theorists contend that the
participative features of gainsharing change the traditional workplace
environment by making workers less likely to hold back on useful ideas,
thus generating more critical information for operational reform.[44]
   Also, it must be remembered that expecting physicians to help with
hospital quality improvement can cost them economically. The time
and effort that they spend on working with hospitals to develop better
care pathways for patients is not necessarily compensated under traditional reimbursement systems. Some quality improvement reforms can
end up imposing costs on the medical staff. At HealthSystem Minne-
sota, which is a large integrated delivery system, officials were concerned about the delays that patients had to endure before receiving a
confirmatory diagnosis of breast cancer. A quality-improvement initiative attempting to reduce the diagnosis time led to the decision to have
the institution's radiologists perform the majority of biopsies using

stereotactic methods. This reform, although helpful for patients, cost the hospital surgeons approximately $40,000 (U.S.) a year in lost revenues under fee-for-service reimbursement that they could no longer generate.[45] Gainsharing can partially offset such quality-reform losses by rewarding physicians economically for contributing to the overall success of the institution.

A gainsharing boost may be needed for hospital quality improvement because of the limited success of other efforts. It is hard to overcome the natural presumption of physicians to prefer their own practice patterns, even when confronted with clinical trial data that suggest the need for significant revision.[46] For example, efforts by U.S. hospitals to introduce total quality management (TQM) and quality improvement (QI) initiatives in the 1990s encountered serious problems.[47] Physicians resisted TQM/QI reform initiatives that they viewed as management-led, without sufficient physician input, and regarded with suspicion many TQM/QI efforts as intrusions onto their clinical autonomy.[48] Gainsharing may have a better chance of jump-starting physician interest in operational reform, including quality improvement. Gainsharing, at least, seems capable of addressing the baseline hospital management-medical staff divide that plagues so many hospitals' efforts at operational reform.

Avoiding Gainsharing Imposes Its Own Costs

Clinical Evidence and the Cost vs Quality Trade-off

Much of the governmental concern over gainsharing relates to a perceived cost versus quality trade-off. The OIG implicitly assumes that reforms that seek to improve hospital productivity will seek to lower costs by an overall reduction in the level of hospital services. It is further assumed that this will inevitably lead to a correspondingly lower quality of patient care.

The cost versus quality position relies on false assumptions. Clinical evidence has demonstrated, perhaps counter-intuitively, a non-linear correlation between cost and quality in health care allocation decisions. In other words, reduction of health care costs can be associated with improved quality as well as lower quality. Donna Greschner (chapter 2, in this volume) has explained well the benefits of evidence-based decision-making. Evidence-based medicine research has demonstrated that considerable clinical variation exists among physicians, even when

treating patients with very similar clinical symptoms.[49] Despite variations in intensity and cost of services between physicians, often no clear
therapeutic difference can be seen in terms of patients' overall health
outcomes.

Evidence-based medicine suggests that some not insignificant level
of current medical care is wasteful. But the problems go deeper than
that. Overutilization of services is not costless. Excessive services not
only drain resources but can also increase the risk of patient injury.
Thus, studies have shown a quality concern related to recurring patterns of inappropriate hospitalization.[50] Indeed, quality improvement
initiatives based on evidence-based medicine may lead hospitals to try
to reduce the level of particular services to certain patients receiving
clinically inappropriate amounts of care.[51] Most likely, many physicians
both underutilize and overutilize services as their practice patterns
develop independently of evidence-based medicine.[52]

Although clinical data on hospital gainsharing in the United States
are limited, they are nevertheless instructive as they help illustrate the
fallacy of the cost-versus-quality trade-off. In the early 1990s the U.S.
government conducted the Medicare Participating Heart Bypass Center Demonstration Project as an effort to test new reimbursement methods for paying for coronary artery bypass graft (CABG) surgery. The
government invited a limited number of hospitals and physicians to
participate. Rather than pay the physicians under the traditional fee-
for-service system and the hospitals under the PPS, Medicare paid the
providers a single, fixed global sum for all hospital and physician
services related to CABG surgery. The hospitals and physicians could
then divide up the single payment any which way that they chose to do
so.[53]

Because it was a demonstration project, ordinary Medicare rules
were lifted for the participating hospitals and physicians – including
the statutory restrictions on gainsharing. At least two of the hospitals
introduced gainsharing plans with their medical staff, and this resulted
in several interesting reforms. The gainsharing hospitals designated a
clinical nurse specialist to be in charge of each CABG patient's stay in
the intensive care unit (ICU), and this led to more coordinated patient
care and shorter and less costly ICU stays. Other reform measures
under the Demonstration Project included the use of less expensive
contrast media, standardization of the surgical kits used, more efficient
use of operating room time, fewer medical consultations, and earlier
discharges from hospital. The participating institutions arranged to

have some patients receive their diagnostic catheterizations elsewhere before arriving at the hospital, thus obviating the need for an extra day in hospital.[54] Overall, the Demonstration Project was a success. The average cost per CABG patient was reduced, and Medicare saved an estimated 10 per cent in payments to these hospitals during the five-year demonstration. Quality of care stayed the same or actually improved for the CABG patients compared with national data for Medicare patients not participating in the Demonstration Project. Indeed, CABG inpatient mortality rates both at discharge and at one year postdischarge declined for the participating hospitals.[55] The Demonstration Project confirms that hospital gainsharing programs need not threaten quality of patient care. On the contrary, it shows that, if properly designed and monitored, gainsharing plans can actually have a beneficial therapeutic impact.

Such examples are not meant to gloss over the fact that gainsharing can pose real concerns about quality. While hospitals are showing increasing sophistication in measuring costs per patient case, measuring quality is much more problematic given the information problems confronting patients and providers. Gainsharing reforms could produce cost savings and at the same time have a negative impact on therapeutic care in ways not readily detected or understood. This means that the target measures that gainsharing programs use to monitor the effect on quality may not offer very strong protection.

Nonetheless, it seems unhelpful and overly rigid to resist any form of gainsharing whatsoever largely on the basis of theoretical harms. Focusing in the abstract on whether any particular level of hospital service may be reduced is a crude and unsophisticated way of protecting quality. Medical care is much more complicated in clinical practice. As studies from evidence-based medicine and the Medicare Participating Heart Bypass Center Demonstration Project demonstrate, reductions in hospital services do not automatically correspond to a lower quality of patient care. Indeed, some service reductions may be therapeutically motivated, and other service reductions may be accompanied by increased utilization of other lines of service. A better way of approaching the problem is not to effectively ban all forms of gainsharing simply whenever any service reductions may result. Quality concerns suggest, instead, the need to proceed cautiously and to ask whether a particular gainsharing initiative, viewed in its specific context, offers sufficient incentives to the institution and its physicians to adopt a clinically sound level of care.

Implications for Disease Management Programs

Overregulating gainsharing presents its own set of dangers, such as the likely detrimental impact on hospital-based disease management programs (DMs). A typical DM targets patients with chronic conditions such as asthma, diabetes, or heart failure and tries to identify optimal care pathways for a person with that disease based on clinical outcomes data. DMPs involve a thorough review of all health care services consumed by patients with chronic conditions, in an effort to establish common care patterns that would be more optimal for patients who can be expected to experience the natural history of a chronic disease.[56] An important goal of DMs is to decrease individual episodes of care, such as visits to the emergency room, by proactively anticipating the progression of the chronically ill patient's disease and coordinating care better, including identifying more opportunities for case management, self-monitoring, and self-care.[57]

For example, a DM instituted at University Hospitals in Cleveland for congestive heart failure (CHF) involved active oversight of staff physicians by a DM committee. The committee counselled individual physicians to increase the use of angiotensin-converting enzyme (ACE) inhibitor medications for CHF patients, as well as to follow other care pathways for treatment of CHF, as recommended by a national cardiac society. As is typical at many institutions, the staff physicians were well aware of the recommended care pathways, but they were not actively following the guidelines – underscoring the basic problems with a voluntary guideline approach to quality improvement. Thus, the hospital designed the hands-on program to change the behaviour of medical staff. The intervention produced cost savings for the institution and fewer days in hospital for the CHF patients, and at the same time the targeted quality-of-care measures actually improved.[58]

But further growth and development of such hospital-based DMPs is likely to encounter significant obstacles because of the gainsharing restrictions. Under the OIG's current, broad regulatory position, a hospital violates the law against gainsharing if it pays a physician with the payment intended to induce the reduction of any hospital service to a Medicare/Medicaid patient.[59] A hospital that pays staff physicians to participate in hospital-based DMPs risks running afoul of the law. The natural outcome of DMPs is to limit certain episodes of care, such as additional lengths of stay or subsequent readmissions. The standardization emphasis of DMPs will inevitably lead to a reduction or elimination of non-standardized care. Thus, a hospital that pays its physicians to participate in DMPs knows that it is likely inducing the reduction of certain hospital services. Accordingly, this implicates the gainsharing law.

If hospitals are restricted in their ability to use monetary rewards to generate physician interest in DMPs, many institutions will have trouble introducing them in comprehensive fashion. Financial incentives are a powerful motivator for participation.[60] DMPs that have used financial incentives in combination with education, feedback, and data collection have been the most successful.[61]

It may be wishful thinking and somewhat naive to expect physicians to actively participate in DMPs under current conditions. Some experimentation with paying physicians to do so may be necessary to accomplish the broader health policy goals associated with disease management.

Ethical and Fiduciary Concerns

The conflict-of-interest concerns that have been voiced about gainsharing assume implicitly that physicians somehow violate their ethical and fiduciary obligations when they participate in gainsharing. This objection probably overstates and oversimplifies the issues. Full analysis of the fiduciary and ethical implications of gainsharing cannot be accomplished in the space limitations of this chapter. The brief discussion that follows merely makes the more limited point that gainsharing should not be subject to a prophylactic ban based on ethical and fiduciary concerns because participation in gainsharing is not per se incompatible with a physician's ethical and fiduciary roles.

First, the concerns that gainsharing bonuses will inevitably and perniciously tempt physicians to stint on care and undertreat patients must be evaluated in their proper context. Financial incentives for physicians can vary considerably in their scope and intensity depending upon the specific circumstances in which they are deployed.[62] Gainsharing bonuses may be experienced with more or less intensity depending upon the number of patients and physicians who are grouped together under the bonus program, the length of time over which the performance measurements are made, and the amount of bonus that can be earned compared with a physician's base compensation, as well as other key factors. A gainsharing program with more modest financial incentives and other safeguards, combined with physicians' own sense of ethics and professional obligations (and the threat of medical malpractice actions) should counter, to an extent, the dangers of extreme and overzealous cost cutting.

Second, gainsharing is hardly unique in posing conflict-of-interest problems. Indeed, Choudhry et al. (chapter 11, this volume) discuss some of the related concerns raised by kickback and self-referral schemes. But the basic point, which should be more explicitly acknowledged by opponents of gainsharing, kickbacks, self-referral, and other newly developing practices, is that no financing scheme is optimal and none is free from the potential for abuse. All payment systems can encourage physicians to either overtreat or undertreat their patients. Fee-for-service payment encourages physician to work up their patients and provide greater levels of higher-reimbursed services, all of which can expose patients to unnecessary and even inappropriate and dangerous care. Flat rate or prospective payment systems can encourage physicians to reduce costs by simply withholding needed services. Even paying physicians fixed salaries can set the wrong incentives. Fixed salaries discourage diligence and greater work effort, particularly with sicker and chronically ill patients, as physicians will find that they can often earn the same fixed salary even when doing less for their more needy patients.[63]

With regard to fiduciary concerns more specifically, the presumable objection is that the physician, owing a level of fidelity to the patient because of the fiduciary nature of the doctor-patient relationship, cannot receive a financial bonus for limiting services to a patient. However, in many different settings, fiduciaries can engage in conflict-of-interest transactions and pursue some degree of self-interest when they fully disclose the conflict and obtain the principals' advance consent,[64] suggesting that there may be a role for informed consent partially to ameliorate the fiduciary concerns about gainsharing. More specific to the doctor-patient relationship, the exact contours of the physicians' fiduciary obligations to their patients are, in fact, not well-defined. U.S. courts, for example, have applied fiduciary principles to the doctor-patient relationship more clearly in limited situations such as the requirements for informed consent or to maintain patient confidentiality,[65] but they have not consistently imposed the same strict fiduciary standards on physicians with respect to financial conflicts of interest.[66]

Fiduciary concerns need not necessarily ban outright the financial bonuses associated with gainsharing. Instead, fiduciary concerns should more probably urge that the arrangements be regulated to make sure that the physician's position of trust as a fiduciary is not being abused.[67] Moreover, the fiduciary issues become more complex when one considers that the physician has multiple patients and therefore multiple fiduciary relationships to deal with concurrently. Arguably, physicians may receive some form of financial incentive for engaging in reform of hospital productivity because this is a socially important activity that most patients would want undertaken ex ante before they themselves may come to experience illness.[68]

Medical ethics concerns would seem to present the more significant obstacle for gainsharing. The AMA's *Code of Medical Ethics* advises that under no circumstances may physicians place their own financial interests above the welfare of their patients and that all such conflicts must be resolved to the benefit of the patient.[69] As well, traditional medical ethics guidance cautions that physicians should not make rationing decisions for the patients they treat directly.[70] However, the orthodox view that physicians must do all that is best for any one patient, shielded from all other considerations of the cost and larger societal considerations of providing care of only limited marginal benefit, no longer finds uniform support. Patients would not necessarily consider it unethical for a physician to try to conserve resources to benefit the largest number of patients.[71] More modern medical ethics considerations have allowed, at least on a very limited basis, that physicians should take into consideration the efficient allocation of resources as they make treatment decisions. Indeed, other professional societies, in their own ethical codes, have stated more forcefully than has the AMA that it *is* ethical for treating physicians to consider efficient resource allocation.[72]

If well-designed, gainsharing programs can encourage thoughtful, careful collaboration between hospitals and physicians in improving productivity as well as quality of patient care. Certainly, more ethical guidelines would be welcome to help physicians navigate and manage the conflicts inherent in gainsharing, with the hope of preserving as much as possible the important levels of trust that patients place in their physicians. But this is just a reason to proceed cautiously and to think of better ways to manage the conflicts – as opposed to consigning gainsharing to oblivion.

Implications for Canadian Health Care

Does the U.S experience with gainsharing have direct relevance for governmental health care reform in Canada? Gainsharing need not be confined to private health care markets and U.S.-style, for-profit managed care entities. As previously noted, the very recent track record with hospital gainsharing in the United States comes from the Medicare Participating Heart Bypass Center Demonstration Project, which involved the federal government as purchaser of hospital and physician services and the participation of non-profit hospitals.

Moreover, some prominent recent Canadian health care reform proposals, such as the *Kirby Report*, have advocated greater use of service-based (or case-mix-based) approaches to funding hospital services.[73] Part of the appeal of such reimbursement systems is to encourage greater hospital efficiency and better performance on the part of hospitals.[74] However, the regulatory framework must be flexible enough to accommodate such innovation. Choudhry et al. acknowledge that self-referral prohibitions may need to be modified if service-based funding reform efforts are to encourage the development of specialized, stand-alone facilities, particularly in rural areas, where avoiding self-referrals seems simply impractical.

I suggest that many more modifications and exceptions will likely be necessary if Canadian regulators hope to find the right balance in regulating physician conflicts of interest, both within the public Medicare program and the increasingly complex private health care system. Gainsharing is a prime example of the need to proceed cautiously in restricting conflict-of-interest activities. Based on the U.S. experience, there is every reason to suspect that health care reforms that tinker with hospital and physician reimbursement, without sufficiently coordinating the incentives of the providers, will prove disappointing. The Medicare prospective payment system (PPS) introduced for U.S. hospitals in the 1980s, which is a form of service-based funding, has not produced the large, dramatic efficiency gains anticipated by its proponents. This is largely because of the inability of U.S. hospitals to influence or control their staff physicians' practice patterns, compounded by the extremely complex, non-aligned nature of hospital organization and service delivery.[75]

Because of such difficulties many U.S. hospitals have looked with renewed interest to gainsharing. Health care reform in Canada will similarly need to address how best to align incentives between hospitals and physicians; this issue is critical to any revised hospital funding scheme, as well as to hospital quality reform initiatives. Gainsharing, therefore, is an intriguing illustration of a practice that raises serious conflict-of-interest concerns – but valid reasons exist to tolerate it, nonetheless, through regulatory exceptions and safe harbours. Gainsharing could serve as a flexible and pragmatic vehicle to support and supplement broader reform in Canada's health care system, whatever direction that may take, because it can be deployed within several different types of hospital and physician reimbursement schemes.

Conclusions

Gainsharing is not the holy grail of hospital operational reform. Deeper structural problems in fragmented, non-unified health care delivery systems cannot be addressed by gainsharing alone. Gainsharing does remain a pragmatic vehicle for experimentation with health care reform on an incremental level. Nonetheless, to date it has been avoided and shunned largely because of broad-based and overly rigid conflict-of-interest concerns.

Can health law and policy encourage gainsharing in its more optimal forms, while avoiding its dangers? Developing a sufficiently balanced regulatory framework for gainsharing will present significant challenges that should not be underestimated.[76] But this regulatory experiment seems well worth it when compared with the status quo. At present, the law's near-complete ban on gainsharing reflects a misleading view that gainsharing's gains always come at the expense of patients. In fact, well-designed gainsharing programs can benefit patients as a whole, through cost *and* quality improvements. Many fears about gainsharing are premised simply upon a misunderstanding of the complex relationship between cost and quality in delivering hospital services. The gainsharing experience in non–health care settings fails to support quality-related concerns. Finally, the ethical and fiduciary concerns about gainsharing do not support a categorical ban.

Because of well-intentioned efforts to avoid conflict-of-interest problems, gainsharing has been subject to a near-ban. But this desire to avoid troubling conflicts of interest in health care allocation decisions has led to many missed opportunities for achieving significant hospital operational reform. The reluctance even to allow experimentation with modest forms of gainsharing is imposing its own costs.[77] In particular, it threatens the viability of therapeutically important hospital-based disease management programs. At some point, we must ask whether living with certain conflicts of interest, such as those inherent in gainsharing, would not be better than trying to avoid the conflicts altogether?

NOTES

My special thanks to Colleen Flood, the Canadian Institutes for Health Research, and the other event sponsors for the opportunity to participate in the National Health Law Conference 2004 and in this book project.

1 See Marc A. Rodwin, *Medicine, Money and Morals: Physicians' Conflicts of Interest* (Washington: Oxford University Press, 1993). This chapter summarizes current health law and policy debates regarding gainsharing, with a particular focus on the conflict-of-interest aspects. For a more comprehensive discussion of gainsharing generally, see Richard S. Saver, 'Squandering the Gain: Gainsharing and the Continuing Dilemma of Physician Financial Incentives' (2003) 98 Northwestern Univ. L.R. 145.

2 OIG Advisory Opinion No. 01-1, at 6 (11 Jan. 2001), http://oig.hhs.gov/fraud/docs/advisoryopinions/2001/ao01-01.pdf (accessed 1 Sept. 2005) [*OIG Advisory Opinion 2001*]; D. McCarty Thornton and Kevin McAnaney, 'Recent Commentary Distorts HHS IG's Gainsharing Bulletin' 4 (1999), http://oig.hhs.gov/fraud/docs/alertsandbulletins/bnagain.htm (accessed 1 Sept. 2005). The authors were counsel in the Department of Health and Human Services (DHHS) OIG.

3 See David Hames, 'Productivity Enhancing Work Innovations: Remedies for What Ails Hospitals?' (1991), 36 Hosp. and Health Services Admin. 545 at 552–3.

4 See Brian Graham-Moore and Timothy L. Ross, *Gainsharing and Employee Involvement* (Washington: BNA Books, 1995).

5 This clinical scenario is based largely on the gainsharing program developed by St Joseph's Hospital in Atlanta. The hospital was one of the few in the United States to receive regulatory approval for implementing a gainsharing program. See OIG Advisory Opinion 2001, *supra* note 2. I have modified and expanded the St Joseph's Hospital example to include other reform idéas that are representative of the types of improvement initiatives that gainsharing programs can generate.

6 Dong-One Kim, 'Determinants of the Survival of Gainsharing Programs' (1999) 53 Industrial. and Lab. Rel. Rev. 21.

7 Carol Kleiman, 'A Way to Make Pay Gains while the Sun Shines,' *Chicago Tribune*, 22 October 1995.

8 The *Social Security Act* is the quite lengthy federal statute that covers, in part, the Medicare and Medicaid programs. For simplicity's sake, this chapter refers to the particular *Social Security Act* provisions that regulate the Medicare and Medicaid programs as the 'Medicare/Medicaid statute.'

9 42 U.S.C. s. 1320a–7a(b)(1).

10 *Ibid*. s. 1320a–7a(b)(2).

11 *Special Advisory Bulletin on Gainsharing Arrangements and CMPs for Hospital Payments to Physicians to Reduce or Limit Services to Beneficiaries*, 64 Fed. Reg. 37985 (1999).

12 See OIG, *supra* note 2. Although the advisory opinion did not name the hospital, its identity became public knowledge anyway. See Amy Miller, 'St Joseph's to Reward Surgeon for Savings,' *Atlanta Journal and Constitution*, 20 January 2001. The OIG more recently issued several additional advisory opinions approving a very limited number of other hospitals' gainsharing plans. See OIG Advisory Opinions No. 05-01 to 05-06 (2005), available at http://oig.hhs.gov/fraud/advisoryopinions/opinions.html (accessed 1 Sept. 2005).

13 The major reforms included (1) limiting the use of Aprotinin; (2) opening surgical trays, cell saver equipment, and comparable items only as needed rather than opening them in advance on a stand-by basis when they might get discarded unused; and (3) substituting less costly surgical equipment and supplies. See OIG, *supra* note 2. It is not surprising that limitation of Aprotinin was chosen as one of the reform measures. Studies indicate that this expensive drug may not always be worth its considerable cost and should be limited to certain cardiac patients who are at higher risk of hemorrhage. See, e.g., Michael J. Ray *et al.*, 'Economic Evaluation of High-Dose and Low-Dose Aprotinin Therapy during Cardiopulmonary Bypass' (1999) 68 Annals of Thoracic Surgery 940, at 944, for a demonstration of cost savings that can be achieved through lower dosage of the drug without compromising therapeutic benefit.

14 For example, in the initial advisory opinion the OIG (*supra*, note 2) felt that quality of care was protected because the St Joseph's plan allowed for terminating a physician's participation if the physician had significant changes in historical patient mix in terms of severity of illness, age, and health care coverage (to guard against the physician cherry-picking only healthier, less costly patients to operate on at that hospital). However, it can be quite expensive for a hospital to develop such historical measures about each medical staff member's previous practice patterns. Also, the

St Joseph's plan's primary cost-reduction proposal – limiting the use of Aprotinin – was well supported in the medical literature, making the overall program more palatable to the OIG. Nevertheless, many other gainsharing programs will involve consideration of good-faith reform proposals by physicians about new, expensive technology where there is an absence of clear clinical indicators in the medical literature. A time lag often exists between the emergence of clinical opinion about a technology and the release of definitive published studies. See, e.g., Lars Noah, 'Medicine's Epistemology: Mapping the Haphazard Diffusion of Knowledge in the Biomedical Community' (2002) 44 Ariz. L. Rev. 393–4.

15 The 2005 OIG Advisory Opinions (*supra*, note 12) have still not significantly expanded potential exceptions to the gainsharing prohibitions. Even under the new guidance, gainsharing programs present numerous legal problems. See D. McCarty Thornton et al., 'Gainsharing: Regulatory Breakthrough, But Challenges Remain' (16 June 2005) BNA Health Law Reporter at 834. Indeed, the Medicare program's recent attempt to allow a pilot gainsharing program by certain hospitals in New Jersey on a demonstration basis has been bogged down by litigation. See *Robert Wood Johnson University Hospital v. Thompson* (D.N.J. 2004), 2004 U.S. Dist. LEXIS 8498.

16 OBRA 1986, Pub.L. No. 99–509, s. 9313(c), 100 Stat. 1874 (1986).

17 The initial PPS applied only to hospital inpatient services. In 2000 the U.S. Medicare program phased in a comparable prospective payment system for hospital outpatient services as well. See 'Health Care Industry Market Update: Wall Street's View of Hospitals' (2002) 7, http://cms.hhs.gov/reports/hcimu/hcimu_04292002.pdf (accessed 1 June 2005).

18 Different hospitals generally receive the same amount for each DRG. However, the payment can vary because a hospital's actual payment under the PPS is determined not only by the DRG, but also by standardized sums for the hospital's labour, non-labour, and capital costs, all of which the PPS recognizes can vary across regions. See Barry Furrow et al., *Health Law: Cases, Materials, and Problems*, 4th ed. (St. Paul, MN: West, 2001). Also, the PPS provides for rare 'outlier' payments that offer extra reimbursement to a hospital for particularly costly cases within a DRG. See 42 C.F.R. s. 412.80(a).

19 42 U.S.C. s. 1395w-4(a) to 4(j).

20 Bruce Spivey, 'The Relation between Hospital Management and Medical Staff under a Prospective-Payment System' (1984) 310 New Eng. J. Med. 984.

21 Health Committee, House of Representatives, *Medicare Incentive Payments*

by Hospitals Could Lead to Abuse (1986) 10, http://161.203.16.4/d4t4/
130544.pdf (accessed 1 Sept. 2005).

22 The legislative record indicates that Congress was concerned that 'such
incentive payments may create a conflict of interest that may limit the
ability of the physicians to exercise independent professional judgment in
the best interest of his or her patients' *H.R. Report* No. 99-727 (1986) at 444,
reprinted in 1986 U.S.C.C.A.N. 3607, 3841.

23 'Reports of the Judicial Council of the American Medical Association'
(1985) 253 J.A.M.A. 424, at 425.

24 See OIG, *supra* note 2; Thornton and McAnaney, *supra* note 2.

25 Timothy Stoltzfus Jost, 'Oversight of the Quality of Medical Care: Regula-
tion, Management, or the Market?' (1995) 37 Ariz. L. Rev. 825 at 856; David
A. Hyman, 'Regulating Managed Care: What's Wrong with a Patient Bill
of Rights' (2000) 73 Southern California L. Rev. 221 at 233; William M.
Sage, 'Regulating through Information: Disclosure Laws and American
Health Care' (1999) 99 Colum. L. Rev. 1701 at 1771–7.

26 John Cotton, 'Does Employee Involvement Work?'(1997) 12 J. Nursing
Care Quality 2 at 33, 38.

27 George Milkovich, 'Gain Sharing and Profit Sharing as Strategic Considerations,' in Myron J. Roomkin, ed., *Profit Sharing and Gain Sharing* (London
and Metuchen. NJ: IMLR Press / Rutgers University Press, 1990). But see
also Woodruff Imberman, 'Gainsharing: A Lemon or Lemonade?' Business
Horizons (Jan./Feb. 1996) at 36, 37 discussing the American Management
Association's 1989 survey and its follow-up survey suggesting that approximately only one-third of companies have had success with
gainsharing.

28 U.S. General Accounting Office (GAO), 'Productivity Sharing Programs:
Can They Contribute to Productivity?' GAO/AFMD-81-22 (3 March 1981).
Later studies found average productivity increases of 16–17% in the years
following a company's initial implementation of gainsharing. Peter
Scontrino, 'Using Gainsharing as an Effective Productivity and Quality
Improvement Tool,' J. Quality & Participation (July/Aug. 1995) 90 at 93
(summarizing previous studies).

29 Denis Collins, *Gainsharing and Power* (Ithaca: Cornell University Press,
1998) at 216–21.

30 See *supra* note 3.

31 See, e.g., Joseph Newhouse, 'Why Is There a Quality Chasm,? Health
Affairs (July/Aug. 2002) 13, at 16–17, 21–2. This can make it more difficult
to design hospital gainsharing formulas with workable, meaningful
quality measurements.

32 Douglas O'Bannon and Craig Pearce, 'An Exploratory Examination of Gainsharing in Service Organizations: Implications of Organizational Citizenship Behavior and Pay Satisfaction'(1999) 11 J. Managerial Issues 363, at 366.

33 Richard S. Saver, 'Squandering the Gain: Gainsharing and the Continuing Dilemma of Physician Financial Incentives' (2003) 98 Northwestern Univ. L. Rev. 145 at 184 & note 143.

34 *Supra* note 29.

35 Imberman, *supra* note 27 at 36–7.

36 *Supra* note 29, at 62, 68–9.

37 Charles DeBettignies, 'Putting Teeth Into Your Quality Reward Efforts' (1992) J. Quality and Participation (Jan./Feb) at 70, 72.

38 Indeed, the corporate practice of medicine doctrine makes it illegal in many states for a hospital to employ a staff physician. See generally *Berlin v. Sarah Bush Lincoln Health Center*, 688 N.E. 2d 106, 110–12 (Illinois 1997), summarizing cases from many jurisdictions and reasons for the corporate practice of medicine doctrine.

39 Mark Hall, 'Institutional Control of Physician Behavior: Legal Barriers to Health Care Cost Containment' (1988) 137 Univ. Pennsylvania L. Rev. 431 at 505–6.

40 David Orentlicher, 'Paying Physicians More to Do Less: Financial Incentives to Limit Care' (1996) 30 U. Richmond L. Rev. 155 at 170, 179–83 [*Orentlicher*].

41 Philip G. Peters, 'The Role of the Jury in Modern Malpractice Law' (2002) 87 Iowa L. Rev. 909 at 953.

42 Barry R. Furrow, 'Incentivizing Medical Practice: What (If Anything) Happens to Professionalism?' (1996) 1 Widener Law Symposium J. 1, at 5.

43 *Ibid.*, discussing studies showing that greater physician involvement in hospital decision-making correlates with lower costs and better quality of patient care.

44 Jeffrey Arthur and Lynda Aiman-Smith, 'Gainsharing and Organizational Learning: An Analysis of Employee Suggestions Over Time' (2001) 44 Academy Management J. 737, at 740.

45 Elizabeth A. Fischer and Dean C. Coddington, 'Integrated Heath Care: Passing Fad or Lasting Legacy?' Health Care Financial Management (Jan. 1998) at 47.

46 See John Johansson, 'Outcomes Research, Practice Guidelines, and Disease Management in Clinical Gastroenterology' (1998) 27 J. Clinical Gastroenterology 306 at 309–10; Edward Philbin et al., 'The Results of a Random-

ized Trial of a Quality Improvement Intervention in the Care of Patients with Heart Failure' (2000) 109 Am. J. of Med. 443 at 448.

47 The TQM/QI movement in hospital care sought to apply quality improvement strategies modelled after Japanese management practices. The TQM/QI movement included, among other features, a focus on meeting the needs of external and internal customers within an organization and making significant use of outcomes data to guide reform efforts. See generally Donald Berwick et al., *Curing Health Care: New Strategies for Quality Improvement* (San Francisco: Jossey-Bass, 1990).

48 Valerie Weber and Maulik Joshi, 'Effecting and Leading Change in Health Care Organizations,' 26 J. on Quality Improvement 388 at 391 (2000).

49 Evidence-based medicine attempts to apply the results of clinical trials and comprehensive outcomes data to inform decision-making about how to treat individual patients. It favours gathering and disseminating clinical trial data to guide clinical decision-making to a much larger degree than how physicians currently make treatment decisions. See Noah, supra n14 and Donna Greschner (chapter 2, this volume).

50 Furrow, *supra* note 42.

51 Neil MacKinnon *et al.*, 'Disease Management Program for Asthma: Baseline Assessment of Resource Use' (1996) 53 Am. J. Health-Systems Pharmacy 535, clinical study detailing how approximately 6% of hospitalized asthma patients receive excessive amounts of beta-agonist drug therapy, leading to higher admissions and emergency room visits and higher total care costs.

52 See, e.g., E. Haavi Morriem, *Holding Health Care Accountable: Law and the New Medical Marketplace* (London and New York: Oxford University Press, 2001).

53 U.S., Health Care Financing Administration, *Extramural Research Report: Medicare Participating Heart Bypass Center Demonstration* (1998).

54 *Ibid.* at 11–13, 17–19.

55 *Ibid.* at 11–12, 13–15, 21–2.

56 See Alicia Fernandez et al., 'Primary Care Physicians' Experience with Disease Management Programs' (2001) 16 Journal General Internal Medicine 163; Gillian Fairfield and Andrew Long, 'Measuring the Outcomes of Disease Management' (1997) 10 Int. J. of Health Care Quality Assurance 161.

57 Daniel Mark, 'Economics of Treating Heart Failure' (1997) 80 Am. J. Cardiology 33H, at 34H; Patrick Rivers and Kai-Li Tsai, 'Managing Costs and Managing Care' (2001) 14 Int. J. Health Care Quality Assurance 302 at 304–6.

58 See Ottorino Costantini *et al.*, 'Impact of a Guideline-Based Disease Management Team on Outcomes of Hospitalized Patients with Congestive Heart Failure' (2001) 161 Archives Internal Med. 177, 178–82.

59 The OIG has framed the central inquiry when evaluating the legality of a gainsharing program as whether there is the potential for services to be reduced. If so, that is enough for finding a violation of the gainsharing law. See *supra* note 11.

60 Alan Hillman, 'Financial Incentives for Physicians in HMOs: Is There a Conflict of Interest?' (1987) 317 New Eng. J. Med. 1743, 1747; see Jost, *supra* note 25.

61 Neil MacKinnon *et al.*, 'Disease Management Program for Asthma: Baseline Assessment of Resource Use' (1996) 53 Am. J. Health-System Pharmacy 535 at 536.

62 Anne Barry Flood *et al.*, 'The Promise and Pitfalls of Explicitly Rewarding Physicians Based on Patient Insurance' (2000) 23 J. Ambulatory Care Management 55 at 67–9; Stephen Magnus, 'Physicians' Financial Incentives in Five Dimensions: A Conceptual Framework for HMO Managers' (1999) 24 Health Care Management Rev. 57.

63 See generally David A. Hyman and Charles Silver, 'You Get What You Pay For: Result-Based Compensation for Health Care' (2001) 58 Washing and Lee L. Rev. 1427 at 1442–3 (discussing the strengths and weaknesses of many leading payment systems).

64 For example, research subjects may consent to participation in a clinical trial, even though, because it is a research study, the physician-investigator may take actions to advance the scientific merits and overall success of the trial rather than the care of the individual patient. See Richard S. Saver, 'Critical Care Research and Informed Consent' (1996) 75 North Carolina L. Rev. 205, 223–25. Similarly, corporate officers and directors, despite their fiduciary roles, may engage in self-interested transactions as long as they disclose the conflict in advance and get disinterested director or shareholder approval. See Delaware General Corporation Law § 144.

65 Mary Anne Bobinski, 'Autonomy and Privacy: Protecting Patients from Their Physician,' (1994) 55 Univ. Pittsburgh L. Rev. 291 at 352.

66 Mark Hall, 'Law, Medicine, and Trust' (2002) 55 Stanford Law Rev., 463 at 503–4; Rodwin, *supra* note 1.

67 William Sage, 'The Lawyerization of Medicine' (2001) 26 J. Health Policy Politics & Law 1179 at 1191; Mark Hall, 'Arrow on Trust' (2001) 26 J. Health Politics, Policy & Law.

68 See Orentlicher, *supra* note 40.

69 'America Medical Associations Code of Medical Ethics' § 8.03 in Baruch

Brody *et al.*, eds., *Medical Ethics: Codes, Opinions and Statements* (Washington: BNA Books, 2000).

70 See Orentlicher, *supra* note 40.

71 See Hillman, *supra* note 60.

72 For example, the relatively new Physician Charter for Medical Professionalism in the New Millennium, a joint project of the American Board of Internal Medicine, the American College of Physicians/American Society of Internal Medicine, and other professional groups advises that physicians have a professional responsibility to work to make the best use of finite resources. The Physician Charter advises that physicians should commit to working with hospitals to develop guidelines for cost-effective care and that '[t]he physician's professional responsibility for appropriate allocation of resources requires scrupulous avoidance of superfluous tests and procedures.' 'Medical Professionalism in the New Millennium: A Physician Charter' (2002) 136 Annals Int. Medicine 243 at 245.

73 Standing Senate Committee on Social Affairs, *The Health of Canadians – The Federal Role: Final Report.* vol. 6, § 2.1.8, 2.3 (2002).

74 *Ibid.;* Jean-Luc Migue, 'Method for Funding Hospitals and Doctors Flawed,' Fraser Forum (March 2003), at 27–8.

75 David M. Frankford, 'The Medicare DRGs: Efficiency and Organizational Rationality' (1993) 10 Yale J. Reg. 273.

76 One possible starting point is to allow gainsharing bonuses only where productivity targets are measured over a sufficiently large group of patients and physicians, the bonus measurement periods are for sufficiently long periods (such as no less than annually), and quality targets must be achieved in addition to productivity targets for bonus payments to be made. These safeguards reflect the assumption that financial incentives for cost-effective care are more moderate when based on groups of patients and groups of physicians and when cost-savings are measured over a sufficiently long period. The basic idea is to avoid incentives that bring too much economic pressure to bear on the treatment decisions made for any one patient. This avoids tempting any one physician to engage in zealous cost-cutting with any one patient over a short period of time in order to reap a bonus. These safeguards are discussed in detail in a 1986 GAO *Report on Physician Incentive Plans.* See *supra* note 21. The Department of Health and Human Services followed many of the Report's recommendations in developing the current regulations for financial incentives used by Medicare managed care plans. See 42 C.F.R. s. 417.479. For more extensive recommendations of how best to regulate gainsharing, see *supra* note 33.

77 See *supra* note 15.

PART FIVE

Free Trade Agreements: Strengthening or Undermining Access to Health Care?

13 The Agreement on Trade-Related Aspects of Intellectual Property Rights and Its Implications for Health Care

ROXANNE MYKITIUK AND MICHELLE DAGNINO

Ours is a world where knowledge and information have increasingly replaced goods and services as the ultimate source of power. Although global restructuring has led academics to examine the genesis and nature of 'intellectual property,' at least one area of the diverse study of intellectual property rights (IPR) – the implications of IPR for health-care delivery, access, and benefits – remains underresearched. This chapter addresses the role of the *Agreement on Trade-Related Aspects of Intellectual Property Rights*[1] (TRIPs) in health-care arrangements focusing, first, on its relevance for developing countries and, second, on its impact within Canada. The TRIPs may not seem to be an obvious subject for inclusion in a collection on fairness in the context of health care; however, in a political economy that favours 'innovation,' international trade agreements have become an important site where the fair allocation and distribution of health care benefits is played out.

There are a number of international trade agreements that deal with aspects of health,[2] but the TRIPs is particularly important in its implications for health care. TRIPs is a responsibility of the World Trade Organization (WTO). The WTO liberalizes trade and alters global governance by its impact on national policies and laws. WTO agreements arise from trade negotiations among countries that come to the bargaining table from vastly different positions of power and economic strength and that often are more of a response to business interests than to social welfare interests.[3] President of the International Council of Médecins sans Frontières, James Orbinski, has said: 'There is no question that WTO decisions have wide-ranging implications for health.'[4] We are concerned with two questions here: How do market-oriented norms and priorities encapsulated in TRIPs usurp social values in relation to the development and utilization of international property rights and biotechnology research? How do these norms and priorities, in turn, affect the way in which we understand the role of health and health care within our political economy?

The Political Economy of Biotechnology

Biotechnology – the use of biological organisms and processes for technological, and often commercial, ends – is one result of a postindustrial information society, which is characterized by the role that capital has in guiding the state to support productivity and innovation to bolster the competitiveness of the national economy.[5] Our discussion of biotechnology adopts a critical perspective that 'stands apart from the prevailing order of the world and asks how that order came about ... [It] does not take institutions and social power relations for granted but calls them into question by concerning itself with their origins and how and whether they might be in the process of change ... [It] is a theory of history in the sense of being concerned not just with the past but with a continuing process of historical change.'[6]

In taking this approach, we view biotechnology as an industry *and* as a social relation. The information society is fundamentally a capitalist society. Although forms of economic restructuring are affected by the vast changes in information technology (IT), they are not caused by it.[7] Contrary to claims that the state has been marginalized by globalization, the importance of the state in creating national policy has been strengthened, even as globalization has fundamentally altered the latter's direction. Although globalization has led to a decline in social welfare programming and a strengthening of capital, ultimately states continue to retain responsibility for legislating to support further economic development.[8] Creating forceful intellectual property laws to support biotechnology productivity is one such key activity of the state.[9]

Biotechnology affects the international political economy in a number of ways. The genetic modification (GM) of plants has increased farming capacities, for example, allowing crops that had been previously limited to certain climates to now be grown worldwide, and GM has created infestation-resistant strains of organisms.[10] Advanced technologies may broaden the gap between developing and developed states, as developed states adopt superior technologies. The increased appropriation of agricultural breakthroughs by private companies, versus public institutions, has constrained the ability of others to replicate or access such new resources because of patents and regulations concerning intellectual property. We suggest that the current global regime for intellectual property rights serves specific interests and creates a power relationship that is rooted in the commodification of knowledge. TRIPs commodifies social goods that were previously non-commodified and creates property out of goods that historically were never considered in such terms.[11]

Thus, the TRIPs represents a watershed in the history of intellectual property rights. The creation of this agreement as the guideline for the management of IPR worldwide reveals the essential role that global institutions have in creating new cultures of regulation that 'act as powerful vectors for the transmission of specific, culturally determined systems for codifying knowledge and as self-appointed arbiters of the 'normative' bases of global regulatory regimes.'[12] It also highlights the north-south divide over IPR, particularly concerning private and public benefits.

Globalization and capital interests have changed how the political economy of health is conceptualized. Innovations in biotechnology succeed because of three major assumptions about medicine and health:[13] (1) The determinants of health and illness are assumed to be almost entirely biological, having little or no relation to the socioeconomic circumstances. Solutions to health problems are therefore seen to lie entirely in the purview of medical treatment, while broader questions about social change towards health promotion are ignored. (2) medicine is presented as science – and therefore assumed to be all but infallible. More importantly, medicine is seen as capable and competent of producing a set conclusion, one that is purely 'scientific' and completely removed from the broader social setting. (3) Medicine is inherently assumed to be good for the health and well-being of society – the only problem being there is not enough of it to go around. Moreover, insufficient access, as a result of market restraints or other causes, is assumed to be solvable through the normal processes of democracy and pressure politics.[14] Problems of health care are thus normatively represented purely as science-based, generally ignoring that there are problems that are intertwined with socioeconomic circumstances and capital interests.

TRIPs in a Global Context

What Is TRIPs and What Are Patents?

The granting of pharmaceutical and biotechnological patents has been formally settled by the TRIPs. Yet, the agreement remains mired in controversy. TRIPs emerged from the Uruguay Round of the negotiations on the General Agreement on Tariffs and Trade (GATT), predecessor of the WTO, and is one among a series of agreements administered by the WTO. Accordingly, TRIPs sets out the rules for IPR that all member-countries of the WTO must accommodate in their own domestic legislation. Among the things that the TRIPs requires are exclusive patent rights; a minimum twenty-year patent term on pharmaceuticals; and non-discrimination, meaning that countries are not allowed to treat national and foreign inventions differently. All WTO countries are bound by TRIPs, although developing countries have been given a longer period than developed countries to change their laws so that they comply with their obligations under the TRIPs.[15] Should a country not meet its TRIPs obligations, others can take it before a trade tribunal. If it is determined that TRIPs has been breached, the complainant country can request authorization from the WTO to impose trade sanctions on the offending country in retaliation, including in other areas of trade.[16]

Any discussion of the TRIPs necessarily involves a definition of patents. A patent is a limited-term monopoly that prohibits anyone else from making, using, selling, or importing the patented invention without explicit permission or compensation. An invention is a thing, a way of making a thing, or way of doing something that is new, non-obvious and useful, and does not exist in nature in the same form. Patents are granted because a reciprocal relationship is imagined – the patentee makes full disclosure of the invention and in return acquires a very valuable monopoly right.[17] The largest incentive to patent an invention is to make money, which a patent holder can do in two ways: make and sell the invention to the public, insofar as the law permits and/or 'licence' the right of the patent to someone else. Patents are seen to be an important incentive to reward innovation.[18] At present, patents usually have to meet the specifications as outlined in national patent legislation and policy. Traditionally, patents, and IPR in general, have been the domain of national legislation.[19] The state balances the monopoly interests bestowed on the private holder of a patent with the social welfare interests of the public at large by, for example, limiting the life of a patent and sometimes allowing for compulsory licensing. But there are wide variations to patent laws from country to country, depending upon the countries' development objectives and economic strategy. Generally this means that intellectual property rights have been stronger in developed and weaker in less developed countries (LDCs). Forcing developing countries to adhere to IPR protection may have the effect of reducing global welfare overall.[20]

The origins of TRIPs as an international regime for the regulation of intellectual property rights can be traced to the late 1970s.[21] As a response to the growth in the trade of counterfeit goods, a hundred multinational corporations formed an anticounterfeiting coalition and, in 1979, the 'Agreement on Measures to Discourage the Importation of Counterfeit Goods'[22] was drafted. The Draft Code was picked up at the 1982 GATT meeting of trade ministers. The United States had been hoping for its belated adoption at that time. Instead, developing countries, led by India and Brazil, continued to dismiss any need for such a code. They argued that the World Intellectual Property Organization (WIPO) was an efficient multilateral forum for the protection of intellectual property standards and that the GATT had no jurisdiction over trademark counterfeiting. These differences were the result of a fundamental divergence in how to conceptualize intellectual property law. Developing countries held that intellectual property is a public good that should be used to promote economic development. Developed countries interpreted intellectual property to be a private right that should have the same rights to protection as granted in law to tangible property.[23] This conceptual divergence was at the core of the debate regarding protection of intellectual property regimes from the 1970s onwards. At the negotiations revising the *Paris Convention for the Protection of Industrial Property* (1883), which had established an international union for the protection of industrial property, the developing and developed countries divide became more pronounced. Developed countries pushed hard for effective enforcement mechanisms to protect trademarked goods; developing countries sought to retain the use of compulsory licensing, by which the government can allow someone other than the patent owner to produce the product or process without consent of the patent owner. This operates as a sanction against patent owners who do not actively use their registered patents, to protect against abuses arising from a large number of unused patents. With positions entrenched along these lines, signatories to the *Paris Convention* met at Geneva (1980), Nairobi (1981), and again in Geneva (1982 and 1984), but were unable to overcome their differences.[24]

It was clear to the developed countries that they were not making any headway in the negotiations. Meanwhile, the United States was becoming more adamant about the need to protect its national industries abroad. It turned away from the consensus-based WIPO towards bilateral trade measures linking access to U.S. markets with IPR compliance. In 1985 the GATT Council directed the Preparatory Committee of the GATT to identify issues for the forthcoming Uruguay Round. The United

States proposed the inclusion of all IPR in the GATT, over the objections, again, of Brazil and India. Other newly industrialized countries, however, in South East Asia in particular, supported the inclusion of IPR. They saw the GATT as providing a proper forum for dispute resolution not available within bilateral trade agreements.[25] Thus, on 30 July 1986, the Swiss and Colombian ambassadors to the negotiations presented a proposal that had the support of forty other delegations and, as a result, IPR was on the agenda at the Uruguay Round. From the 1987 negotiating plan to the 1994 adoption of the final text of the TRIPs, the biggest obstacle that the U.S.-led push for TRIPs faced was the objections of the developing countries. On the face of it, WTO member-countries were representing their own national interests. But these national interests were becoming increasingly aligned with business interests, most prominently so in the case of the United States:

> The official Uruguay Round negotiators were greatly concerned with reflecting the interests of multinational business and negotiations were conducted against the background of bilateral trade legislation introduced by the United States. With representatives of global corporate actors close to official negotiators throughout the Uruguay Round and particularly active once the details of the Agreement came to be discussed, the role of business representatives behind the scenes during the negotiations was crucial both in terms of providing the stimulus for making the link between intellectual property and trade in the GATT and bilateral context, and, at a practical level, in terms of providing the knowledge and drafting expertise that was often lacking among national delegations.[26]

This representation of corporate interests lay at the core of the negotiations from 1987 on. Faced with constant opposition to the TRIPs from the developing countries, the United States decided to bypass continuing multilateral discussions and, instead, threatened bilateral trade sanctions.[27] Making an example of India, the United States suspended the Generalised System of Preferences (GSP) tariff exemptions previously granted to Indian pharmaceutical products. This was costing India, the chief opponent of TRIPs, close to $60 million annually in lost exports. Cowed by such devastating losses, India weakened its resolve.[28] Throughout the TRIPs negotiations, access to U.S. markets, especially for agricultural countries that relied heavily on export to American markets, was central in the minds of delegates opposed to broader protection for intellectual property. By the end of the Uruguay

Round, therefore, the majority of developing countries no longer opposed the TRIPs.

The TRIPs negotiations bring the tension between developed and developing countries to the fore.[29] The Uruguay Round was monumental not only for IPR but for international trade as a whole: it was this round that led to the creation of the World Trade Organization. Although it emerged from GATT negotiations, the WTO holds responsibility for TRIPs, and as such, the WTO guides the current TRIPs climate. That the TRIPs negotiations may be categorized as pitting developing and developed countries against each other is significant, and betrays the core criticism of the WTO – that the agreements that emerge from it are the result of a process of bargaining away democratic sovereign rights. The WTO describes itself, however, as an institution that:

> is run by its member governments. All major decisions are made by the membership as a whole ... Decisions are normally taken by consensus. In this respect, the WTO is different from some other international organizations such as the World Bank and International Monetary Fund. In the WTO, power is not delegated to a board of directors of the organization's head. When WTO rules impose discipline on countries' policies that is the outcome of negotiations among WTO members. The rules are enforced by members themselves under agreed procedures that they negotiated, including the possibility of trade sanctions. But those sanctions are imposed by member countries, and authorized by the membership as a whole. This is quite different from other agencies whose bureaucracies can, for example, influence a country's policy by threatening to withhold credit. [30]

Such a description betrays the WTO's promise as being the bastion of embedded liberalism.[31] Rather, the WTO is guided by the interests of its most wealthy and powerful member-states. In the above quote, the WTO portrays itself as an institution of globalization. But critical scholars of globalization theory argue that the notion of state cooperation among developed and developing countries is unlikely, because globalization is fundamentally a continuance (even an acceleration) of capitalist social relations aided by state policies.[32] TRIPs is a particularly poignant example of how market norms guide state interests. TRIPs saw the emergence of multinational companies securing global trade regulation to the benefit of their own interests to an extent not previously witnessed in the history of IPR. Duncan Matthews argues that pharmaceutical company alliances linked with government action, and a distinct advantage on the part of the United States and the European Union over developing countries vis-à-vis IPR expertise have led to 'successful outcomes in the ... negotiations as far as business interests were concerned.'[33] The TRIPs negotiations were unique in the history of IPR for their emphasis on the role of national governments in promoting private business interests in a desire by states to increase innovation and maintain their competitiveness.

As established earlier, developing countries relinquished control over the regulation of intellectual property rights out of fear of U.S. trade sanctions, particularly in agriculture. The TRIPs was part of a package that conferred 'greater' agricultural rights on the developing countries, although arguably it only allowed them to keep what they already had.[34] Even more ironically, as patents are increasingly extended to seeds, agricultural countries are paying more for patented agricultural inputs.[35]

A frequently cited example of the inequality caused by IPR agreements such as TRIPs are the inordinate costs of some pharmaceuticals – costs that are completely out of reach for most people in developing countries. The enormous socioeconomic inequalities between developing and developed countries are further exacerbated when patent protection in accordance with TRIPs increases the inaccessibility of essential drugs.[36] One of the major issues of division during the TRIPs negotiations was the question of patents for pharmaceutical drugs. The European Union and the United States sought an extension of patent protection to twenty years, while others, including the developing nations, proposed that patents expire after fifteen years. The right to health and patents on medicines, particularly in developing countries, are becoming increasingly linked.[37] For example, in March 2001, the U.N. Commission on Human Rights found that access to drugs is one of the fundamental components of the right to health.[38] Prior to the Uruguay Round, few developing countries offered patent protection on pharmaceutical drugs, arguing that access to pharmaceuticals was a fundamental human right.[39] The introduction of patents in developing countries was presented as something that would provide greater incentives to the private sector pharmaceutical industry to undertake more research in tropical and other diseases common to developing countries. Yet, if patent protection may encourage further development, it can also support higher prices. The Commission on Intellectual Property Rights found that research and development takes place almost entirely with respect to diseases whose remedies have a large market in the developed world and that it has almost no impact on diseases that occur predominantly in developing countries.[40] For developing countries aiming to keep health care costs manageable, the widespread introduction of patents has led to significant tensions. Where life-saving drugs do exist – as in the case for HIV/AIDS – their costs are so high that in developing countries they are only available to the wealthy few.[41] The political economy of patenting becomes all the more significant when one considers that patents are at the core of the expansion of biotechnology, currently the twenty-first century's most pervasive technology.

Why TRIPs Is Relevant to Public Health Access: The Doha Round

Alongside disputes over national treatment laws, copyright issues, and neighbouring rights,[42] TRIPs negotiations proved to be contentious, but they did result in a comprehensive agreement. G10 and developing countries eventually agreed to sign on because they hoped that they would be able to benefit from greater access to advanced technologies and to win some trade concessions over the export of their agricultural and textile products.[43] As a result, many of the controversial issues – such as moral rights, rental rights, and parallel importation – were resolved largely in favour of the United States or held over for future negotiations. Issues that were resolved in favour of the developing countries were, for the most part, related to timelines for implementation, such as providing developing countries five years to comply with the terms of TRIPs.[44] Although TRIPs negotiations largely focused on pharmaceutical patents, the context of trade negotiations was generally seen as neglecting urgent public health needs with regard to questions of access.[45] In response to these criticisms, the issue of access to medicines was tabled at the WTO's ministerial meeting in Seattle in 1999. There the trade ministers became deadlocked primarily over the question of access to medicines being closely linked to patents. Two years later, in November 2001, the ministers met in Doha, Qatar, where they were able to conclude a declaration on the relation between TRIPs and public health. This declaration stands on its own, separate from the WTO Development Round that was initiated at Doha.[46]

To date, there are four nested texts – the original Agreement on Trade-Related Aspects of Intellectual Property Rights,[47] the 2001 Ministerial Declaration on the TRIPs Agreement and Public Health,[48] the Decision on Paragraph 6 of TRIPs (see below),[49] and the Chairman's

Statement[50] – that regulate the production and export of generic medicines and their importation and are directly related to public health interests. Options within a particular country are also circumscribed by that country's legislation; furthermore, participation in bilateral or regional trade agreements may limit rights that a country might otherwise have under the WTO.

The *Doha Declaration* was seen to be highly significant for a number of reasons, not least because it brought security and clarity to many developing countries in their efforts to develop sustainable health policies.[51] The most important issues were: (1) the least developed countries (LDCs) can refuse pharmaceutical patents in their national legislation promulgated before 2016 and (2) the Decision on Paragraph 6, on instructing the Council for TRIPs to find an expeditious solution to the problem of the difficulties faced by WTO members with insufficient or no manufacturing capacities in the pharmaceutical sector in making effective use of compulsory licensing under TRIPs. The Council for TRIPs was to report its progress to the General Council before the end of 2002.[52] Although pre-Doha most of the WTO member-countries had already recognized the need for compulsory licensing,[53] the Doha Round was the first time that the WTO members formally turned their attention to the issue of manufacturing capacity in relation to pharmaceuticals. This essentially involved two issues: (1) a confusing restriction in Article 31 of TRIPs, which allowed for the granting of compulsory licensing, but contained statement 31(f) that compulsory-licensed drugs must be limited almost exclusively to supplying the country's domestic market,[54] and (2) the widespread recognition that the right to use a compulsory licence was almost useless because most LDCs have little or no manufacturing capacity.[55] This motivated the Decision on Paragraph 6 of the Doha Declaration which brought attention to the circumstances of countries lacking domestic capacity.

The three major issues related to lack of domestic capacity are the lack of manufacturing capacity, a small domestic demand, and finding a source of supply. The 30 August 2003 decision of WTO members on Paragraph 6 was meant to overcome these three issues, through the clear granting of compulsory licensing capabilities for non-domestic markets. Briefly, the Decision on Paragraph 6 waived the obligations of an exporting member under Article 31(f) of TRIPs and a compulsory licence was granted to a country to the extent necessary for the purposes of producing the necessary pharmaceutical product(s) and its export to an eligible importing member.[56] A compulsory licence does not solve the problem, though. For example, no country has extensive experience using compulsory licences to deal with national emergencies. Past experience, however, leads one to believe that rather than issuing a compulsory licence, governments will negotiate with the patent holder for a reduced price.[57] Ultimately, although compulsory licensing can potentially solve an immediate health crisis, it will not address development objectives such as technology transfer.

Freedom to Produce?

This discussion has largely involved issues surrounding patents; however, not all countries in the world are obliged to patent holders. First, countries that are not members of the WTO can produce and export medicines without WTO complications because of their non-membership status. Second, under the Doha Declaration LDCs do not have to provide patent protection for pharmaceutical products or processes until 2016. But some LDCs have already begun to provide patent protection for pharmaceutical products either under trade agreements with the United States, or as part of negotiations with U.S. companies. Third, Brazil did not start granting patents on medicines until compelled to do so by the TRIPs. Thus, Brazil can make generic versions of pre-1995 drugs, with no need for a licence. Fourth, India only extended protection to pharmaceutical 'processes' (versus the normally granted patents on 'products'), and there is no requirement until 2005 for it to become compliant with TRIPs (and in the meantime India can make medicines not yet patented as products). Finally, there are other countries in which the patent-holder has not yet filed a patent application.[58]

It is clear that by itself the Decision on Paragraph 6 will not significantly improve access to medicines. A pressing problem will come in 2005, when drug-producing developing countries must comply with WTO rules, making it harder for them to export. Developing countries have so far been exempt from WTO drug-trade rules, and although LDCs will continue to be exempt until 2016, from 2005 developing countries without adequate drug production capacity will no longer have access to cheaper generic medicines.[59] This points to the hierarchy among developing countries that have sufficient funds to buy large quantities and possess negotiating power to achieve the best possible price quantities (that is, China, Egypt, Brazil, and India).[60] Although these countries form a distinct minority, they are often held up as the example of the drug-producing capacity of the developing world.

OXFAM has pointed out that the Decision on Paragraph 6 effectively replaces one double standard with another.[61] The original double standard that the WTO trade ministers were attempting to solve was the problem of insufficient drug production capacity that prevents developing countries from making effective use of compulsory licensing. The new double standard that results from the Decision on Paragraph 6 is the requirement that both the importing and the exporting country issue a compulsory licence. This effectively leaves most poor countries dependent upon a political decision made in another country to trigger the Paragraph 6 decision and meet their health needs. TRIPs has essentially stripped developing countries of their public health governance autonomy because their ability to rely on or create a source of affordable medicines for their population is restricted or even prohibited by an agreement created by the rich countries with little or no approval from the developing countries.[62]

TRIPs represents a far greater intrusion on national sovereignty than was the case with past multilateral trade agreements.[63] Benefits of TRIPs accrue mainly to the European Union countries and the United States. Thus, the WTO's capacity to maintain the 'embedded liberal compromise' appears weakened. This compromise is the basis upon which the WTO has built its promise of maintaining welfare states while liberalizing international trade. As such, this retreat to economic interests over social welfare has great implications for the future of international trade.

The TRIPs in Canada: Creating a Policy Tension

The impact of TRIPs is not limited to the distribution of affordable medicines worldwide and the exacerbation of the gap between the health care standards of the the developed and developing world. Even a developed country such as Canada faces important challenges to its publicly funded health care system as it struggles to cope with monopoly pricing by pharmaceutical and multinational companies. The remainder of this chapter will explore the policy tension between the social goal of ensuring a sustainable health care system that equitably distributes limited health care resources to produce the greatest health benefits across the population of Canada and the economic goals of promoting innovation and commercialization.

Over the past decade, in Canada and in other developed countries, vast public funds have been devoted to biotechnology research. Three of the most significant funders of biotechnology research in Canada – Genome Canada, the Canada Foundation for Innovation, and the Canadian Institutes of Health Research – have policies that either require or actively encourage grant applicants to partner with the private sector and obtain at least equivalent funding from there. These measures are part of a larger governmental strategy to develop biotechnology as a cornerstone of the Canadian economy.[64] The development of a Canadian biotechnology strategy is a key component of an overall industrial strategy aimed at reaping the benefits of a 'knowledge-based economy' to meet the challenges of globalization. The Organization of Economic Cooperation and Development (OECD) defines 'knowledge' in the 'knowledge-based economy' as 'the acquisition of intellectual property through learning or research.'[65] It is therefore important to recognize that the appropriation of research as intellectual property is an integral aspect of the knowledge-based economy, in general, and industrial strategy focused on biotechnology, in particular.

The federal government promotes biotechnology claiming that it will be basic to the new economy and that this in itself will be a social good as a result of Canada's enhanced competitiveness in a global economy. The government also emphasizes the *health benefits* that biotechnology will produce. Policy literature emphasizes that 90 per cent of the current uses of biotechnology worldwide are related to human health and that it is projected that this proportion will not go down. Thus, biotechnology is being promoted as a strategy that will help to develop the tools to improve the health and well-being of Canadians through, 'improved disease surveillance, diagnosis, treatment and prevention.'[66]

Patent protection plays a significant role in Canada's new biotechnology strategy.[67] The standard defence of the current expansive approach to gene patenting, for example, is that private investment in research is essential because of the high costs involved in conducting therapeutically useful research and in transferring research findings to the marketplace.[68] Investors, it is argued, demand strong protection for their intellectual property before they are willing to commit the required resources. Therefore, failure to provide strong IPR protection will result in a loss of jobs, a brain drain, and a loss of revenues, as investment flows to jurisdictions with more favourable regimes. A further loss will be the failure to realize the health benefits associated with technological advances in the biosciences. [69] This argument raises a number of important questions. For example, what constitutes 'strong' IPR protection, and would investors actually disinvest or fail to invest should Canada not provide 'strong' IPR protection? Also, is the primary goal of bio-technology patent policy a concern with better health through promot-ing research or is it about innovation?

Note that the availability of public, rather than private, support for scientific research is not constrained by scarcity but rather by compet-ing political priorities. In Canada governments have chosen to tie avail-able research support to the needs of industry. An example of the distorted impact that a public policy tied to the patent regime has on innovation is that many laboratories have avoided developing and offering diagnostic tests because of fears of patent infringement [70] or have stopped actively communicating their research results. [71] A study of all laboratory directors in the United States who were members of the Association for Molecular Pathology or listed on the *GeneTests.org* website found that 25 per cent had stopped performing a clinical genetic test because of a patent or licence, and 53 per cent had decided not to develop a new clinical genetic test because of a pre-existing patent or licence.[72] A survey about the licensing of genetic tests found that 20 per cent of 2,100 life science researchers delayed publishing their results for at least six months in order to file patent applications, deal with pos-sible patent liability, and/or resolve problematic intellectual property issues.[73] Where the research conducted was part of a university-corpo-rate partnership, publication delays were even greater. But, some ar-gued that without intellectual property protection, the tests would never even have been developed at all.[74]

Uncertainty about the legal reach of upstream patents means that risk-averse researchers must negotiate with multiple patent holders. This raises questions about the capacity of governments to shift the terms of the social contract represented by the granting of a patent by limiting economic returns to investors and inventors in favour of access to knowledge and products that benefit human health. International trade agreements – and TRIPs specifically – create barriers for those wanting to alter established patent rules with their strong emphasis on harmonization and patent protection.

TRIPs promotes a globally uniform regime of intellectual property laws and rights, whether in Tanzania, Germany, or Canada.[75] One of the most important aspects of the reach of this international trade law on intellectual property rights is the internationalization of Euro-American values. Regulatory regimes begin as local, culturally based systems of determining knowledge. Adoption of TRIPs was forced on the majority of the world's countries. TRIPs as an internationalized regime rests on a very particular form of regulation – one that follows traditional Euro-American intellectual property rights law. TRIPs has faced considerable controversy regarding its legitimacy as a global system of law and given rise to charges of cultural hegemony and 'bio-colonialism.'[76] Yet Canadian debate has been muted, although the federal government was an enthusiastic partner on the TRIPs negotiations. It was with the Myriad case that many Canadians became aware of the true effect of the current IPR regime in their own backyard.

Myriad Genetics is an American biotechnology firm that obtained patents on the *BRCA1* and *BRCA2* genes – genes related to some forms of breast and ovarian cancer. In summer 2001 Myriad informed publicly funded testing laboratories in Canada that their tests for *BRCA1/2* were in violation of Myriad's patent rights. Myriad demanded that any future testing be done through Myriad's affiliated genetic testing laboratories. The consequences are far-reaching. For example, in Ontario laboratories these tests cost approximately $1,150 per patient. In Myriad laboratories, this testing costs $3,800.[77]

In one case, Fiona Webster was a participant in a research study conducted at the Breast Cancer Research Unit of Women's College Hospital in Toronto. Webster had a significant family history of breast cancer. The issue that propelled her case into the newspaper headlines was one of timing. Webster was 6 months into the study and anxious to know her results. To that point only 60 per cent of the genetic mutations that could increase her susceptibility to breast cancer had been screened for. Webster had earlier indicated that, were it determined that she had a mutation, she would immediately seek a double mastectomy – a service that is fully publicly funded through the Ontario Health Insurance Plan (OHIP). She was informed that the genetic testing through the research study was going to take about a year, whereupon Webster found out from a genetic counsellor that Myriad Genetic Laboratory in Salt Lake City, Utah – a private commercial laboratory – could deliver test results within a number of weeks for a fee of U.S.$2,400. Webster requested that OHIP pay for the costs of her testing in Utah and was refused on the ground that OHIP 'does not pay for an experimental procedure.' OHIP would, however, pay for the double mastectomy, a procedure that would be unnecessary should the genetic test show no indication of a mutation.[78] As Flood, Stabile, and Tuohy discuss in chapter 1 (this volume), Ontario has an independent administrative board that citizens can appeal to in the event of a decision made by the government not to publicly fund a particular service or treatment.

Webster appealed to the Health Services Appeal and Review Board of Ontario in 1998.[79] But before her appeal was heard she received a donation allowing her to pay for the commercial genetic testing from Myriad. Subsequently, in 1999, the Board found in her favour, and this created an important precedent for other women in Ontario seeking access to the *BRCA1* and *BRCA1* genetic tests.[80]

The Webster case shows that the normative debate of needs versus rights has been transformed into one of needs over rights. The basis of OHIP's refusal to Webster was that a (new) genetic test was not a medically necessary service. OHIP policy promotes efficient social allocations of the health care budget and the best possible health care outcome for the largest possible number of people. Webster understandably approached the issue from her own perception of her health care needs. By entrenching in public policy a model of (intellectual) private property and private appropriation, TRIPs contributes to the promotion of a view of health care as a consumer good in preference to the social good implicit in the Canadian model of health care delivery.

A number of chapters in this volume (for example, those by Greschner and Jackman) focus on the increasing challenges to the limits of publicly funded health care. In some cases the failure of governments to serve particular patients will prove to be discriminatory. The overall pattern of increased challenges to government-imposed limits on publicly funded Medicare, however, is evidence of a shift towards a new concept of rights to health care. Such a conception of rights is in sympathy with the concept of property rights as promoted by TRIPs. In *A Philosophy of Intellectual Property Rights*, Peter Drahos argues that property is now understood to be 'the embodiment of a rights relationship between one person and another, or one person and many others ... a contest for the control of objects that people need or want.'[81] Through such conceptions of property, Canadians are beginning to believe that their access to health care is not only a basic need but also a fundamental proprietary right. This has emerged from a regime of IPR that is globalizing certain regulatory systems in order to facilitate the pursuit of particular interests or sustain relations of domination. Furthermore, as den Exter highlights in the next chapter, cross-border health care mobility may not seem to be the site of egalitarianism that we expect it to be. Although conceptually we imagine 'access' to mean 'without limits,' in the case of health care agreements, unlimited patient mobility rights seem to only serve short-term interests and may have irreversible repercussions for long-term health care.

Conclusion

We looked at TRIPs in two different contexts and at two different levels of analysis. In determining the allocation of pharmaceuticals and other forms of patented medical goods between developed and developing countries, we examined the TRIPs as an international regime of legally mandated obligations that have direct effects on the allocation of medical goods. TRIPs prioritizes a property rights regime as a matter of public policy, a priority that not only constrains health care budgets and health care allocations, but it also conditions a particular way of looking at health care goods. Distributive 'fairness' must contend not only with entrenched property rights. Now it must also incorporate into the social debate on the allocation of health care resources an outlook that favours a private appropriation regime. Both globally and locally, TRIPs undermines the case for health care as a public good. In any debate over fair allocation, TRIPs predisposes arrangements that favour capital accumulation in the guise of promoting innovation – for the public good.

NOTES

The support of the Health Law Institute of the University of Alberta, Genome Canada, and the Ontario Genomics Institute is gratefully acknowledged.

 1 Being Annex 1C to the Agreement Establishing the World Trade Organisation concluded during the Uruguay Round of GATT in 1994, http://www.wto.org/english/docs_e/legal_e/27-trips.pdf (accessed 12 May 2005).
 2 For a discussion of international trade agreements affecting health in the Canadian context, see E. Richard Gold, 'Health Care Reform and International Trade,' in Timothy A. Caulfield and Barbara von Tigerstrom, eds., *Health Care Reform and the Law in Canada* (Edmonton: University of Alberta Press, 2002) 223; Jon R. Johnson, 'How Will International Trade Agreements Affect Canadian Health Care?' (2002) *Commission on the Future of Health Care in Canada* [Romanow Commission], Discussion Paper No. 22.
 3 For support of this view, see generally Duncan Matthews, *Globalising Intellectual Property Rights: The TRIPs Agreement* (London: Routledge, 2002).
 4 James Orbinski, 'Health, Equity, and Trade: A Failure in Global Governance' in Gary P. Sampson, ed., *The Role of the World Trade Organization in Global Governance* (Tokyo: U.N. University Press, 2001) 223 at 235.

5 Roxanne Mykitiuk, 'Public Bodies, Private Parts: Genetics in a Post-Keynesian Era,' in Brenda Cossman and Judy Fudge, eds., *Privatization, Law, and the Challenge to Feminism* (Toronto: University of Toronto Press, 2002) 311.

6 Robert Cox with Timothy J. Sinclair, *Approaches to World Order* (Cambridge: Cambridge University Press, 1996) at 88–90.

7 See Christopher May, *A Global Political Economy of Intellectual Property Rights: The New Enclosures* (London and New York: Routledge, 2000).

8 *Ibid.*

9 *Ibid.* at 4.

10 *Ibid.* at 102.

11 See generally, *supra* note 7 at ch. 1.

12 Bronwyn Parry, 'Cultures of Knowledge: Investigating Intellectual Property Rights and Relations in the Pacific' (2002) 34:4 Antipode 679, at 680.

13 The following conceptions of medicine and health draw their inspiration from the work of Lesley Doyal, *The Political Economy of Health* (London: Pluto Press, 1981).

14 *Ibid.* at 13.

15 WTO, 'Fact Sheet: TRIPs and Pharmaceutical Patents – Developing Countries' Transition Periods' (Sept. 2003), http://www.wto.org/english/tratop_e/trips_e/factsheet_pharm04_e.htm (accessed 29 August 2005).

16 WTO, *Ministerial Declaration on the TRIPs Agreement and Public Health*, adopted 14 Nov. 2001, Doha, WT.IN(01)/DEC/02, 20 Nov. 2001 [*Doha Declaration*]; Carlos Maria Correa, *Intellectual Property Rights, the WTO and Developing Countries: The TRIPs Agreement and Policy Options* (London: Zed Books, 2000) at 1–21ff.

17 See generally, Michael J. Trebilcock *et al.*, 'Chapter Nine: Competition Policy and Intellectual Property Rights,' in *The Law and Economics of Canadian Competition Policy* (Toronto: University of Toronto Press, 2002) 573; Timothy A. Caulfield, E. Richard Gold, and Mildred K. Cho 'Patenting Human Genetic Material: Refocusing the Debate' (2000) 1 Nature Reviews Genetics 227 at 228–30.

18 Ted Schrecker, 'Benefit Sharing in the New Genomic Marketplace: Expanding the Ethical Frame of Reference,' in Bartha Maria Knoppers, ed., *Population and Genetics: Legal and Socio-Ethical Perspectives* (The Hague: Martinus Nijhoff, 2003) 405; Peter Drahos, 'Negotiating Intellectual Property Rights: Between Coercion and Dialogue,' in Peter Drahos and Ruth Maynes, eds., *Global Intellectual Property Rights: Knowledge, Access and Development* (Oxford/Houndsmill: Oxfam/Palgrave, 2002) 161 at 162; Sol Picciotto, 'Defending the Public Interest in TRIPs and the WTO,' in Drahos

and Maynes, ibid., 224, at 225; Ikechi Mgbeoji and Byron Allen, 'Patent First, Litigate Later! The Scramble for Speculative and Overly Broad Genetic Patents: Implications for Access to Health Care and Bio-Medical Research' (2002) 2 Can. J. of Law and Technology 83 at 83–6.

19 Ann Capling, 'Trading Ideas: The Politics of Intellectual Property,' in Brian Hocking and Steven McGuire, eds., *Trade Politics*, 2nd ed. (London: Routledge, 2004) 179 at 180.

20 *Ibid.* at 181.

21 The following section on the history of TRIPs and the TRIPs negotiations is drawn from Matthews, *supra*, note 3, ch. 2, 'The Origins of the TRIPs Agreement,' and from Michael Blakeney, *Trade-Related Aspects of Intellectual Property Rights: A Concise Guide to the TRIPs Agreement* (London: Sweet and Maxwell, 1996).

22 *Supra* note 3 at 9.

23 *Ibid.* at 11.

24 *Ibid.* at 12.

25 *Ibid.* at 17.

26 *Ibid.* at 29.

27 *Ibid.* at 3.

28 Blakeney, *supra* note 21 at 6.

29 *Ibid.* at 185.

30 WTO, 'Understanding the WTO: The Organization – Whose WTO Is It anyway?' http://www.wto.org/english/thewto_e/whatis_e/tif_e/org1_e.htm (accessed 29 August 2005).

31 See John Gerrard Ruggie, 'International Regimes, Transactions and Change: Embedded Liberalism in the Postwar Economic Order' (1982) 36 International Organization 379.

32 See generally, Ellen M. Wood, 'Labor, Class and State in Global Capitalism,' in Ellen M. Wood, ed., *Rising from the Ashes* (New York: Monthly Review Press, 1998) 3; Manfred Bienefeld, 'Capitalism and the Nation State in the Dog Days of the Twentieth Century,' in Leo Panitch and Ralph Miliband, eds., *Between Globalism and Nationalism: Socialist Register 1994* (London: Merlin Press, 1994) 94; Leo Panitch, 'Globalisation and the State,' in Panitch and Miliband, ibid. 60; Greg Albo and Jane Jenson, 'Remapping Canada: The State in an Era of Globalization,' in Wallace Clement, ed., *Understanding Canada: Building on the New Canadian Political Economy* (Montreal: McGill-Queen's University Press, 1997) 215.

33 *Supra* note 3 at Introduction.

34 *Ibid.*

35 *Ibid.* at 11.

36 Richard Elliot and Marie-Helene Brown, 'Patents, International Trade Law
and Access to Essential Medicines,' 1, www.accessmed-msf.org (rev.
version, May 2002) (accessed 15 January 2004).
37 See Philippe Cullet, 'Patents and Medicines: The Relationship between
TRIPs and the Human Right to Health' (2003) 79:1 International Affairs
139, where he states: 'Human rights law, in particular through the International Covenant on Economic Social and Cultural Rights, has made a
significant contribution to the codification of the human right to health
and our understanding of its scope.' See also Joseph, infra n41 at 438, and
M. Gregg Bloche, 'WTO Deference to National Health Policy: Toward an
Interpretive Principle' (2002) 5:4 J. of International Economic Law 825 at
827.
38 U.N. Commission on Human Rights, Resolution 2001/33, 'Access to
Medication in the Context of Pandemics such as HIV/AIDS,' in *Report on
the 57th Session*, 19 March to 27 April 2001, UN Doc. E/2001/23-E/CN.4/
2001/167.
39 Cullet, *supra* note 37 at 141.
40 Commission on Intellectual Property Rights, *Integrating Intellectual Property Rights and Development Policy* (London: CIPR, 2002) at 33.
41 This is not to say that the major pharmaceutical companies have not been
under intense pressure to lower prices in developing countries, a pressure
to which they have somewhat responded. As Sarah Joseph argues, we are
still to see whether the change being made by the big pharmaceutical
companies as to how they operate in developing countries is sincere: 'it
is fair to note that a number of pharmaceutical companies have become
involved in programs aimed at delivering patented drugs to poor countries at discounted prices, such as the U.N. "Accelerating Access" initiative. However, the programs have had limited success due to a number of
conditions attached to country participation by drug companies, such as
the surrender of any rights a state might have, even under the TRIPs, to
approve compulsory licenses, and Big Pharma's refusal to supply the
private as opposed to public sectors in target countries. It also seems that
the discounts have simply not been deep enough to facilitate access, and
were certainly not as low as the prices offered by generic drug makers.
Chronic shortages of the discounted drugs have also been reported.' Sarah
Joseph, 'Pharmaceutical Corporations and Access to Drugs: The "Fourth
Wave" of Corporate Human Rights Scrutiny' (2003) 25 Human Rights
Quarterly 425 at 436–7.
42 Neighbouring rights generally refers to relations arising from the programs of broadcasting or cable distribution organization.
43 Drahos, *supra* note 18.

44 *Supra* note 19 at 188.

45 Phillip McCalman, *The Doha Agenda and Development: Prospects for Intellectual Property Rights Reform* (Manila: Asian Development Bank, 2002). McCalman argues that 'a need for a special Declaration was not driven so much by a lack of clarity within the TRIPs Agreement, but rather the difficulty that many countries had in exploiting the flexibility contained within it,' at 3.

46 *Ibid.*

47 *Supra* note 3.

48 [*Doha Declaration*], *supra* note 16.

49 *Ibid.* at para. 6.

50 GATT doc. no. MTN.GNG/NGG11/W/76 (18 July 1990).

51 Richard Elliot and Marie-Helene Brown, 'Patents, International Trade Law and Access to Essential Medicines' 8, www.accessmed-msf.org (revised version, May 2002) (accessed 15 January 2004); Shinzo Kobori, 'TRIPs and the Primacy of Public Health' (2002) 9 Asia-Pacific Review 10; *supra* note 38, at 139.

52 WTO, 'Implementation of Paragraph 6 of the Doha Declaration on the TRIPs Agreement and Public Health. Decision of the General Council of 30 August 2003,' http://www.wto.org/english/tratop_e/trips_e/implem_para6_e.htm (accessed 29 August 2005) [Decision on Paragraph 6].

53 A licence granted pursuant to a court order requiring a patent holder to allow a third party to use a patented product or process, where the patent holder has failed to exploit it, or has exploited it on overly restrictive terms. www.austlii.edu.au/au/other/alrc/publications/issues/27/Glossary.doc.html (accessed 29 August 2005).

54 Frederick M. Abbott, 'The Doha Declaration on the TRIPs Agreement and Public Health: Lighting a Dark Corner at the WTO' (2002) 5 J. of International Economic Law 469 at 486–8.

55 *Ibid.*

56 Lena Sund, 'Intellectual Property Protection and Public Health' (2003) 201 Courier ACP-EU 201 at 28, http://europa.eu.int/comm/development/body/publications/courier/index_201_en.htm (accessed 29 August 2005).

57 In late 2001, in response to biological warfare threats, Canada and the United States considered the option of compulsory licensing. Ultimately neither of these countries pursued this option, instead getting the drug provided by the manufacturer at half-price. *Supra* note 54 at 486–8.

58 Elliott and Brown, *supra* note 51.

59 Ruth Mayne, 'The Recent Agreement on WTO Patent Rules' (2003) 201 Courier ACP-EU at 31, http://europa.eu.int/comm/development/body/publications/courier/index_201_en.htm (accessed 29 August 2005).

60 Frederick M. Abbott, 'Canada and the Decision on Implementation of Paragraph 6 of the Doha Declaration on the TRIPs Agreement and Public Health' (21 Oct. 2003). http://www.aidslaw.ca/Maincontent/issues/cts/patent-amend/Implement-Paragraph6-Waiver.ppt (accessed 29 August 2005).

61 *Supra* note 56.

62 *Ibid.*

63 *Supra* note 19 at 180.

64 Ontario Ministry of Health and Long-Term Care, 'Genetics, Testing and Gene Patenting: Charting New Territory In Healthcare' (Jan. 2002) 4, at 44, www.health.gov.on.ca./english/public/pub/ministry-reports/geneticsrep02/report_e.pdf (accessed 29 August 2005).

65 OECD, *Biotechnology: Economics and Wider Impacts* (Paris: OECD, 1989).

66 Canadian Biotechnology Strategy Task Force, *Health Sector Consultation Document: Renewal of the Canadian Biotechnology Strategy* (Ottawa: Industry Canada, 1998) at 3.

67 *Supra* note 9.

68 The argument and discussion that takes place over the following page borrows heavily from: Schrecker, *supra* note 18.

69 *Supra* note 7.

70 Mildred K. Cho *et al.*, 'Effects of Patents and Licences on the Provision of Clinical Genetic Testing Services' (2003) 5:1 Journal of Molecular Diagnostics 3 at 3.

71 *Ibid.*

72 *Ibid.*

73 Jon F. Merz et al., 'Diagnostic Testing Fails the Test' (2002) 415 Nature 577.

74 *Ibid.*

75 Matthews, *supra* note 21, generally at ch. 1.

76 *Ibid.*

77 R. Benzie, 'Ontario to Defy U.S. Patents on Cancer Genes,' *National Post*, 20 September 2001 at A15.

78 C. Abraham, 'The Politics of Hope,' *Globe and Mail*, 17 July 1998 at A2.

79 Decision on file with the author.

80 See C. Abraham, 'Tenacious Woman Scores Medical Victory,' *Globe and Mail*, 27 August 1999 at A1; see also P. Kaufert, 'From the Laboratory to the Clinic: The Story of Genetic Testing for Hereditory Breast Cancer,' in Penny van Esterik, ed., *Head, Heart and Hand: Partnerships for Women's Health in Canadian Environments* (Toronto: National Network on Environments & Women's Health, 2003) 487 at 499–501

81 P. Drahos, *A Philosophy of Intellectual Property Rights* (Aldershot: Dartmouth, 1996) at 4.

14 Patient Mobility in the European Union

ANDRÉ DEN EXTER

In the European Union (EU) issues of access to and allocation of health care services are primarily under the jurisdiction of individual national governments. Recently, however, EU institutions such as the European Court of Justice (ECJ) have intervened and exerted their own influence upon this otherwise national endeavour. This can be seen in the Court's rulings on the cross-border mobility of patients and, thus, on the portability of health care rights. The provisions in the European Communities Treaty (*EC Treaty*) relating to mobility and portability are based on free market principles and were not originally intended to encompass health care. Since the *Decker* and *Kohll* rulings, however, it is now settled that health care services do fall within the scope of the *EC Treaty*.[1] With respect to both these and more recent rulings on cross-border health care, one may wonder what will be the consequences for patient mobility in the European Union and what will be the consequences for the future sustainability of social health insurance in Europe.

This chapter examines the influence of European Community law, particular with regard to the role of the ECJ, and argues that common market principles have strengthened the rights of patients looking for health care abroad. This development affects national decision-making on access to and allocation of health care resources, including the purchase of health care services by social security institutions. The borders between countries are increasingly disintegrating, and this may have dramatic consequences for a country like Canada, adjacent as it is to the United States, which has no apparent aspirations in the direction of universal health insurance and which allows a much greater role than Canada for the private sector. As Canada reflects on its participation in international agreements such as the North American Free Trade Agreement (NAFTA), there may be lessons to be learned from experiences in the European Union regarding what are likely to be future sources of pressure for liberalization of Canada's health care system. The great challenge for Canada, as it is for the European Union, will be how to balance individual rights to health care with the goal of ensuring universal access for all.

First, this chapter examines aspects of health care policy that are directly governed by the EU, namely, public health. Then it turns to an examination of how the goal of trade liberalization within the EU has affected the management by EU countries of their own health insurance systems.

EC Law and Public Health

According to the *EC Treaty*'s provision regarding public health (article 152),[2] the Union has supranational competence to oversee a public health policy of preventing disease and promoting health. Other health care services fall within the jurisdiction of the member-states' national governments. With the ratification of the *Treaty of Amsterdam* (1997) special emphasis has been placed upon certain areas important to public health, for example, in the veterinary and phytosanitary fields. Article 152 describes measures in relation to the quality and safety of organs, substances of human origin, and blood and blood derivates.[3]

The public health provision excludes the organization of health services and the delivery of medical care from EU policy. As a result of the subsidiarity principle, this remains the explicit responsibility of member-states.[4] Although national authorities have in theory exclusive competencies vis-à-vis the organization, financing, and delivery of health care services, this jurisdiction is affected by policy decisions made at the European level and by provisions of EU law designed for the benefit of the internal market. The impact of these provisions on the health sector, however, is incomplete and differs from provision to provision. In an attempt to achieve a more coherent and effective approach to health issues across all different policy areas, the European Commission has proposed a new public health approach that would set out a broader health strategy for the EU.[5] The Commission's proposal emphasizes links with health-related initiatives in other policy areas and encompasses the free movement of articles, consumer protection, the environment, and agriculture. Within these sectors, there are a significant number of legislative norms related to health protection, for example, the legislation on consumer protection.[6]

EU consumer protection legislation includes a number of directives related to public health.[7] In terms of protecting consumers from potentially harmful medical products, the *Directive on Product Liability 85/374/ EEC (Directive 85/374)* may be applied, as it gives consumers the right to claim compensation from the producer of defective products.[8] *Directive 85/374* aims to harmonize to a large extent national law on producer liability[9] and acknowledges the difficulties inherent in the harmonization process for (candidate) member-states where consumers already benefit from advanced protection and thus allows for the principle of minimum harmonization. Member-states may, in the areas covered by *Directive 85/374*, maintain or introduce more stringent consumer protection measures, as long as they are compatible with the *EC Treaty*, especially with Articles 28 and 30. Several applicant countries have taken *Directive 85/374* as a model to define their own national product liability legislation.[10]

EC Internal Market Law and Access to Health Care

Notwithstanding the significance of Article 152 and the provisions that relate to public health, the most important treaty provisions in this regard are those that concern the internal market rules and how they affect health-related rights. According to Article 14(2), the internal market 'shall comprise an area without internal frontiers in which the free movement of goods, persons, services and capital is ensured in accordance with the provisions of this *Treaty*.' Under certain circumstances, EU citizens may even derive specific rights emanating from the 'free movement' provisions. For patients, the most relevant provisions here are for the free movement of goods, persons, services.[11]

With regard to the free movement of persons, relevant *EC Treaty* provisions include the freedom of movement for 'workers' (art. 39–42) and the rights of 'establishment' (art. 43–44). These have, in turn, been further substantiated by secondary legislation.[12] The free movement for workers entails, inter alia, the right to stay in a member-state for the purpose of employment in accordance with the provisions governing the employment of nationals of that state as laid down by law, regulation, or administrative action. As regards the right of establishment, this includes the right to take up and pursue activities as self-employed persons and to set up and manage undertakings under the conditions laid down for a state's own nationals. Interpreted in EU law, this includes a right of access to the territory of the member-states in order to carry out the economic activity in addition to a right to remain on the territory for that purpose.[13] An exception to the free movement of persons is granted in article 39(3), which permits member-states to limit the free movement of persons 'on grounds of public policy, public security and public health.' The application of the derogation in article 39(3) is governed by *Directive 64/221/EEC* (*Directive 64/221*).[14] The only diseases or disabilities that justify a refusal of entry of workers, self-employed people, and recipients of services are those listed in an annex, article 4 of *Directive 64/221*.

The provisions relating to the free movement of persons are primarily relevant for health professionals who want to enter the employment markets of the European Union. In view of the barriers erected to the mobility of (health) professionals, the European Council issued various directives regulating the mutual recognition of professional qualifications. The guiding principle is that the host member-state cannot refuse access to membership in a regulated profession if the applicant is fully qualified for that profession in his home member-state. Consequently, nationally accredited parties competent to authorize health professionals to practise within their own territory are obliged to recognize qualifications obtained in another member-state.[15]

The free movement provisions are relevant not only to health professionals, but also to patients. Free movement is not restricted to 'workers,' and relatives, tourists, and other categories of EU citizens can also make an appeal to benefit from this provision. Article 22 of *Coordination regulation 1408/71* (*Regulation 1408/71*), in conjunction with article 39, entitles cross-border workers to access the health care system in their country of residence; emergency care in case of temporary residence abroad; and care abroad that is pre-authorized by the patient's insurer or the competent (national) health authority. *Regulation 1408/71* aims to coordinate the different social security systems in the member-states, but the free movement of patients remains problematic. A major problem with cross-border health care is how to regulate and finance it. Some member-states fear an influx of patients from those member-states that lack facilities and/or provide lower-quality care. Rulings from the European Court of Justice, simplifying cross-border health care, have only strengthened this fear.[16]

The regulation of patient mobility is provided for in article 22 of *Regulation 1408/71*. Although member-state authorities are authorized to define the conditions for entitlements, an overrestricted interpretation of article 22(1)(a) would 'cause a significant obstacle to the freedom of movement of persons whose conditions necessitate continuous and

· regular medical treatment such that they will be likely to require immediate benefits in the event of a stay in the territory of another member-state.'[17] Regulating patient mobility requires an adequate authorization policy adopted by (secondary) law, that includes the relevant procedures to be used when citizens incur health care in another member-state.

Since precedents set in *Decker* and *Kohll*, the ECJ has been confronted with a growing number of cases questioning the legitimacy of pre-authorization, in view of internal market principles.[18] In the joint case of *Smits* and *Peerbooms*, Mrs Smits suffers from Parkinson's disease.[19] The Dutch social insurance fund (*Ziekenfonds*) refused reimbursement for specific multidisciplinary hospital treatment costs that she incurred in a German clinic. Unlike in Canada, the Dutch equivalent of Medicare is comprised of several social insurance providers. Justifying its decision, the social insurer in question said that satisfactory and adequate treatment for Parkinson's disease was available in the Netherlands and that the specific clinical treatment offered in Germany provided no additional advantage. Thus, it was deemed not 'medically necessary' that Mrs Smits undergo treatment at the German clinic.

The second claimant, Mr Peerbooms, fell into a coma after a road accident. He was transferred to a hospital in the Netherlands and then transferred, in a vegetative state, to the university clinic in Innsbruck, Austria, where he received special intensive therapy using neurostimulation. In the Netherlands that technique was considered experimental and to be used only in certain circumstances. Pursuant to guidelines in effect in the Netherlands, Mr Peerbooms would not have qualified for such experimental treatment because of his age. Thus, his sickness insurance fund refused to pay the costs of his treatment.

In both cases, the ECJ had to make a determination based on the pre-authorization rule, and whether such a rule in the particular circumstances constituted a barrier to the freedom to provide services. In contrast to *Decker* and *Kohll* (dealing with non-hospital care within a reimbursement system), *Smits/Peerbooms* concerned access to hospital care services for which the sickness fund had not contracted, and which, within the Netherlands, is provided on a 'benefit-in-kind' basis.[20] The Court agreed that sickness funds should not be exposed to the cost of hospital services for which they have not contracted. However, the pre-authorization condition, as applied by the authorities in the Netherlands, was criticized for its potentially discriminatory effect. In the Netherlands, the general legal rule under which the costs of medical treatment are covered is in instances where the treatment is found to be 'normal in the professional circles concerned.'[21] This expression, however, is open to a number of interpretations, depending in particular on whether what is 'normal' is considered as such in Dutch medical circles (this narrow interpretation being favoured by the national court in the Netherlands). In contrast, the ECJ decided that to allow only treatment that is habitually carried out on national territory, and based on scientific views prevailing in national medical circles and which determine what is or is not 'normal,' does not offer sufficient guarantees to patients that the treatment guidelines in place are objective, non-discriminatory, known in advance, and not used arbitrarily. Moreover, such a focus on national conceptions of 'normal' will make it likely that Dutch providers will always be preferred in practice.[22] The ECJ found that where treatment is sufficiently tried and tested by international medical science, refusal of the prior authorization cannot be justified. Further, to satisfy the 'normal' criterion, a member-state 'must take into consideration all the relevant available information, including, in particular, existing scientific literature and studies, the authorized opinions of specialists and the fact that the proposed treatment is covered or not covered by the sickness insurance system of the member-state in which the treatment is provided.'[23]

From this case, it became clear that member-states must apply the pre-authorization procedure consistently and that patients cannot be denied health care abroad arbitrarily (that is, there have to be non-discriminatory, transparent procedures and appeal mechanisms). For patients entitled to benefit-in-kind services, such as in the Dutch system, this ruling means that it should be just as easy to receive medical treatment from a foreign non-contracted provider as it is to obtain it from a non-contracted provider in the country of insurance. As such, the ECJ's interpretation of communal pre-authorization conditions creates new opportunities for extended access to health care abroad.[24]

Subsequent to *Smits/Peerbooms*, the ECJ ruled on two more or less identical situations in the Dutch mixed case of *Müller-Fauré/Van Riet*.[25] Here, the Court consolidated and clarified its previous reasoning on prior authorization, at least concerning inpatient hospital care. However, the Court also confirmed that there are several reasons that may justify requiring prior authorization where social health insurance funds cover benefits provided in another member-state. These reasons include: the protection of public health in as much as the system of agreements is intended to ensure that there are high-quality, balanced medical and hospital services open to all; to guarantee the financial balance of the social security system; and, finally, to enable managing authorities to control expenditures for, and the planning of, health care services. The Court noted that concerns regarding undermining the financial balance of the social security system were particularly valid vis-à-vis hospital care. In the case of hospital services, according to the ECJ, it is well known that to ensure sufficient access to a wide range of hospital services and to contain costs, careful planning is required regarding the number of hospitals, their geographic distribution, the mode of their organization, and the equipment with which they are provided.[26] Nonetheless, the conditions attached to the grant of authorization must be justified and satisfy the requirement of proportionality, and such a prior authorization scheme must likewise be based on a procedural system that is easily accessible and capable of being challenged in judicial or quasi-judicial proceedings.[27]

With respect to outpatient (non-hospital) health care, however, as in *Müller-Fauré* (that is, dental care), the Court was not convinced that abolishing prior authorization would have a system-undermining effect. According to the Court, 'there was no evidence that indicated that the removal of the prior authorization requirement for that type of care would give rise to patients travelling to other countries in such large numbers, despite linguistic barriers, geographic distance, the cost of staying abroad and lack of information about the kind of care provided there, and that the financial balance of the social security system would be seriously upset.'[28] Therefore, applying the free movement principles, in case of non-hospital services, there was no justification for requiring prior authorization.

Consequences for Patients and Member-States

Although the questions raised in these proceedings concerned individual cases, the implications of the ECJ rulings are nevertheless considerable, both for patients and for member-states of the European Union.

First, the Court's rulings enable patients to search for non-hospital services that are not available in their home country or, if available, are not available in a timely fashion. One should keep in mind, however, that without prior authorization, social health insurance providers are still fully entitled to reimburse only costs up to the maximum amount applicable in the claimant's country of residence. For that reason, the Court did not consider the removal of the administrative prior authorization condition to be a serious threat to the financial balance of the social security system, since it had to bear the cost of treatment when received in the patient's home country anyway. Patients seeking non-hospital care in other EU nations without prior authorization must bear any additional costs above and beyond the relevant tariff provided for in their own country.

The ECJ has specified the conditions that member-states must meet when restricting citizens' claims on social security (including health care) entitlements abroad. Although the individual rulings seem prima facie clear, general conclusions on the effects on cross-border care in the EU, as such, are much less so given that social security systems vary by country. Nonetheless, one can derive some general conclusions relevant to member-states. First, it has now been established that medical services fall within the scope of the EC treaty provision on free movement of services, even hospital services. Consequently, national social security rules cannot be used to exclude implementation of the free-movement provision.[29] This applies to insurance arrangements, such as those in the Netherlands, that provide benefits in kind, but also to hospital services provided by a national health service such as exists in Canada. The U.K. government unsuccessfully attempted to exempt its National Health Service from the ambit of Article 50 of the *EC Treaty* since the NHS provides services directly rather than reimbursing the cost of services received.[30] The ECJ noted 'that a medical service does not cease to be a provision of services because it is paid for by a national health service or by a system providing benefits-in-kind.'[31]

Second, the ECJ has also, on occasion, made explicit that EU law does not undermine the power of the member-states to organize their respective social security systems.[32] In the absence of harmonization at the EU level, each member-state may pass legislation pursuant to which citizens have a right or duty to be insured with a social security scheme, and, second, the conditions for entitlement to benefits.[33] Moreover, it is not incompatible with EU law for a member-state to establish, with a view towards achieving its aim of limiting costs, a negative list excluding certain products or services from reimbursement.[34] It follows that EU law cannot, in principle, have the effect of requiring a member-state to extend the list of medical services paid for by its social insurance system.[35]

Nonetheless, in exercising its powers, the member-state must not disregard EU law. It follows from this that the list of insured medical treatments must be drawn up in accordance with objective criteria, which are known in advance, and without reference to the origin of the service (non-discrimination). In the Netherlands, the health insurance system is not based on a pre-established list of types of treatment for which payment will be guaranteed; rather the legislature has enacted a general rule providing that all costs of medical treatment will be assumed provided that the treatment is 'normal in the professional circles concerned.'[36] It is thus largely up to the discretion of the social health insurers to decide which types of treatment satisfy that condition; however, in applying that criterion, these insurers must now interpret it on the basis of what is sufficiently tried and tested by *international* medical science. This may mean that where a certain treatment has sufficiently been tried and tested by international science, authorization by the sickness fund could not be refused on the grounds that it is not presently provided in the Netherlands. The only justifiable reason for refusal of authorization would be where, given the need to maintain an adequate supply of hospital care and to ensure the financial stability of the sickness insurance system, the 'same or equally effective treatment can be obtained without undue delay' at a contracted provider.[37]

It should be noted that in determining whether 'the same or equally effective treatment can be obtained without undue delay,' the mere fact that a person is on a waiting list does not necessarily mean that the treatment is unavailable. 'Undue delay' should be determined as the period within which medical treatment is necessary with respect to the patient's medical condition and history (or, perhaps in countries like the United Kingdom that have maximum waiting times, where a patient has had to wait longer than this guaranteed time). Moreover, those member-states, like the Netherlands, that use the 'normal criterion' in determining entitlements to coverage will not be required to allow their citizens to obtain treatment in any hospital in any EU country unless that treatment is both accepted in international medical circles and is not sufficiently available in the home country (medical necessity criterion).

Third, as mentioned above, the larger public interest in maintaining a sustainable social insurance system may be accepted as justifying barriers to freedom to provide medical services in the context of a hospital infrastructure.[38] Member-states need to determine whether their respective national rules can be legitimately justified in the light of such overriding reasons. In accordance with settled case law, it is necessary to ensure that they do not exceed what is objectively necessary for the given purpose and that the same result cannot be achieved by less restrictive rules. As determined in *Müller-Fauré/Van Riet*, these requirements apply regardless of the type or nature of the health care system (for example, whether a social insurance system as in the Netherlands or a national health service as in the United Kingdom).[39]

Fourth, and finally, the various ECJ rulings leave some unsettled questions, particularly given that the difference between hospital (in-patient) and non-hospital (outpatient) care is not always that clear. For example, some surgical services may be provided in a hospital or in an outpatient clinic. Moreover, certain types of care are only partly hospital-based, for example, hospital treatment combined with admission to an outpatient clinic. Disagreement about the nature of the provided care concerned may give rise to legal uncertainty among the insured and lead to more litigation. Patients need to be particularly aware of whether the provided service will be classified as a hospital service. In such a case if a patient has not obtained prior authorization before receiving treatment in another member-state, then he or she may be denied reimbursement.[40] In a recent ruling, the ECJ confirmed the nexus between the need for prior authorization and hospitalization, finding that where the 'multidisciplinary treatment of pain which the claimant envisages [...] involves her hospitalization,'[41] then this necessitated the patient obtaining prior authorization. In contrast, the District Court in Maastricht concluded that a special type of physiotherapy, which requires hospital admission, should not be considered to be hospital care, since it is generally qualified as non-hospital care.[42] These contrasting cases show that the difficult question of what constitutes hospital or non-hospital care is decisive for determining whether prior authorization is required and thus whether patients will be reimbursed for the costs of treatment received in other member-states. However, in some cases there may be no *communis opinio* among medical professionals about whether or not hospitalization is necessary. Such patients searching for alternative treatment options in other member-states without prior authorization take a considerable financial risk. Arguably, at least, hospitalization should be interpreted in the patient's favour (as opposed to that of the national authorities), meaning that the place of actual treatment should be decisive in interpreting whether hospitalization is required.[43] Any other interpretation may create a perverse incentive for social insurance providers to organize outpatient care in a hospital sphere for merely opportunistic reasons.[44]

Given the continuous organizational changes and innovations in health care arrangements, one may question whether the criterion of hospital or non-hospital care is appropriate in combination with the authorization requirement. This raises the question of alternative approaches, including the removal of the authorization procedure for inpatient care.

Future Approaches to Patient Mobility

The ECJ's approach to patient mobility has been both welcomed and criticized. Patients welcomed the rulings on cross-border health care. The governments of several member-states, however, responded with apocalyptic predictions about the future financial viability of their social security systems. There was also a concern expressed over losing what some viewed as the last bastion of sovereignty.[45] The reality is, however, that while the ECJ rulings have certainly eroded the 'territoriality' of member-states' social security systems in theory, this has not yet resulted in massive flows of patients crossing national borders.[46] Indeed, one may question whether the large-scale movement of patients from member-state to member-state will ever happen, given that patients prefer to be treated just 'around the corner' and that extralegal barriers exist for border-crossing patients (such as language or culture).

Apart from the ECJ's role in removing barriers to patient mobility, we see that national sovereignty in the field of health care is being challenged by the practice of improving transnational mobility, notably in border areas. Several countries already collaborate in 'Euregios in health care,' which are pilot projects designed to remove impediments to the free flow of patients and health services. Neighbouring health institutions and purchasers in border areas have concluded agreements regarding access to border-crossing patients. Often, these agreements concern highly specialized types of health care, requiring very expensive equipment and specialized staff. The flourishing of these 'centres of excellence' throughout the European Union would not only eliminate the need for member-states to duplicate investment in the same type of care, but at the same time they would also ensure a more optimal use of these centres (given that higher quality care in certain highly technical fields is often associated with high turnover).[47]

These cross-border arrangements are now expanding highly specialized centres of excellence. Pilot projects in Belgium, Germany, Luxembourg and the Netherlands have promoted complementarity for existing medical services (for example, regular interventions in the fields of surgery, ophthalmology, rehabilitation, and ambulance transportation).[48]

Such experiments are particularly interesting given the potential that better and more strategic use of resources could result in reduced waiting times and also help better address the fluctuating demands associated with tourist areas.[49]

Cross-border contracts are appropriate instruments for guaranteeing patients a *certain* level of quality of care, as agreed upon, and for arranging the level of remuneration for the contracted care. These contracts do not respond to variations in quality of care as provided in different member-states. These differences are even more apparent since enlargement of the European Union in 2004,[50] and they make painfully clear that contractual arrangements also require legal measures at the EU level to regulate and ensure minimum safety and quality standards. Because these collaborative initiatives in health care are mainly based on *Regulation 1408/71*, updating the regulation would be a further contribution to simplifying patient mobility.

Updating EU law requires, first of all, adequate information about various matters such as the diversity of provided services, tariffs, qualitative differences in services, and waiting lists. At the EU level, this could be realized by permanent mechanisms that collect data on tariffs, patient flows, quality issues, and so forth. These data may enhance collaboration in the purchase of cross-border health care, subsequently enhancing patient mobility. Such an approach would be based on the exchange of best practices; the 'open method of co-ordination' (OMC). To increase coordination and convergence of social security systems, OMC introduces a strategy of common goals and/or guidelines to be laid down at the EU level. Progress is measured against jointly agreed upon indicators, pursuant to which best practices are identified and compared.[51] The OMC is a political process that supplements EU legislative procedures.[52] Its 'process-driven' approach aims to enhance the convergence of the diverse national systems.

In the field of health care, common policy goals and/or guidelines include, among others, solidarity, access to high-quality care, financial sustainability of social security schemes, and non-discrimination. Identified indicators include, inter alia, the level and quality of care, and accessibility. Measuring outcomes of national health policies enables member-states to compare differences in outcomes and, consequently, to discuss and formulate uniform EU standards regarding best practices of patient care.

Modernizing EU regulations and introducing OMC may provide the initial impetus towards more fundamental change, that is, changing the *EC Treaty*. This has been discussed during a reflection process initiated by the European Commission.[53] Apart from improving patient mobility, a change to the *EC Treaty* could improve legal certainty regarding the application of European rules to health care. Although the European Commission has not gone into much detail, such a change should not only be in line with the underlying principles of the ECJ's rulings on cross-border care, but also recognize the member-states' sovereignty in organizing and financing health care services. Recognition of the right to health care abroad at the level of EC principles could be considered as a first step towards an 'internal market of health care.' But harmonization at the level of principles is not enough. As well as recognizing patients' right to mobility, the *EC Treaty* must also guarantee a minimum set of common standards of quality for health services, taking into account the more political approach of the OMC. This could lead to a 'European standard of due care.'[54]

A change to the *EC Treaty* could be incorporated into the draft text of the *European Union Charter on Human Rights*.[55] In this European 'bill of rights,' article II-35 stipulates that 'everyone has the right of access to preventive health care and the right to benefit from medical treatment under conditions established by national laws and practices. A high level of human health protection shall be ensured in the definition and implementation of all Union policies and activities.' According to the explanatory text, the principles set out in Article II-35 are based on the current provision for public health (art. 152) and the health provision in the *European Social Charter* (art. 11). As such, it reaffirms existing rights. But apart from consolidating existing law, it should also embrace innovative rights, such as patient mobility as established by the ECJ. To do this, measures need to be taken at both the EU and member-state levels to enhance patient mobility, and new legal measures are required to ensure 'European standards of due care.' This would enhance the meaning of the rights and obligations as enshrined in EU law and, therefore, enhance legal certainty.

Patient Mobility in an Enlarged Union

On 1 May 2004, ten new countries entered the European Union.[56] Prior to accession, however, the new member-states had to transpose the *acquis communautaire*, that is, the legal framework of EC law, into their national law. This *acquis* covers the entire framework of EU law (*EC Treaty* provisions, regulations, directives, and decisions, and the juris-prudence of the ECJ), focused on the internal market provisions, but not exclusively. In fact, the full *acquis* covers thirty-one chapters of EU policy to be incorporated in national law, comprising the entire body of EU legislation that has been accumulated and revised over the past forty years.[57]

Preparing for accession, the European Council developed a pre-accession strategy. In so-called partnerships, the Council assisted appli-cant countries in setting principles, priorities, and general conditions for accession.[58] The intent was that these bilateral partnerships would support each country in developing both a national program for taking up the *acquis* and a timetable for its realization. Given the magnitude of the 'approximation of laws' process, the strict timetable for incorpora-tion and the fact that new member-states are just finishing the 'first wave of health system reforms,'[59] it will not come as a surprise that these countries are facing serious problems incorporating EU law, at least in the field of health care. The new member-states' respective legal frameworks on health care policy are not fully 'Europe compatible' (at least not yet).[60] Given the fledgling state of both their health insurance systems and the legal frameworks supporting them, one must question the effects of enlargement on patient mobility and the possible implica-tions of the ECJ's rulings on cross-border care.

Regulation 1408/71 oversees the coordination of social security sys-tems in the European Union. This regulation, covering the right to health care abroad, has been identified as part of the 'hard core' *acquis*. This means that new member-states, from 1 May 2004, must fulfil the (legal and administrative) conditions with respect to border-crossing patients. Will there be a significant outflow of patients from these new member-states to 'old' Europe?

First, there have been several 'waves of accession' (for example, the accession of Spain and Portugal in 1986 and Austria, Finland, and Sweden in 2000). EU accession to the East has been often compared with that of the Mediterranean countries, which were at that time confronted with more or less similar economic development. Even then, politicians point out, EU accession did not initiate major flows of border-crossing patients. However, this comparison is not quite appro-priate, because the patient mobility rulings from the ECJ have emerged only recently. Patients have become more mobile and more assertive in claiming health care entitlements. Nonetheless patient mobility is restricted by the conditions defined in Article 22(1) and (2) of *Regulation 1408/71* (in case of medical necessity, and included in the benefit package of the home and guest country). According to the latest ECJ rulings, pre-authorization of the competent national authority is still required at least vis-à-vis hospital care.

In the case of ambulatory care, it can be expected that particularly in border areas, patients may look for trans-frontier health care. Since the ECJ cases establish that the level of reimbursement paid in the absence of pre-authorization is to be based on national tariffs (see *Decker, Kohll*, and *Müller-Fauré*), this is not likely to seriously affect the financial balance of the health insurance funds in the new member-states. There is, however, the problem of cross-border hospital care where there has been 'undue delay.' In that case, new member-states may not refuse treatment abroad and will have to reimburse according to the applicable tariffs in the country of stay.[61] Because there is a large discrepancy between the tariffs of treatment in border-sharing countries such as Germany and Poland or Austria and the Czech Republic, this means that recently established health insurance funds will be confronted with major financial claims from German or Austrian providers who are treating Polish and Czech patients.[62] Given the weak financial position of these funds, it can be expected that they will interpret the authorization condition very strictly, and, therefore, limit patient mobility to more expensive health care systems. Such a development will threaten the right to cross-border care in new member-states and may create a new distinction between EU citizens based on developed and developing health care systems. Moreover, based on the ruling in *Smits/Peerbooms*, further limitation of patient mobility may be allowed on the part of countries with fledgling health insurance systems on the basis that allowing cross-border care will pose a serious threat to the financial security of that country's social security system.

Despite these rather gloomy prospects, one should not forget that also several positive border-crossing developments are occurring between Germany and Poland and the Austrian-Hungarian-Czech border. Since the privatization trend started in the new member-states, numerous private practices (for example, dentistry or pharmacy) have been established, notably in border areas. Many German and Austrian patients, attracted by high-quality services at reasonable prices, are crossing the borders to obtain these services. This is even more attractive where ambulatory services are not covered by the social insurance scheme, and patients have to pay these services out of pocket.

In spite of the fact that such a development may improve the financial position of several health professionals in these new member-states, one should be concerned about this 'one way' patient mobility. Such an unbalanced patient mobility requires adequate action to improve conditions for the benefit of patients in the new member-states. Establishing 'Euregios in health care' in new border areas may function as 'laboratories for accession.' As mentioned before, such experiments could include agreements on the level and quality of care and the applicable tariffs, and as such, improve the portability of health care rights in the new member-states.

Conclusion

More than EU public health law, EU market rules have had a significant influence on the organization and provision of health care services in the EU member-states. Health care is now considered a service that falls within the scope of the *EC Treaty*, and the resulting consequences are considerable, both for patients and member-states. For patients the principle of free movement has enhanced their right to search for health services (particularly non-hospital services) across borders. Member-states, however, in theory if not in practice, have lost part of their sovereignty in organizing and providing health services.

In the absence of an EU health care policy, the ECJ based its rulings on patient mobility primarily on the free movement provisions in the *EC Treaty*. Interpreting these in the health care sector, the ECJ has challenged the ways that member-states define their respective benefit packages. This is particularly so for countries that employ rather vague criteria such as 'normal treatment' or 'medically acceptable.' Canada, if it were part of the European Union, would find its reliance upon terms like 'medically necessary' similarly restricted. As pointed out by Flood, Stabile, and Tuohy (chapter 1, this volume), the tendency across Canadian provinces is to exclude from public funding all services deemed 'experimental.' In the EU context such exclusion can now be justified only when supported by international evidence. Evidence that such a service is not presently provided within a country or not yet generally accepted among that country's medical profession would not be enough.

By extending the scope of health care benefits to what is internationally usual or accepted among health professionals, the ECJ has made it impossible for EU countries to limit entitlements on the basis of national understanding only. More and more, national decision-making in health care is based on international (legal) norms. This is an important observation, given concerns about the impact of new technologies on the sustainability of publicly funded health care systems, which, muta-tis mutandis, similarly affect countries such as Canada, a participant in multinational agreements such as NAFTA and the Agreement on Trade-Related Aspects of Intellectual Property Rights (TRIPs). Nevertheless, major differences in perception can be noted. For instance, whereas the TRIPs agreement in relation to health is largely oriented to property rights (see Mykitiuk and Dagnino, chapter 13, in this volume), the *EC Treaty* considers access to health care more as a fundamental human right based on insurance entitlements as defined by law. The EU ap-proach allows the Court to balance public health interests (including financial sustainability) with individual claims to health care services.

One may welcome the ECJ's progressive approach towards patients. Nevertheless, the ECJ casuistic approach does have limitations and does raise further questions about the extent of the influence of EU law in health care. Because of the critical importance of the health insurance and health care delivery sectors, legislative intervention is needed at the EU level, with a focus on access to and allocation of health care services. In this respect, revision of the *EC Treaty* and the *EU Charter of Human Rights* should be considered, with amendments regarding pa-tient mobility. This could stimulate the convergence of health care sys-tems in the EU, at the level both of principles and policy.

The need for intervention will become even more manifest after the 2004 enlargement of the EU. Facing major differences in health status, new member-states will not be able to solve this problem by themselves at the national level, supra-national measures will be required. Such an approach by the EU may contribute to overcoming major discrepancies in the provision and quality of health care services in the new member-states, which is one of the main justifications for eased patient mobility.

NOTES

1 *Decker v. Caisse de Maladie des Employés Privés* C-120/5, [1998] E.C.R. I-1831 [*Decker*] and C-158/96 *Kohll v Union des Caisses de Maladie*, [1998] E.C.R. I-1931 [*Kohll*].

2 Article 152 of the *EC Treaty*. References to article numbers are references to provisions in the *EC Treaty*, unless otherwise noted. When I refer to the *EC Treaty*, I mean the consolidated version of the original Treaty of Rome,

including all the latest amendments: *Consolidated versions of the Treaty on European Union and of the Treaty Establishing the European Community* (2002) OJ [Official Journal] 2002 c 325 at 01, available at http://www.europa.eu.int/eur-lex/pri/en/oj/dat/2002/c_325/c_32520021224en00010184.pdf (accessed January 2004)

3 *Ibid.*

4 *EC Treaty, supra* note 2 at Article 152(5).

5 Decision No. 1786/2002/EC of the European Parliament and of the Council, 23 Sept. 2002, adopting a program of Community action in the field of public health (2003–8) *Commission Statements* O.J. 2002 L 271 at 1–12.

6 *EC Treaty, supra* note 2.

7 Because of the lack of a specific legal basis prior to the adoption of the *Maastricht Treaty* in 1992, most of the Union's initiatives in the field of consumer protection were based on Articles 95 and 308 (internal market provisions).

8 O.J. 1985 L 210 at 29, as amended by *Directive 99/34/EC* to include primary agricultural products. O.J. 1996 L 141 at 20.

9 The primary reason that approximation of national product liability laws are necessary is that the existing divergences may distort competition and affect the movement of goods within the common market.

10 In the safety field, the *Directive on General Product Safety (92/59/EEC)* functions as the 'counterpart' of the *Product Liability Directive*, O.J. 1992 L 228, at 24. The Directive aims to give an incentive to producers to pay particular attention to the safety aspects of the products they want to market within the European Union. Apart from this general 'horizontal' directive prior ('vertical') directives lay down technical standards for specific sectors, e.g., toys, cosmetics, and foodstuffs.

11 EC competition rules fall out of the scope of this chapter since these principles are primarily of relevance in the context of competition among health providers and social health insurance funds. See, e.g., T.S. Jost, D. Dawson, and A.P. den Exter, 'The Role of Competition in Health Care: A Western European Perspective,' J. Health Politics, Policy and Law (in press).

12 See, for instance, social security coordination Regulation 1408/71 O.J. 1971 L 149, as amended by *Regulation 859/2003* PB 2003 L 124, at 1.

13 *Reyners*, C-74 [1974], E.C.R. at I-631.

14 O.J. 1964 B56 1964 at 850.

15 In addition to these specific branch directives, other health professionals may rely on the general 'new approach' directives that facilitate a general system for the recognition of diplomas: *Directives 89/48/EEC and 92/51/*

EEC, O.J. 1989 L 19, at 16; O.J. 1992 L 209, at 25. *Directive 89/48* has now been supplemented by *Directive 94/38* O.J. 1994 L 217, at 8. Directive 89/48 applies when the diploma requires the equivalent of at least three years' full-time study at a university or similar institution, whereas Directive 92/51 applies when the profession requires a postsecondary course equivalent to at least one year's full-time study. Implementing both directives means, *inter alia*, that member-states' competent authorities set up a procedure for examining an applicant to pursue a regulated profession. Instead of attempting to harmonize by profession, known as the sectoral or 'vertical' approach, the Commission decided to adopt henceforth a general or 'horizontal' approach, based not on harmonization but on the mutual recognition of qualifications.

16 E.g., *Decker* and *Kohll, supra* note 1. The European Court of Justice overruled the pertinent Luxembourg regulations, which made reimbursement by the social security system of medical services provided in another member-state – respectively orthodontic treatment and the supply of spectacles – conditional on prior authorization.

17 Administrative Commission, quoted by Herbert E.G.M. Hermans and Philip Berman, 'Access to Health Care and Health Services in the European Union: Regulation 1408/71 and the E111 Process,' in Reiner Leidl (ed.), *Health Care and Its Financing in a Single European Market* (Amsterdam: IOS Press, 1999) 329.

18 E.g., *Geraets-Smits/Peerbooms* C-157/99 [2001] E.C.R. I-5473 [*Smits/ Peerbooms*]; *Müller-Fauré/Van Riet*, C-385/99, [2003] E.C.R. I-4409 [*Müller-Fauré*]; *Van der Duin v. Onderlinge Waarborgmaatschappij ANOZ Zorgverzekeringen* and *Onderlinge Waarborgmaatschappij ANOZ Zorgverzekeringen v. Van Wegberg-van Brederode* C-156/01, [2003] E.C.R. I-7045; *Leichtle v. Bundesanstalt für Arbeit*, C-8/02, 28 March 2004 n.y.p. On the same day as the *Smits/Peerbooms* case, the Court also ruled on the peculiar case (C-368/98) of *Vanbraekel and Others v. Alliance nationale des mutualités chrétiennes*, [2001] E.C.R. I-5363 [*Vanbraekel*]. The issue in question concerned the tariff that should be reimbursed in case of incorrectly refused authorization to receive hospital treatment in a member-state other than the state in which the individual is insured. The Court ruled that the reimbursement must be at least the same as the amount that would have been granted had the insured person received hospital treatment in the member-state in which he or she is insured. Otherwise, this could hinder free movement. Strangely enough, this could mean a profit for the insured in cases where tariffs are higher in the country where he or she is insured!

19 *Geraets-Smits/Peerbooms, ibid.*

20 In a benefit-of-kind system, the insured is entitled only to statutory benefits, provided by health providers having an agreement with health insurance funds. This is different from a reimbursement system in which health insurers reimburse the costs of treatment to the insured. In such a model there is no contractual relationship between the health insurer and the health provider.

21 Based on settled case law of the Central Court of Appeal in social security matters (*CR v. B*) 23 May 1995, RZA 1995, No. 126.

22 *Smits/Peerbooms, supra* note 18 at para. 96.

23 *Ibid* at para. 98.

24 H.A.G. Temmink, 'Kroniek van het Europees recht' (2001) 31 Nederlands Juristenblad 1502.

25 *Müller-Fauré, supra* note 18.

26 *Ibid.* at para. 77.

27 *Ibid.* at para. 85. Under the proportionality test, if a less invasive alternative measure or arrangement could perform an assigned task under the same conditions as the arrangement being challenged, the less invasive alternative should be chosen.

28 *Ibid.* at para. 95.

29 *Smits/Peerbooms, supra* note 18 at para. 54.

30 *Müller-Fauré, supra* note 18 at para. 59.

31 *Ibid.* at para. 103.

32 *Duphar and Others*, C-238/82, [1984] E.C.R. I-523 at para. 16 and C-158/96; *Kohll*, supra note 1 at para. 17.

33 E.g., *Kohll, ibid.* at para. 18.

34 *Duphar and Others, supra*, note 32 at para. 16. Nevertheless, the member-states must comply with Community law when exercising that power. This means, e.g., that they should respect basic community principles, including the non-discrimination principle. *Ferlini* v *Centre hospitalier de Luxembourg*, C-411/98 [2000], E.C.R. I-8081. In this case, the Court ruled that the application, on a unilateral basis, by a group of health care providers to EC officials of scales of fees for medical and hospital maternity care that are higher than those applicable to residents affiliated to the national social security scheme constitutes discrimination on the ground of nationality prohibited under Article 12(1) EC, in the absence of objective justification.

35 *Smits/Peerbooms, supra* note 18 at para. 87.

36 *Supra* note 24.

37 *Smits/Peerbooms, supra* note 18 at para. 103.

38 *Kohll, supra* note 1 at para. 41; *Müller-Fauré, supra* note 18 at para. 72.

39 *Müller-Fauré, ibid.*
40 Also suggested by Advocate General Colomer in his opinion on *Smits/ Peerbooms, supra* note 18 at 61.
41 *Inizan v. Caisse Primaire d' Assurance Maladie des Hauts-de-Seine,* C-56/01, [2003] E.C.R. I-12403 at para. 55.
42 Maastricht District Court, 26 Sept. 2003, AL3183, Netherlands.
43 See also Gareth Davies, 'Health and Efficiency: Community Law and National Health Systems in the Light of Müller-Fauré' (2004) 67:1 Mod. L. Rev. 103.
44 A similar interpretation – mutatis mutandis – was used by Court in *Vanbraekel, supra* note 18, when ruling that the level of reimbursement for foreign hospital services should have been the same had the same services been received in the home country.
45 E.g., Vassilis G. Hatzopoulos, 'Killing National Health and Insurance Systems but Healing Patients? The European Market for Health Care Services after the Judgements of the ECJ in Vanbraekel and Peerbooms' (2002) 39:4 Common Market L. Rev 683.
46 Willy Palm et al. (2000) 'Implications of Recent Jurisprudence on the Co-ordination of Health Protection systems.' Summary Report, published by Association Internationale de la Mutualité (AIM) for the European Commission Directorate General for Employment and Social Affairs. All AIM publications are available at the AIM website www.aim-mutual.org (accessed January 2004); see also Werner Brouwer et al., 'Should I Stay or Should I Go? Waiting Lists and Cross-Border Care in the Netherlands' (2003) 63:3 Health Policy 289.
47 Jean Hermesse, Henri Lewalle, and Willy Palm, 'Patient Mobility within the European Union' (2003) 3:supplement Eur. J. Public Health 9.
48 E.g., Herbert E.G.M. Hermans and André P. den Exter, 'Cross-Border Alliances in Health Care: International Co-operation between Health Insurers and Providers in the Euregio Meuse-Rhine' (1999) 40:2 Croatian Med. J. 266.
49 Elias Mossialos and Willy Palm, 'The European Court of Justice and the Free Movement of Patients in the European Union' (2003) 56:2 International Social Security Rev. 25.
50 'EU Commission Staff Working Paper on Health and Enlargement SEC' (1999) 713.
51 Originally, the OMC was introduced in the field of economic and financial policy. By decision of the European Council (Lisbon Summit) in March 2000, it was later transferred to the field of social policy, starting with employment and social exclusion.

52 This concept has been adopted into the draft of the European Constitution in the fields of social and health policy, by stating that 'the Commission may take any useful initiative to promote co-ordination, in particular initiatives aiming at the establishment of guidelines and indicators, the organisation and exchange of best practice, and the preparation of the necessary elements for periodic monitoring and evaluation.' Article III-107 and Article III-179 of the *Draft* Treaty *Establishing a Constitution for Europe*, O.J. 2003 L (C 169).

53 E.g., EC, 'High Level Process of Reflection on Patient Mobility and Health Care Development in the European Union; Outcomes of the Reflection Process.' European Commission Health and Consumer Protection Directorate General (2003), HLPR 16, at 10.

54 Herman Nys, 'The Harmonisation of Patient Rights in Europe and Its Consequences for the Accession Countries,' in André P. den Exter (ed.), *EU Accession and Its Consequences for Candidate Countries' Health Care Systems* (Rotterdam: Erasmus University Press, 2004) at 40.

55 Officially, the *Charter of Fundamental Rights of the European Union*, O.J. 2000 C C-364/01. The *Charter* has been incorporated into the *Draft* Treaty, *supra* note 52.

56 Accession of Cyprus, the Czech Republic, Estonia, Latvia, Lithuania, Hungary, Malta, Poland, Slovenia, and Slovakia. *Treaty of Accession*. OJ 2003 L 236. At the time of writing, these countries had not yet entered the EU.

57 The chapters cover, inter alia, the free movement principles, competition law, agriculture, transport policy, economic and monetary union, social policy and employment, telecommunication, and the environment.

58 Council *Regulation (EC) No. 622/98*, O.J. 1998 L. 85 at 1.

59 I.e., the transformation from a 'socialist' health care system into a more 'western' market-oriented social insurance system.

60 Den Exter has examined the difficulties that accession countries face in the field of health. Serious problems have occurred, inter alia, in the field of social security, regulated by coordination Regulations *1408/71* and *574/72*. *Health Care Law-Making in Central and Eastern Europe: Review of a Legal-Theoretical Model* (Antwerp: Intersentia, 2002).

61 Article 22(2) of Regulation 1408.

62 Most of these funds are already facing major deficits because of weak premium collection mechanisms and the perverse and uncontrolled expansion of the services that are provided.

PART SIX

Manufacturing Demand for Access:
The Role of the Media and the
Commercialization of Research

15 The Power of Illusion and the Illusion of Power: Direct-to-Consumer Advertising and Canadian Health Care

PATRICIA PEPPIN

Issues of access and allocation of health care resources are intertwined with the processes by which demand for health care is determined. This chapter and those that follow explores how demand or 'need' for health care is manufactured. Canada permits advertising of prescription drugs directed to physicians but like most developed countries prohibits advertising directly to consumers. Direct-to-consumer advertising (DTCA) is permitted in only two countries in the Organization for Economic Cooperation and Development (OECD) – the United States and New Zealand. Advertising is a powerful means of creating demand for products and perceptions about diseases, treatments, and patients and, as a result, is an important contributor to the spiralling costs of health care. The power of advertising is derived from the methods used by advertisers to construct the images and text that draw on the underlying values of the target audience. I will examine these means of creating perceptions through illusion in the first part of this chapter. Following this, I will examine the impact of direct advertising on patients, doctors, and access to health care. The claim that patients are empowered through direct-to-consumer advertising is critically examined against my assertion that advertising creates only the *illusion* of consumer power.

History of Regulation

Canadian state involvement in controlling messages related to drug therapies began in the early twentieth century in response to developing concerns about excessive claims made for patent medicines, which are those medicines available without a prescription.[1] At the time, these secret formula medicines often included addictive and/or dangerous ingredients such as alcohol, narcotics, and derivatives of coal-tar. To control these medicines, in 1908 Canada's Parliament enacted the *Proprietary or Patent Medicine Act* (PPM), which contained a list of prohibited ingredients and a prohibition on offering for sale any patent medicine that contains a prohibited ingredient.[2] This legislation also prohibited door-to-door sales of patent medicines and handouts of samples to the public. In 1919 the Act was amended to prohibit false, misleading, or exaggerated claims in advertisements, labels, and circulars for patent medicines.[3]

Prescription drugs have been subject to federal regulation since 1875, when the first portions of what became the *Food and Drugs Act* were enacted as part of other legislation.[4] In 1927, the *Food and Drugs Act* was amended to prohibit false, misleading, and deceptive advertising for prescription drugs. In its current form, the Act continues to prohibit false, misleading, or deceptive advertising.[5] A prohibition on advertising prescription drugs directly to the public is contained in section 3(1): 'No person shall advertise any food, drug, cosmetic or device to the general public as a treatment, preventative or cure for any of the diseases, disorders or abnormal physical states referred to in Schedule A.'

Schedule A lists diseases for which products aimed at treatment, prevention, or cure must be prescribed by a physician and includes such ills as heart disease and cancer. The *Food and Drug Regulations* have prohibited direct-to-consumer advertising of prescription drugs since 1949.[6] This prohibition was amended in 1978 to provide that no representation other than the name, price, and quantity of prescription drugs (Schedule F drugs) may be advertised directly to the public.[7] This provision was added to permit pharmacists to advertise comparative prices.[8] The name-price-quantity exception to the prohibition on direct-to-consumer advertising has provided a means for advertisers to expand into consumer-directed advertising without further policy debate or legislative change. Since 'education' of consumers is not prohibited, the sometimes ambiguous difference between advertising and education is a second means to expanded advertising.[9] Further, 'help-seeking advertisements' and reminder advertisements provide a third way for advertisers to advertise directly to consumers.

Restrictions are ineffective where advertising crosses geographic jurisdictional boundaries. Multinational pharmaceutical companies operate in a global environment subject to few effective global restrictions on their promotional activities. The World Health Organization (WHO) adopted the *Ethical Criteria for Medicinal Drug Promotion*, and Canada, as a signatory, has an obligation to adhere to and apply these standards.[10] But although advertising may be subject to domestic regulation and enforcement, such regulation has no impact on advertising generated in other jurisdictions and conveyed by the mass media across permeable borders. In the view of Health Canada, 'The TPD [Therapeutic Products Directorate] has jurisdiction over advertising originating in any country but no effective means of ensuring compliance for advertising that originates outside of Canada. This limitation applies to all forms of advertising, including the Internet.'[11]

Broadcast advertising has required pre-broadcast clearance since 1936, when the *Canadian Broadcasting Act*[12] gave the Canadian Broadcasting Corporation (CBC) authority to make regulations regarding advertising time and to control the character of advertising on radio.[13] Under the authority of the *Food and Drug Regulations*,[14] inspectors acting on behalf of the Canadian Radio-Television and Telecommunications Commission (CRTC) currently pre-clear radio and television advertising of any item that falls under the *Food and Drugs Act* or the *Proprietary or Patent Medicine Act* for advertising containing recommendations for prevention, treatment, or cure of a disease or condition.

Pre-clearance of prescription drug advertising directed to health professionals is carried out by the Pharmaceutical Advertising Advisory Board (PAAB). The PAAB applies its own *Code of Advertising Acceptance* as well as the federal statute and regulations, provides a dispute resolution mechanism, declines misleading advertising, reviews comparative claims against scientific evidence, requests labelling changes, and refers non-compliant advertisements back to the government when all other appeals have failed.[15]

The PAAB is an organization that operates outside government and consists of representatives of the pharmaceutical industry organizations, the health professions, medical publishers, advertising agencies, and the Consumers Association of Canada (CAC), among others. Health Canada's Therapeutic Products Directorate (TPD) has an *ex officio* adviser/observer on the PAAB, and TPD retains ultimate jurisdiction over regulatory compliance and enforcement. However, Health Canada considers that responsibility for case-by-case voluntary pre-clearance, and the review of advertising to health professionals has been largely 'delegated' to the PAAB and its counterpart for over-the-counter drugs, Advertising Standards Canada.[16]

The *Canadian Charter of Rights and Freedoms*[17] applies to all legislation, regulations, and other forms of government activity that might limit freedom of expression. The arm's length mechanism adopted to review advertisements, the infrequent use of criminal law powers provided under the *Food and Drugs Act*, and government's preference for voluntary compliance make constitutional challenges by the pharmaceutical industry unlikely – and unnecessary.

The Power of Illusion

Novelist J.M. Coetzee has written about the process of signifying meaning in a passage in *Elizabeth Costello*: 'Supply the particulars, allow the significations to emerge of themselves. A procedure pioneered by Daniel Defoe. Robinson Crusoe, cast up on the beach, looks around for his shipmates. But there are none. "I never saw them afterwards, or any sign of them," says he, "except three of their hats, one cap, and two shoes that were not fellows." Two shoes, not fellows: by not being fellows, the shoes have ceased to be footwear and become proofs of death, torn by the foaming seas off the feet of drowning men and tossed ashore. No large words, no despair, just hats and caps and shoes.'[18]

The same process of signification operates in advertising. Values that the audience correlates with the images used in advertising are transferred to the product to be consumed. As Judith Williamson explained in her groundbreaking work, *Decoding Advertisements*, advertising draws upon the 'system of differences'[19] or 'distinctions existing in social mythologies'[20] to distinguish between products: 'Images, ideas or feelings, then, become attached to certain products, by being transferred from signs out of other systems (things or people with "images") *to* the products, rather than originating in them. This intermediary object or person is bypassed in our perception; although it is what gives the products its meaning, we are supposed to see that meaning as already there, and we rarely notice that the correlating object and the product have no inherent similarity, but are only placed together (hence the significance of form). So a product and an image/emotion become linked in our minds, while the process of this linking is unconscious.'[21]

For example, the advertising campaign that created the Marlboro man in the mid-1950s grew out of the failure of the genteel Marlboro woman to sell the product to women, the target audience.[22] The new image of the cowboy repositioned the cigarette as the ultimate in masculinity, and made its most successful dimensions for the targeted youth audience the 'separation from restraints (the tattoo) *and* a sense of belonging (Marlboro Country).'[23] The Marlboro man epitomized the romanticized version of independence and freedom that had already been distilled into the movie and television imagery of such heroes as Roy Rogers and Gene Autrey.[24] These meanings were read into the man's image, transferred over to the cigarettes in the red and white flip-top cigarette box, and further transferred over to the viewer, who would become like the Marlboro man through consuming the product. The sources of meaning, known as the referent systems, are found in the social system in which the viewer is located.

Advertising agencies attempt to tap into these underlying myths to give meaning and power to the advertisements. The classical mythology drawn upon in advertising Paxil (paroxetine) adds a layer of legitimacy and heroism to the drug's image, just as the morality plays of westerns were repackaged as lures for young people to seek maturity and independence through smoking. Roland Barthes stated in 1957 that myths naturalize connections that are 'falsely obvious'[25] and existing outside the reality of history: 'what allows the reader to consume myth innocently is that he does not see it as a semiological system but as an inductive one. Where there is only equivalence, he sees a kind of causal process: the signifier and the signified have, in his eyes, a natural relationship. This confusion can be expressed otherwise: any semiological system is a system of values; now the myth-consumer takes the signification for a system of facts: myth is read as a factual system, whereas it is but a semiological system.'[26]

The appropriation and transformation of such meanings occurs with the participation of the viewer but without the viewer's consciousness of the process.[27] Judith Williamson has noted that '[t]he obvious ideological function of this is to make the subject feel *knowing* but deprive him of *knowledge*.'[28] This insight is significant for the process of direct-to-consumer advertising of pharmaceutical products. The viewer is seemingly empowered by knowledge but actually disempowered in several ways: through lack of real knowledge, through the use made of the viewer's referent systems, and through the inaccuracy of the patient's sense of power. The spurious empowerment created by advertising is more dangerous in the context of health care than in commercial contexts such the purchase of, say, running shoes, where the stakes are low and the information simple.

We acquire the values extolled in the advertising process through a process of objectification of ourselves; we exchange our own selves for commodified versions acquired through buying.[29] We complete our personalities through consumption of particular products. Advertisements create social groups of consumers by persuading us that we belong to these groups already and that we merely indicate our membership by consuming the product. Williamson notes: 'If you use Chanel No. 5, you are signified as a different kind of person from someone who uses Babe,'[30] products signified by Catherine Deneuve and Margaux Hemingway, respectively. Further, says Williamson, 'you do not simply buy the product in order to *become* a part of the group it represents; you must feel that you already, naturally, belong to that group and *therefore* you will buy it.'[31]

The lifestyles that sell such consumer products are part of drug advertising as well. Lifestyle indicators such as social popularity, material success, and achievement in sports are associated with particular medications. For example, the happy man skips along the street in front of the white picket fence of middle class North America, while we hear the music 'Good Morning!' He has become Viagra man, easily recognizable by adults, signifying sexual happiness, after a remedy that the advertisement suggests is legitimate in such neighbourhoods peopled by middle-aged men like him. Now a man showers while singing that he's doing it 'myyyy way' (an oddly solitary approach to a two-person activity). The earliest advertisements for Prozac used the same legitimization technique to normalize the experience of depression – along with the remedy.

Williamson discusses advertisers' use of 'magic,' defining it as 'the production of results disproportionate to the effort put in (a transformation of power – or of impotence *into* power).'[32] Drug advertisements persuade us that drugs possess magical powers – the very magical powers that we seek in order to overcome the impotence of disease. Buying, Williamson argues, is a spell or short cut; the individual's passivity increases along 'with the ability to plug into a vast source of external power' though, like Faustus, the individual never experiences control.[33] The perception of this magic link is so potent that caveats about risk act as unwelcome intrusions from the world of reality that infringe on the normalization of the magic link. Such a view is consistent with Goldman and Papson's observation that the amount of text in print and television advertising has shortened over time, starting in the 1930s, both because it had become 'redundant and unnecessary' and because viewers resented its overdirectedness.[34]

As Goldman notes in *Reading Ads Socially*, desire is the common factor in commodity advertising.[35] When drug advertising is directed to physicians, such desire is referred through the intermediary. Doctor-directed advertising must appeal to different desires of doctors, such as the role of the doctor as the heroic battler of disease, imagery that is quite common in drug advertising.[36] A desire for patient compliance – a political concept – has also been used by advertisers to promote the product; for example, advertising for Premarin exhorted doctors to bring patients back into line when they stopped taking hormone replacement therapy after they had sought information outside the doctor-patient relationship.[37] The positioning of Prozac as a one-a-day pill is a further measure designed to help doctors achieve greater patient compliance with the therapeutic regime. A desire to be able to offer a remedy to patients is a powerful motivator for doctors.

When advertising is aimed at patients directly, and the doctor's desires are no longer the key target, the nature of advertising changes to focus on fostering desire among patients for the services or treatments. This process occurs within the context of western medicine, which itself conceptualizes disease as something external that happens to people and healing as something for which the individual bears responsibility.[38] Advertising uses these perceptions by reinforcing the view of disease as an individualized rather than a socially determined event and by offering treatment in an individualized form that promotes personal responsibility for cure.[39] Direct advertising permits the advertiser to establish connections with these patient desires directly, and then propel the patient back to the doctor. The path to consumption requires a stop in the doctor's office to obtain a prescription. While such an interaction may have the appearance of patient autonomy and participation in responsible health care, desire is its defining characteristic. As Barthes indicates, the artificial connections appear to the viewer to be natural and causal. The apparent knowledge possessed by the patient is illusory and seductive.

Existing laws and regulations protecting patients conceive of a hierarchy of information transfer from the manufacturer to the doctor and, in turn, to the patient. The addition of direct-to-consumer marketing complicates the information flows and allows the manufacturer to appeal directly to both. The reduction of the doctor's role completes the transformation in the locus of power from the physician to the drug itself. Early advertisements depicted doctors as healers while subsequent advertisements showed the healing power in the drugs themselves.[40] As John R. Neill describes it, 'The therapeutic task of the early advertisements [for psychotropic drugs] was to convince the psychiatrist that he or she was, with the help of medication, potent, able to perform those careful interpersonal maneuvers which would help or cure his patient. Later the therapeutic function of the advertisements was to reassure the psychiatrist that his medication, rather than he himself, is powerful.'[41] Deborah Lupton observed this theme in two Australian advertisements depicting doctors: 'the traditional healing properties of the doctor's caring relationship with his or her patient have been transferred to the drug: it is Zocor that inspires confidence, not the doctor himself. It is as if the doctor is only a mediator between patient and drug, a shadowy figure lurking in the background, the necessary authority who signs the prescription but provides little else of relevance to the patients' relationship with drug therapy.'[42] Direct-to-consumer advertising has effected the transition from caring healer to healing drug.

The Illusion of Power

The impact of direct-to-consumer advertising on the provision of health care is being debated vigorously in Europe, New Zealand, the United States, and Canada. Industry advocates maintain that such direct advertising serves an educational purpose; patients are empowered and public health is improved through the use of beneficial prescription drugs.[43] In examining this argument, I will look first at the economic context of advertising communications, then at the standard for communication established by the Supreme Court of Canada, and finally at the literature on advertising of pharmaceutical products to consumers.

The processes of drug advertising have an impact on access to appropriate and necessary health care. Since 1997, when the guidelines on DTCA in the broadcast media lowered the requirements in the United States,[44] advertising expenditures have increased exponentially. Palumbo and Mullins note that from 1989 to 1996 spending increased from U.S.$12 million to U.S.$595 million annually and that it quadrupled (after the relaxation of the relevant regulations) to $2.38 billion in 2001.[45] The independent National Institute for Health Care Management (NIHCM) Foundation found that spending on prescription drugs in the United States in the year 2000–1, increased by 17.1 per cent[46] as follows: the number of prescriptions increased (6.7 per cent), while price increases (6.3 per cent) and switches to higher priced drugs (4.1 per cent) made up the remainder.[47] Global figures compiled by IMS Health indicate that pharmaceutical sales grew in constant dollars by 12 per cent from 2000 to 2001, from U.S.$321.8 billion to U.S.$364.2 billion. North

America contributed 17 per cent to this growth figure and made up 50 per cent of the global sales.[48]

Although Canada has also had to address rising prescription drug costs, spending increases at rates similar to those in the U.S. context would result in potentially unbearable pressures on Canada's Medicare system. The Canadian health care system has no national universal plan for prescription drugs, and drug treatments are not covered as necessary services under the *Canada Health Act* unless provided within a hospital or other institutional setting. Although not required to do so, most provincial governments do provide insurance for prescriptions drugs, at least to the elderly and to those on welfare or to those who incur catastrophic costs. Consequently, public financing of health care at the provincial level could be severely affected by the much higher sales resulting from increased DTCA.

Direct-to-consumer advertising is itself expensive and these costs are passed on to consumers. One must thus ask whether these additional costs are outweighed by a significant improvement in public health. Research carried out by the NIHCM Foundation on the degree of innovation in drugs newly approved by the U.S. FDA from 1989 to 2000 found that only 15 per cent of new drug approvals could be considered highly innovative drugs. Most did not contain new active ingredients or provide significant clinical improvements.[49] Charles Medawar has argued that pharmaceutical companies need highly innovative drugs – blockbuster drugs – to make big profits. These profits are necessary to sustain the industry at current levels. These 'blockbuster drugs' are not available to them because research productivity is declining[50] and so they have turned to mergers to obtain capital and products, and towards aggressively attempting to change advertising laws to permit heavier marketing.[51] If blockbuster drugs are not forthcoming, then manufacturers need to promote their existing products more aggressively to expand their markets.[52]

Patient Autonomy

The nature of the relationships between doctors and patients, and among doctors, patients, and the pharmaceutical industry, have been defined in a remarkable series of judgments by the Supreme Court of Canada over the past two and a half decades. These judgments have set a standard against which advertising directed to patients may be measured.

The Supreme Court of Canada radically altered the doctor-patient relationship in 1980 when it decided that doctors owed a duty of disclosure to patients and that the standard of disclosure would be measured by standards relevant to the patient rather than to the custom of the profession.[53] The relationship that the Supreme Court had in mind required enhanced equality of information. These steps mandated a reshaping of the profession in the direction of disclosure to patients as a necessary step in making informed decisions.[54]

The Court returned to the issue of equality in the doctor-patient relationship in 1992 with two decisions: first, in *Norberg v. Wynrib*[55] which underscores the impact of power imbalance and, second, *McInerney v. McDonald*[56] in which they asserted the right of a patient to access his or her own medical information as part of the doctor's fiduciary obligation. In *Hollis v. Dow Corning Corp.*,[57] the Supreme Court addressed the nature of the pharmaceutical manufacturer's duty to warn about product risks. The duty is owed to the patient but in the case of prescribed products, this duty may be discharged by warning the doctor (the learned intermediary), who has an existing duty to disclose risks of treatment at common law and in any provincial consent-to-treatment legislation. The Court in *Hollis* explicitly conceptualized the relationship between manufacturer, doctor, and patient in equality terms.[58] The information possessed by the manufacturer so far exceeds that known to the patient, and even the doctor, that the manufacturer has a very high duty to disclose.

The Supreme Court of Canada has specifically identified communication between doctor and patient as vital to effective health care. In the 1997 case of *Eldridge*,[59] it found that this communication had been prevented by an unconstitutional infringement of the Section 15 equality rights of disabled persons denied access to sign interpreters in attempting to access health care under the *Canadian Charter of Rights and Freedoms*.[60] In these important decisions, the Supreme Court of Canada set out the requirements for communication of treatment information and highlighted the crucial role of effective communication in ameliorating the inherent inequalities of the doctor-patient relationship. Patients are empowered through comprehension of the range of information relevant to health care decisions that affect their lives. To what extent do the claims that direct advertising empowers patients meet the standards set out in this series of Supreme Court of Canada judgments?

DTCA and Patient Autonomy

The literature on doctor-directed advertising provides evidence of the limitations of advertising as a means of education. It is doubtful that patients are better informed by direct-to-consumer advertising. A study conducted by Bell, Kravitz, and Wilkes that analysed 329 consumer advertisements promoting over a hundred drug brands in eighteen popular magazines from 1989 to 1998 supports this conclusion.[61] Coders assessed each advertisement's information about the specific aspects for which the drug was advertised and the treatment. Advertisements generally provided information about symptoms but not about causes, prevalence, or misconceptions, or about the success rate for the treatment, length of treatment, mechanism of action, alternatives, or the behavioural changes that the patient could make. They found that while some advertising was informative, most advertisements were not and that the information contained in advertisements could be improved. A study by Woloshin and co-authors found that advertisements appeal to emotions and rarely quantify the expected benefits of a drug.[62] They thought that the FDA's emphasis on truth and balance, rather than on the means by which the information was conveyed, contributed to this result.

The idea that advertising is informative was fundamentally challenged in a 1992 study by Wilkes, Doblin, and Shapiro.[63] They examined 109 advertisements in ten leading medical journals and found that unbalanced information about side effects and efficacy was presented in 40 per cent; headlines were misleading about efficacy in 32 per cent; and, most significantly, in 44 per cent of cases these advertisements would lead to improper prescribing in the absence of any other information. This study has been widely quoted as evidence of the misleading nature of pharmaceutical advertising.[64] An eighteen-country WHO study analysed 6,710 advertisements in twenty-three leading medical journals over a twelve-month period in 1987–8.[65] It was designed to provide base data for analysis of the impact of the WHO's revised *Ethical Criteria for Medicinal Drug Promotion*. The study found that advertisements provided information about indications for the drugs more often than adverse effects, that half omitted important warnings and precautions, and about 40 per cent omitted side effects and contraindications.[66]

The number of warning letters sent out by the FDA for violations of regulations that require risk and product information provides another sense of the dangers of direct-to-consumer advertising. The U.S. General Accounting Office (GAO) in its report on FDA oversight of DTCA noted that some pharmaceutical companies repeatedly disseminated misleading advertisements for the same product, and that companies do not always submit all their newly distributed advertisements to the FDA for review. [67] Advertising is reviewed after it is disseminated, and, since there is no requirement to pre-clear advertisements, voluntary submission for advice is the only basis for prepublication clearance. If the process of review is lengthy – and procedural and staffing issues have made it so – then the advertising campaign may have ended before a regulatory letter is sent.[68] The GAO reported that FDA issues regulatory letters asking the company to cease disseminating the advertisement in only a small proportion of the advertisements reviewed – between 1999 and 2001, 5 per cent of broadcast advertisements (88 regulatory letters).[69] Advertisements and warning letters may be viewed together on the website.[70] Similarly, Burton indicated that in a November 2002 memo to the New Zealand Pharmac Board reporting on a survey of regulatory compliance by direct to consumer advertisers, carried out by Medsafe in the Department of Health, 'only 1 of the 6 (16.6%) of the television advertisements was compliant with the [Medicines Act] regulations.'[71]

Awareness of the risks of drugs is conveyed in only a truncated form by the broadcast advertisements permissible under the U.S. guidelines.[72] Under the legislation and regulations, advertisements must fairly balance the risks and benefits, provide full disclosure, and contain a brief summary of the risks and benefits. When the guidelines were 'clarified' in 1997 in a set of draft guidelines, which were subsequently formalized, broadcast advertisements were permitted to drop the brief summary and to fulfil this requirement through other means. These means included inserting directions to other sources of information, including doctors or pharmacists, toll-free numbers, websites, or pamphlets. This has meant that, in a broadcast ad, the benefits of the drug are promoted and the major statement of the most important risks given, but without immediate disclosure of the risks or harms. Similarly, broadcast advertisements omit any mention of alternatives to the proposed drug treatment. Inclusion of risk information directly in advertising heightens the general level of awareness that drugs *have* risks. It is hardly surprising that the FDA survey, discussed below, found that doctors perceived that patients lacked an understanding of product risks and the real level of efficacy of the drugs. Margaret Gilhooley recommended that the regulations be changed to incorporate a requirement that direct-to-consumer advertisements mention that consumers should consult their doctors about the range of treatment alternatives that exist and their risks, benefits, and costs.[73] Doing this, she argues, would increase respect for the doctor's role as adviser about a choice of alternative therapies.

As with all advertising, DTCA is structured to draw patients into the interpretive process. Since prescription drugs require the doctor to prescribe the drug, the patient must take the next step of seeing a physician. The number of patients asking their doctors for prescriptions is significant – around one-third (30–35 per cent) of patients who remembered seeing a direct advertisement asked their physicians about a specific drug.[74]

A significant study by Barbara Mintzes and researchers from the University of British Columbia, University of California at Davis, and York University compared patient and doctor groups in Sacramento, California, where DTCA is legal, with those in Vancouver, Canada, where it is not.[75] Patients and doctors were paired, so that exposure to advertisements could be compared with prescriptions for advertised medications. The researchers found that the Sacramento patients, who were significantly more likely to have seen almost all advertised products, were twice as likely to request medicines and twice as likely to request advertised medicines as were the patients in Vancouver.[76] The study found that higher exposure to advertising was linked to increased requests for advertised drugs and that patients requesting DTCA drugs had a seventeen times greater likelihood of receiving a drug prescription of any kind than those who did not make such a request. Fully 90 per cent of patients requesting a specific DTCA drug received a prescription for some drug.[77] This staggering rate of prescriptions and the link established between exposure to advertising and requests for drugs underscores the power of advertising.

This leads to the question of whether patients are benefiting from earlier detection of disease and prescription of appropriate treatment at that point. As Mintzes and co-authors point out in the Sacramento-Vancouver study, many advertised products leading to patient requests were 'lifestyle' drugs or treatments for symptoms.[78] A study, part of the Toop Report, conducted in New Zealand concluded that the evidence does not support advertiser claims that DTCA promotes earlier detection or greater likelihood of taking the drug.[79] In the study of all 3,200

New Zealand general practitioners, over two-thirds of the 1,611 respondents reported feeling pressured to prescribe advertised medicines, almost 80 per cent stated that patients often asked for DTCA drugs, 44 per cent said they had prescribed an advertised drug that they considered offered little benefit over drugs they would normally prescribe, and only 12 per cent thought direct-to-consumer advertising was a useful way of educating patients about risks and benefits.[80]

Bell, Wilkes, and Kravitz found that a doctor's unwillingness to provide a requested drug may lead not only to patients' disappointment but also, according to a quarter of respondents, to attempts to persuade the doctor or to prescription-shop. These patient responses were more common among those with positive attitudes to direct-to-consumer advertising and undue confidence in government regulation.[81] The same study of anticipated responses to refusal found that positive attitudes to DTCA correlated with negative reactions towards doctors.

Doctors feel pressured to prescribe in accordance with patients' requests.[82] A survey of 500 physicians carried out by the FDA in 2002 found that almost half of physicians perceived some pressure from patients: 53 per cent reported feeling no such pressure at all, while 29 per cent reported a little pressure, 13 per cent reported feeling pressure somewhat, and 4 per cent reported very much pressure.[83] Doctors feel that they would like to please their patients and respond to their requests,[84] and they also feel concerned about the possibility of losing patients.

At a public meeting on DTCA held by the FDA in September 2003, Kathryn Aikin presented the FDA physician survey.[85] Ms. Aikin summarized the results by indicating that DTCA increases awareness of possible treatments but does not convey risk and benefit information equally well. Doctors believe that patients understood benefits much better than risks and that the advertisements confused patients about relative risks and benefits.[86] Further, it was found that 'brand-specific requests are likely to be accommodated' as physicians reported feeling pressure to comply with their patients' requests.[87] General practitioners and specialist practitioners were also asked about specific benefits that might be achieved by direct-to-consumer advertising. When general and specialist practitioners were asked to indicate the benefits of DTCA[88,89] and what they thought patients understood,[90] their responses indicated that American doctors perceive that direct-to-consumer advertisements convey information that is weighted in the direction of benefits and have little success in conveying the more balanced information about risks that patients need to make an informed decision.

In addition to the standard means of communicating with doctors through detailers who visit their offices, sponsored seminars, product literature, samples left with doctors, journal advertising, and the industry-produced *Compendium of Pharmaceuticals and Specialties* (CPS), marketing also includes expenditures on lobbying, contributions to political campaigns, and donations to consumer-identified groups.[91] David Healy refers to such patient groups as 'a key pressure point in a market worth billions of dollars ... the perfect conduits for generating views among the 'informed' general public, such as the idea that depression is known to be a chemical imbalance in the brain.'[92] Dr Healy cites the examples of the National Alliance for the Mentally Ill, whose slogan was 'mind illnesses are brain illnesses' and the childhood attention deficit disorder group (CHADD), which lobbied vigorously for Ritalin. DTCA is appealing to the industry because it reaches beyond the doctor, permitting the industry to reach individual consumers. Such advertising can be targeted to specific parts of the market, to specific consumers, through choice of medium and vehicle. It can leave the private space of medical journals and penetrate into the public spaces reached by television, magazines, and billboards. For example, Women's Health Watch reported that in New Zealand at the Americas' Cup race, Eli Lilly used seven different forms of display space to brand their impotence drug, including billboards, banners, boat hulls, sails, bunting, sandwich boards, and free-standing displays.[93]

Advertising creates perceptions of diseases themselves and this, too, has an impact on the level of patient autonomy. For example, efforts have been made to expand the market for the anti-depressant Prozac, which has been repackaged in pink and purple, renamed Sarafem, and promoted by Eli Lilly as a remedy for the symptoms – mood swings, irritability, and bloating – of a new disease known as premenstrual dysphoric disease (PMDD).[94] In an article in the *British Medical Journal*, Ray Moynihan, Iona Heath, and David Henry discuss the pharmaceutical industry's role in constructing diseases, stating: 'The social construction of illness is being replaced by the corporate construction of disease.'[95] The authors give examples of five types of 'disease mongering': identifying ordinary processes, such as baldness, as medical problems; portraying mild symptoms as harbingers of serious disease, as with irritable bowel syndrome; promoting personal or social problems as medical problems, as with social phobia; conceptualizing risks as diseases, as with osteoporosis; and framing disease incidence estimates to maximize the medical problem's apparent prevalence, as with erectile dysfunction. To remedy 'disease mongering,' the authors recommend greater use by doctors of independent sources of medical information and a corresponding decrease in reliance on corporate sources of data and a widening of the scope of informed consent requirements to include disclosure of information about controversies related to disease definitions.[96]

The debate about the purported educational value of direct-to-consumer advertising underlines the need for independent, reliable sources of information about drugs. Regulators rely on the pharmaceutical industry to provide information about the drug at all stages of the drug approval process, and the industry constructs knowledge of the product at each of these stages. Donna Greschner (chapter 2, this volume) has discussed cogently the virtues of evidence-based decision-making. As physicians move increasingly in the direction of evidence-based medicine, their demand for valid and reliable data increases. Economist Uwe Reinhardt has proposed a research institute as a means to assist physicians to evaluate the relative efficacy of drugs.[97] More complete information will help doctors to make better-informed judgments and recommendations about drug treatments and minimize their reliance on the pharmaceutical industry.

Concerns about the impact of direct-to-consumer advertising on an already reduced role played by doctors in the United States managed care system led the New Jersey Supreme Court to find that a manufacturer that had promoted Norplant extensively through DTCA was subject to a direct duty to warn.[98] The court found that the assumptions underlying the learned intermediary rule were no longer valid – patients no longer relied primarily on doctors for information, doctors were no better placed because of patient contact and their own duties, the expenditure of billions on DTCA precluded the company from arguing that they lacked an effective means of communicating directly with consumers, and patient package insert requirements meant that consumers presumably were capable of understanding complex warning information. In my opinion, it is important for a court to examine the messages conveyed to patients through the manufacturer's channel of information and to measure them against a standard of communication in the context of an awareness of the power relationship. Direct advertising downplays the role of the doctor and, as we have seen, the drug has supplanted the physician as the heroic cure. Managed care in the United States adds to this effect as it has led to changes in the dynamics, with patients becoming less involved in choosing doctors and with doctors reacting to managed care pressures by spending less time with patients and often losing the full range of treatment options through insurer decisions.[99] Physicians in Canada already find that too little time is available to educate patients, particularly as pressures on the publicly funded health care system mount, and the additional task of dissuading pre-sold patients is unlikely to be well received. Doctors who are feeling pressured to diagnose and prescribe in particular ways, and who respond to that pressure by prescribing rather than engaging in discussion, deprive their patients of their professional judgment.

From the patient's perspective, DTCA creates the appearance of power. The Supreme Court of Canada's decisions have attempted to remedy the inequality inherent in the power imbalance between doctors, patients, and manufacturers and to enhance patient autonomy, but direct-to-consumer advertising produces the opposite effect. The power of the pharmaceutical industry is reinforced and extended. Through the power of illusion, patients participate in creating their own desires for drugs as magic solutions, and they become identified with the products as Viagra men and Sarafem women. Once patients begin to see the doctor as an impediment to satisfying their desires, the relationship is unlikely to achieve the goal of effective communication as envisaged by the Supreme Court of Canada. Patients have the illusion of power in a consumer relationship created by the power of illusion.

Conclusion

Advertising uses the power of illusion to draw on viewers' values and norms to create desires. Any educational value achieved by pharmaceutical advertising is secondary to the primary purpose of promoting the drugs. As identified by Williamson, the sense of knowing, without real knowledge, characterizes patient consciousness and represents the illusion of power.

Legalizing direct-to-consumer advertising would empower companies much more than it would consumers. The impact of DTCA in creating demand for higher priced and newer drugs creates distortions in health care allocation. Through the cost of DTCA itself, which is passed on to consumers, and through the increased consumption of products that such advertising creates, pharmaceutical companies contribute to unaffordable costs, costs that cannot be sustained within the

Canadian public health care system. In addition, money allocated to prescription drugs is thereby rendered unavailable for expenditures in other parts of the health care system, and this distortion of priorities contributes to further pressures within the system. Appeals to lifestyles and stereotypes, the medicalization of health care, and the normalization of drug-taking are all effects linked to drug advertising. Research on the effects of advertising directly to patients has not demonstrated that such promotion has the beneficial effects claimed for it. Indeed, advertising undermines the comprehension of the relative benefits and risks of drug therapies.

To achieve balanced and informed decision-making, patients and doctors need access to unbiased and reliable sources of information. Government efforts are needed to create such information sources to empower patients by providing full information about the risks, alternatives, and success rates of particular drug (and other) therapies and by avoiding subliminally connecting treatments to new diseases, lifestyles, and stereotypes of patients and diseases. Government must resist the campaign to permit direct-to-consumer advertising. Greater government awareness of the subtle processes through which advertising creates illusions is necessary to protect health care in Canada.

NOTES

I am grateful to Sarah Viau for her research assistance and to the Hampton Fund of the University of British Columbia for their financial support of this research.

1 L.I. Pugsley, 'The Administration and Development of Federal Statutes on Foods and Drugs in Canada' (1967) 23:3 Medical Services J. 387.
2 S.C. 1908, c. 56.
3 Pugsley, *supra* note 1 at 401–2.
4 *Inland Revenue Act of 1875*, R.S.C. 1875, c. 8.
5 'No person shall label, package, treat, process, sell or advertise any drug in a manner that is false, misleading or deceptive or is likely to create an erroneous impression regarding its character, value, quantity, composition, merit or safety.' *Food and Drugs Act*, R.S.C. 1985, c. F-27, s. 9(1).
6 Health Canada, Health Products and Food Branch, *Direct-to-Consumer Advertising* [*DTCA*] *of Prescription Drugs* (6 April 1999) (Discussion Docu-

ment), available at http://www.hc-sc.gc.ca/hpfb-dgpsa/oria-bari/99-04-14_3_e.html (accessed 13 March 2004).

7 C.R.C., c. 870, s. C.01.044.

8 Health Canada, DTCA, *supra* note 6 at 1.

9 Health Canada, Therapeutic Products Programme, *The Distinction between Advertising and Other Activities* (Jan. 1996). Updated Nov. 2000, administrative update Aug. 2005), www.hc-sc.gc.ca/dhp-mps/advert-publicit/pol/actv_promo_vs_info_e.html (accessed 30 August 2005).

10 World Health Organization, *Ethical Criteria for Medicinal Drug Promotion* (Geneva: WHO, 1988), http://www.who.int/medicines/library/dap/ethical-criteria/ethicalen.shtml (accessed 15 March 2004).

11 Health Canada, DTCA, *supra* note 6 at 2.

12 S.C. 1936, c. 24.

13 Pugsley, *supra* note 1 at 413–14.

14 C.R.C., c. 870, s. A.01.025.

15 The roles of the PAAB are specified in the Health Canada document, *Therapeutic Comparative Advertising: Directive and Guidance Document*, issued 6 April 2001, http://www.hc-sc.gc.ca/hpfb-dgpsa/tpd-dpt/ther_comp_adv_mar-2001_e.pdf (Mar. 2001, administrative update Aug. 2005) www.hc-sc.gc.ca/chp-mps/advert-publicit/pol/guide_Idir_ther_comp_e.html (accessed 30 August 2005). See at 6–8 in Part I. Relations among companies are also subject to the *Competition Act*, R.S.C. 1985, c. C-34.

16 Health Canada, DTCA, *supra* note 6 at 2.

17 Part I of the *Constitution Act, 1982*, being Schedule B to the *Canada Act 1982* (U.K.) 1982, c. 11.

18 J.M. Coetzee, *Elizabeth Costello* (London: Knopf, 2003) at 4.

19 Judith Williamson, *Decoding Advertisements: Ideology and Meaning in Advertising* (London: Boyars, 1978) at 26.

20 *Ibid.* at 27.

21 *Ibid.* at 30.

22 James B. Twitchell, *Twenty Ads that Shook the World: The Century's Most Groundbreaking Advertising and How It Changed Us All* (New York: Three Rivers Press, 2000) at 129.

23 *Ibid.*

24 This romanticized version of independence and freedom was already embodied by the Remington oil paintings and Western-genre pulp fiction to which Twitchell refers, *ibid.* at 130.

25 Roland Barthes, *Mythologies*, trans. by Annette Lavers (New York: Hill and Wang, 1972) at 11.

26 *Ibid.* at 131.
27 Robert Goldman, *Reading Ads Socially* (London: Routledge, 1992) at 39.
28 Williamson, *supra* note 19 at 116.
29 See, e.g., Goldman's analysis of fragrance marketing, *supra* note 27 at 37–60.
30 Williamson, *supra* note 19 at 45.
31 *Ibid.* at 47.
32 *Ibid.* at 45.
33 *Ibid.* at 47.
34 Robert Goldman and Stephen Papson, *Sign Wars: The Cluttered Landscape of Advertising* (New York: Guildford Press, 1996) at 29.
35 Goldman, *supra* note 27 at 169.
36 See, e.g., our discussion of heroic and interventionist imagery in Patricia Peppin and Elaine Carty, 'Semiotics, Stereotypes, and Women's Health: Signifying Inequality in Drug Advertising' (2001) 13 *Canadian Journal of Women and the Law* 326, at 343–53.
37 *Ibid.* at 349–53.
38 Emily Martin's work on the conceptualization of immunity, e.g., indicates that the body is seen as having a boundary that is invaded by bacteria and viruses. *Flexible Bodies: Tracking Immunity in American Culture – from the Days of Polio to the Age of AIDS* (Boston: Beacon Press, 1994).
39 Elizabeth Ettore and Elianne Riska, *Gendered Moods: Psychotropics and Society* (London: Routledge, 1995) at 19; Gerry V. Stimson and Barbara Webb, *Going to See the Doctor: The Consultation Process in General Practice* (London: Routledge and Kegan Paul, 1975) at 159.
40 John R. Neill, 'A Social History of Psychotropic Drug Advertisements' (1989) 28 Social Science and Medicine 333 at 337.
41 *Ibid.*
42 Deborah Lupton, 'The Construction of Patienthood in Medical Advertising' (1993) 23 Int. J. of Health Sciences 805 at 816.
43 U.S., General Accounting Office, 'Prescription Drugs: FDA Oversight of Direct-to-Consumer Advertising Has Limitations' (Washington: GAO, 2002) (Report No. GAO-03-177) at 1, http://www.gao.gov (accessed 10 January 2003). ['GAO 2002']
44 U.S., FDA, Draft Guidance for Industry, 62 Fed. Reg. 43171 (Aug. 12, 1997); *Guidance for Industry: Consumer-Directed Broadcast Advertisements* (Washington, DC: FDA, Aug. 1999), 64 Fed. Reg. 43197, www.fda.gov/cder/guidance/1804fnl.htm (accessed 5 July 2003).
45 Francis B. Palumbo and C. Daniel Mullins, 'The Development of Direct-to-Consumer Prescription Drug Advertising Regulation' (2002) 57 Food and Drug L. J. 423 at 423 (Table 1); 'GAO 2002,' *supra* note 43 at 3, 9–10.

provides similar figures noting that over the four-year period 1997–2001 such direct advertising increased by 145 per cent to $2.7 billion.

46 NIHCM Foundation, *Prescription Drug Expenditures in 2001: Another Year of Escalating Costs* (Washington: NIHCM Foundation, 2002).

47 'GAO 2002,' *supra* note 43 at 5.

48 IMS Health, 'IMS Reports 12 Percent Growth in 2001 Audited Global Pharmaceutical Sales to $364 Billion,' http://www.ne.imshealth.com/public/structure/dispcontent/1,2779,1341-1341-144056,00.htm (accessed 10 July 2003).

49 NIHCM Foundation, *Changing Patterns of Pharmaceutical Innovation* (Washington: NIHCM Foundation, 2002) at 3. A drug must satisfy both criteria to be considered highly innovative.

50 *Ibid.* at 1, citing data from Price, Waterhouse Coopers, 2001.

51 *Ibid.* at 2–3. citing *inter alia*, G. Harris, 'Drug Firms Stymied in the Lab, Become Marketing Machines' Wall Street Journal, 6 July 2000.

52 Charles Medawar, 'Health, Pharma and the EU, A Briefing for Members of the European Parliament on Direct-to-Consumer Drug Promotion' (Dec. 2001), http://www.socialaudit.org.uk/5111-005.htm (accessed 12 March 2004).

53 *Hopp* v *Lepp*, [1980] 2 S.C.R. 192; *Reibl v. Hughes*, [1980] 2 S.C.R. 880.

54 In Bernard Dickens's phrase, the term 'informed decision-making' is more appropriate to describe what has become a process within a relationship, in Jocelyn Downie, Timothy Caulfield, and Colleen Flood, eds., *Canadian Health Law and Policy*, 2nd ed. (Scarborough: Butterworths, 2002) at 130–1.

55 *Norberg v. Weinrib* (1992), 92 D.L.R. (4th) 449 (S.C.C.).

56 *McInerney v. McDonald*, [1992] 2 S.C.R. 138.

57 *Hollis v. Dow Corning Corp.* (1995), 129 D.L.R. (4th) 609 (S.C.C.).

58 Justice Robins for the Ontario Court of Appeal had reached a similar conclusion in *Buchan v. Ortho Pharmaceuticals (Canada) Ltd.* (1986), 25 D.L.R. (4th) 658 (Ont. C.A.).

59 *Eldridge v. British Columbia (Attorney General)*, [1997] 3 S.C.R. 624.

60 *Ibid.* at paras. 69–70.

61 Robert Bell, Richard Kravitz, and Michael Wilkes, 'Direct-to-Consumer Prescription Drug Advertising, 1989–1998; A Content Analysis of Conditions, Targets, Inducements, and Appeals' (2000) 49:4 Journal of Family Practice 329.

62 Steven Woloshin, Lisa M. Schwartz, Jennifer Tremmel, and H. Gilbert Welch, 'Direct-to-Consumer Advertisements for Prescription Drugs: What Are Americans Being Sold?' (2001) 358:9288 Lancet 1141.

63 Michael S. Wilkes, Bruce H. Doblin, and Martin F. Shapiro, 'Pharmaceuti-

cal Advertisements in Leading Medical Journals: Experts' Assessments' (1992) 116:11 Annals of Internal Medicine 912.

64 FDA Commissioner David Kessler, e.g., wrote an affirmative article about the study. 'Addressing the Problem of Misleading Advertising' (1992) 116:11 Annals of Internal Medicine 950.

65 Andrew Herxheimer, Cecilia Stalsby Lundborg, and Barbro Westerholm, 'Advertisements for Medicines in Leading Medical Journals in 18 Coun- tries: A 12-Month Survey of Information Content and Standards' (1993) 23:1 Int. J. of Health Services 161.

66 *Ibid.* at 166 (Table 3).

67 'GAO 2002,' *supra* note 43 at 17, 21.

68 *Ibid.* at 22–3.

69 *Ibid.* at 18. Barbara Mintzes reported that in the late 1997 to early 1999 period following the clarification of the guidelines for DTCA, just over half the broadcast advertisements violated the *Food, Drug and Cosmetic Act.* 'An Assessment of the Health System Impacts of Direct-to-Consumer Advertising of Prescription Medicines (DTCA),' *Health Policy Research Unit Research Reports*, vol. 2, *Literature Review* (Vancouver: University of British Columbia, 2001) at 65.

70 Available at www.fda.gov/cder/warn/ (accessed 15 March 2004). Adver- tising for the drug Allegra, e.g., was posted on 14 Jan. 2004, along with the regulatory letter that lists the identified violations.

71 Bob Burton, 'Ban Direct to Consumer Advertising, Report Recommends' (2003) 326 Brit. Med. J. 467, at 467a citing Nov. 2002 memo to the Pharmac board.

72 The legal position is summarized in Palumbo and Mullins, *supra* note 45 and in 'GAO 2002' *supra* note 43.

73 Margaret Gilhooley, 'Drug Regulation and the Constitution after *Western States*' (2003) 37 U. of Richmond L. Rev. 901 at 919.

74 'GAO 2002,' *supra* note 43 at 16 and App. II.

75 Barbara Mintzes, M.L. Barer, R.L. Kravitz, K. Bassett, J. Lexchin, A. Kazan- jian, and R.G. Evans, 'How Does Direct-to-Consumer Advertising (DTCA) Affect Prescribing? A Survey in Primary Care Environments With and Without Legal DTCA' (2003) 169:5 Can. Med. Assoc. J. 405.

76 *Ibid.* at tables 2 and 3.

77 *Ibid.* at table 5.

78 *Ibid.* at 9, citing Joel Lexchin, 'Lifestyle Drugs: Issues for Debate' (2001) 164:10 Can. Med. Assoc. J. 1449.

79 Les Toop, Dee Richards, Tony Dowell, Murray Tilyard, Tony Fraser, and Bruce Arroll. *Direct to Consumer Advertising of Prescription Drugs in New*

Zealand: For Health or for Profit? Report to the Minister of Health Supporting the Case for a Ban on DTCA (Departments of General Practice, Christchurch, Dunedin, Wellington, and Auckland Schools of Medicine: University of Otago 2003): http//www.chmeds.ac.n/report.htm (accessed 2 January 2004).

80 *Ibid*. App. 3.

81 Robert Bell, Michael Wilkes, and Richard Kravitz, 'Advertisement-Induced Prescription Drug Requests: Patients' Anticipated Reactions to a Physician Who Refuses' (1999) 48:6 Journal of Family Practice 446.

82 Toop *et al.*, *supra* note 79 at 19–21, summarizing the literature.

83 Kathryn Aikin, U.S. FDA 'Direct-to-Consumer Advertising of Prescription Drugs: Physician Survey Preliminary Results 1/13/2003,' http://www.fda .gov/cder/ddmac/globalsummit2003/ (accessed 15 March 2004), slide 22. See also, U.S., FDA Talk Paper, 'FDA Releases Preliminary Results of Physician Survey on Direct-to-Consumer RX Drug Advertisements' (13 Jan. 2003), www.fda.gov/bbs/topics/ANSWERS/2003/ANS01189.html (accessed 21 Jan. 2003).

84 Jerry Avorn, Milton Chen, and Robert Hartley, 'Scientific versus Commercial Sources of Influence on the Prescribing Behavior of Physicians' (1992) 93:1 Am. J. of Med. 4; Jill Cockburn and Sabrina Pit, 'Prescribing Behaviour in Clinical Practice: Patients' Expectations and Doctors' Perceptions of Patients' Expectations – a Questionnaire Study' (1997) 315:707 Brit. Med. J. 520. These studies are discussed in Toop *et al.*, *supra* note 79 at 19.

85 Kathryn Aikin, U.S. FDA, 'The Impact of Direct-to-Consumer Prescription Drug Advertising on the Physician-Patient Relationship' (slide presentation to the FDA Public Meeting on DTC Promotion), http://www.fda.gov/ cder/ddmac/DTCmeeting2003_presentations.html (accessed 15 March 2004).

86 *Ibid*. at slide 58.

87 *Ibid*. at slide 60.

88 *Ibid*. at slide 49.

89 *Ibid*. at slide 51 shows the further breakdown into general and specialist practitioners. Just over a quarter agreed that benefits were exaggerated by confusing relative risks and benefits a great deal (26%), while 32% answered a great deal to the idea that patients thought that drugs worked better than they do.

90 *Ibid*. at slides 46, 47.

91 Sheila McKechnie, 'Public Health or Private Profit?' Rapid response to Ray Moynihan, Iona Heath, David Henry, and Peter C Gøtzsche, 'Selling Sickness: The Pharmaceutical Industry and Disease Mongering' (2002) 324

Brit. Med. J. 886, http://bmj.bmjjournals.com/cgi/eletters/324/7342/886#2123, reported that the Consumers' Association in Britain had found many examples of companies forming alliances with patient groups 'to get their marketing messages out to a wider public under the guise of providing patients with much-needed information.'

92 David Healy, *Let Them Eat Prozac* (Toronto: Lorimer, 2003) at 178.

93 Sandra Coney, 'Impotence Drug Marketing Doesn't Stand Up to Scrutiny,' Women's Health Watch Selections from April 2003 http://www.womens-health.org.nz/whwapr03.htm at 7 (accessed 14 March 2004).

94 'Women's Health Issues: Direct-to-Consumer Advertising,' *Our Bodies Ourselves*, posted 4/02; last revised 6/10/03, http://www.ourbodiesourselves.org/dtca3.htm (accessed 15 March 2004).

95 Moynihan et al., *supra* note 91 at 886.

96 *Ibid.* at 890.

97 *Ibid.* at 921; Uwe Reinhardt, 'Perspectives on the Pharmaceutical Industry' (2001) 20 Health Affairs 136, at 147.

98 *Perez v. Wyeth Laboratories Inc.* 161 N.J. 1, 734 A. 2d 1245 (N.J.S.C., 1999).

99 Bernard J. Garbutt III and Melinda E. Hofmann, 'Recent Developments in Pharmaceutical Products Liability Law: Failure to Warn, the Learned Intermediary Defense, and Other Issues in the New Millenium' (2003) 58 Food and Drug L. J. 269 at 274.

16 The Media, Marketing, and Genetic Services

TIMOTHY CAULFIELD

The public gets most of its information about genetics and biotechnology from the popular media. From stories about gene discoveries to the prospect of human cloning, the media have informed the public debate and helped to set the broader research and policy agenda.[1] As a result, the popular media have emerged as tremendously important sources of science information. They not only inform public perceptions about the risks and benefits of a given technology or area of research, but help to shape the discourse around important policy issues.

Often, however, the media seem to get it wrong. Many view press coverage of biomedical stories as 'inaccurate, superficial or sensationalised.'[2] In the context of genetic research, for instance, it has been suggested that 'genohype' – the inaccurate portrayal of genetic research – is having an adverse effect on the public understanding of science, policy development, and the way in which genetic services are utilized.[3] One need only think of the many headlines and magazine covers that have proclaimed the next significant, near future, scientific breakthrough.[4] Although the recent advances in the science of genetics have provided an unprecedented amount of basic scientific information and invaluable research tools, the promised therapies and diagnostic procedures have been slow to materialize. Nevertheless, we continue to see optimistic predictions in the popular press around topics such as pharmacogenomics and gene therapy.[5]

The nature and impact of media representations of science have become a major policy concern.[6] In the context of health care policy, for example, media representations may help to generate a public demand for a given technology that may not be supported by a more dispassionate technology assessment. Many of the suggested reforms in the area of science reporting have, understandably, concentrated on ensuring that researchers learn effective communication skills and that reporters understand basic scientific principles.[7] However, there are reasons to believe that the 'hyping' of research results might be part of a more systemic problem associated with the increasingly commercial nature of the research environment. Indeed, in many ways, this chapter builds on the concerns articulated in the preceding one by Patricia Peppin regarding direct-to-consumer advertising. In that context, the pharmaceutical industry uses specific strategies to generate interest in a given product – often with less than positive social consequences. In this chapter I explore a broader, less explicit, social phenomenon: the role of the commercialization agenda in research in the generation of media hype. I argue, as does Peppin, that the commercialization of science communication may inappropriately distort resource allocation policy.

The chapter begins with a review of the available evidence on the accuracy and nature of media representations of genetics and biotechnology. Next is a consideration of how the tone of media representations may be influenced by the commercialization and innovation agendas that increasingly guide both universities and government. This is followed by an analysis of the social concern associated with the hyping of science. Finally, a few policy recommendations are made.

Are the Media to Blame?

Despite an enduring perception that the media are the primary source of inaccurate claims about science, the evidence suggests that the story is much more complex. There is certainly evidence that the coverage of specific topics, such as the alleged finding of the gay gene and human cloning, has been less than ideal.[8] However, available data show that, in some circumstances, the media reporting of science is surprisingly accurate and portrays a message created by the scientific community. For example, in one study that involved a survey of first authors who had an interaction with the media it was found that most had a generally positive experience and 86 per cent rated coverage of their scientific studies as accurate. Interestingly, only 3 per cent called the coverage inaccurate.[9] Nevertheless, despite their own favourable experience, many of the first authors still had concerns about the accuracy of science portrayed in the media.

Another study that examined how the print media reported 'genetic discoveries' found that only 11 per cent of the newspaper stories could be categorized as inaccurate.[10] The study concluded that, in general, the media uncritically convey messages found in the peer-reviewed science articles. The study, which analysed 627 newspaper articles reporting on 111 papers in scientific journals, also found that few of the newspaper articles (15 per cent) and even fewer of the science articles (5 per cent) dealt with potential risks or social consequences of the genetic discovery.

This latter finding is consistent with the results from other studies. Indeed, a strong preference for positive messages is a constant theme in the literature on the media coverage of biomedical stories.[11] For example, a study by Moynihan et al., of 207 news stories on drugs used for disease prevention found that only 15 per cent of the stories presented both relative and absolute benefits.[12] Such research supports the concern voiced by a number of commentators and policy groups, namely, that media stories overemphasize potential breakthroughs and do a poor job of reflecting the incremental manner in which scientific knowledge usually develops.[13]

This largely positive and, as we will see below, commercially influenced message is picked up by the public. There is a growing body of literature that suggests that the public generally views media coverage of biotechnology as being predominantly positive in tone. And, more importantly, this influences the public perception of the technology.[14]

Commercialization Pressure and the Media

If, in fact, journalists often do a reasonable job reporting science stories, how does the hype find its way into the popular media? One possible source is the research community itself. Researchers and research institutions are under increasing pressure to justify their work in terms of future economic benefits. As noted in the chapters that follow, by, respectively, Trudo Lemmens and Jocelyn Downie, commercialization and economic growth have emerged as a dominant theme for public funding agencies and, as a result, researchers must now frame both grant applications and research results in a manner that reflects this reality. Indeed, in the knowledge-based economy, university research is increasingly viewed as an important part of the economic agenda – at least in the developed world. In the context of Canadian biomedical research, virtually all of the major public funding entities, including the Canadian Institutes of Health Research (CIHR) and Genome Canada, have the promotion of economic growth as an explicit mandate.[15]

In such an environment, it is only natural that research results are portrayed in a manner that emphasizes benefits and possible future therapies. For example, researchers seeking federal funding will want to emphasize how their work may be commercialized and/or have clinical relevance. To do otherwise is to place oneself at a disadvantage in the research-funding game. And for those researchers seeking co-funding – a requirement for some federal funding entities, such as Genome Canada[16] – expressing research in terms of possible products and economic benefits is all but essential. Industrial partners will want to be assured that the partnership has a chance of facilitating a growth in profits. In this regard, a media story that reports a possibly commercializable product can be a wonderful tool in the search for private investors. More broadly, those individuals who lead major funding agencies need to constantly 'sell' the value of research to politicians and high-level bureaucrats to ensure continued public funding.

While systemic commercialization pressures may be a covert causal factor in the perpetuation of science hype, some commentators, such as Dorothy Nelkin, place more direct blame with the scientific community. She has suggested that 'geneticists have become skilled in rhetorical strategies designed to attract the media.'[17] For Nelkin, self-promotion and the forwarding of a particular research agenda underlie the hype found in the popular press, and they are part of the past and ongoing effort to sell the genetic research agenda to both the general public and government research funding entities: 'It was not journalists but geneticists who initially employed attention-seeking metaphors to describe the genome as a "Book of Man" or a "medical crystal ball." Geneticists themselves have promoted the "gene of the week" and promised therapeutic solutions. Courting media attention, scientists have helped to evoke premature enthusiasm and optimistic expectations. And their messages are amplified by the press.'[18]

Whether scientists, themselves, are the instigating force behind science hype or are merely responding to a commercialization trend, growing evidence supports the conclusion that positive messages are the norm for media stories about biomedical research.[19] And, perhaps more importantly, the tone of peer-reviewed publications also seems to be influenced by the commercialization agenda.[20] In a recent Canadian study, for example, it was found that 'industry funded trials are more likely to be associated with statistically significant pro-industry findings.'[21]

Given the trust that the public, policy-makers and the media place in peer-reviewed publications, the fact that these publications may be unduly influenced by industry is particularly worrisome. Peer-reviewed studies found in respected science journals hold particular sway with media reporters. Tom Wilkie notes that 'Journalists depend on the accuracy and relevance of scientific papers published in the academic journals for their regular daily fare. The journals are perceived as trustworthy sources of information which, unlike a company or research institution's press release, is believed to be disinterested.'[22] The reality that reporters rely on studies that appear in trustworthy and prestigious journals was observed by Bubela and Caulfield, who found that the vast majority of the newspaper stories on genetic discoveries came from just a few well-known and respected peer-reviewed journals. The most commonly cited scientific journals were *Science* (31 per cent), *Nature* (19 per cent), *Nature Genetics* (16 per cent), and *Cell* (16 per cent).[23]

Naturally, journalists also view scientists as trusted sources of information. Indeed, 'they rarely go beyond the information presented by scientists themselves, via their professional publications and/or interviews.'[24] As such, newspaper stories are often missing an alternate point of view or an interdisciplinary perspective[25] – both valuable components of a balanced presentation of research results.[26] Given the time constraints imposed on journalists to produce a story quickly, this is hardly surprising. It is time consuming to find credible alternate views. And often journalists do not have the space to include counterarguments or in-depth discussions about risks and possible social consequences. In such circumstances, readers are left with a story that is largely a reinterpretation of the peer-reviewed science article with commentary from one of the primary authors.

In the end, researchers, research institutions, funding entities, and the media can all be viewed as 'complicit collaborators' in the subtle hyping of science stories.[27] Obviously, researchers have long had a variety of reasons to seek media attention. Media coverage brings attention to their research, helps attract funding, and raises the profile of the institution.[28] But the desire for media attention is greatly magnified in an increasingly commercially driven research environment – particularly in relation to potentially commercializable products.

Social Concerns

Why is science hype problematic? What is the relevance of media portrayals to health policy? First, simplistic and overly optimistic portrayals of research results may have an adverse impact on public understanding.[29] This will impact the public's ability to participate in policy discussions and may create unrealistic expectations about the potential benefits and clinical value of a given biotechnological intervention.[30] Media stories that emphasize the genetic basis of disease and downplay the complex and multifactorial nature of most illnesses could help to inappropriately 'geneticize' our health care system.[31] While we need to be careful to not oversimplify the way in which the media may influence the public's attitude and behaviour,[32] simplistic explanations of the role of genes in human health or overly optimistic stories can, at a minimum, be misleading and, over time, may influence how a technology is implemented and utilized.[33] This speculative concern is supported by research that shows that media stories about health generate a high degree of public interest and may affect behaviour.[34]

There is ample evidence that patient demands influence the clinical practices of health care providers. For example, in the context of pharmaceuticals, Mintzes et al. note that '[p]atients' requests for medicines are a powerful driver of prescribing decisions.'[35] There is already a high degree of interest in genetic testing.[36] There is also evidence that, in many countries, the public believes it has a right of access to genetic services.[37] For example, one study found that 95 per cent of women (first degree relatives of women with breast cancer) thought that they should be able to get testing despite a physician's recommendation to the contrary.[38]

This combination of patient interest, positive media coverage, and a strong autonomy-driven (or consumer)[39] conception of access could result in a patient-driven utilization pattern. This is particularly so given that many physicians currently lack a knowledge base about genetics and, therefore, may not be in a position to critically appraise media portrayals or patient requests.[40]

Given what I believe to be a close connection between the nature of media portrayals of biotechnology and the broader commercialization agenda, media representations can be viewed as a subtle form of advertising – albeit often inadvertent. This is not to say that all science reporting is part of a coordinated effort to promote a particular product. On the contrary, in the case of the reporting of genetic discoveries, there is rarely a specific 'product' to promote. However, in the long run, a continued, systemic, trend to report positive media representations may affect health care providers and the public in a manner similar to advertising. There seems little doubt that advertising influences clinical decision-making.[41] For example, recent work on direct-to-consumer advertising of pharmaceuticals has shown 'more advertising leads to more requests for advertised medicines, and more prescriptions.' [42] Consistently enthusiastic stories about the results of genetic research could send a powerful message about the worth of a specific technology, such as a genetic test, or, more broadly, a given area of research in much the same manner as an explicit advertising campaign does.

In fact, in some ways, optimistic media portrayals could be considered a more powerful form of promotion. The message is delinked from an obvious marketing agenda and often includes a trusted voice, a university-based researcher. The public places a good deal of trust in university-based scientists. In part, this is because university researchers are perceived as independent and, for example, removed from the pressures of commerce.[43]

A second concern relates to the potential impact of media representations on pubic funding decisions. Media stories have a role in how a society, as a whole, views the benefits and risks associated with a given technology.[44] Although I am unaware of any specific research on this point, optimistic stories in the popular press also seem capable of influencing policy decisions about what services are covered by the publicly funded health care system. This is particularly so given (as discussed by Flood, Stabile, and Tuohy in the first chapter of this volume), the relatively ad hoc way in which health care services are deemed 'medically necessary.' Absent a robust technology assessment process, political pressure, fostered by a media-informed interest in a particular service, could result in a decision to fund a service that may not otherwise have been funded.[45] Naturally, such a phenomenon would place unnecessary and inappropriate cost pressures on the public health care system. In addition, 'genohype' could pressure us to invest in services, technology, and research areas at the expense of health care strategies that are potentially effective but lacking commercial potential (for example, public health initiatives). As Jocelyn Downie notes (in chapter 18), upstream research policy decisions can have profound downstream health policy implications.

Third, science hype may, eventually, have an impact on both the research environment and the biotechnology industry. Media stories that emphasize unrealistic, near future, benefits will inevitably result in unmet expectations. The markets may grow increasingly suspicious of claims of commercial potential. In addition, the research community may also lose public trust.[46] Currently, university researchers are a tremendously trusted voice. However, if it becomes apparent that their message is influenced by commercial interests, public trust will erode. Without public trust, political support and, perhaps, public funding for research may diminish.

Reducing the Hype

Developing strategies that can meaningfully address these concerns will be challenging. The pressure to justify research in economic and practical terms has created a 'media arms race.' All researchers are competing for a slice of the same funding pie, and so a given researcher or institution has little to gain by moderating the hyperbole. Why should you moderate your message if your colleague in another university is not moderating hers? Why should a university press office withhold or tone down a press release if other universities are not doing the same?

To have any hope of success, communication policies should be national in scope and involve all the major research funding entities. However, there are also major obstacles at this level. In Canada, the public funding research entities, such as the Canadian Institutes of Health Research and Genome Canada, are involved in a never-ending campaign to attract federal funds. This means that they must explain the value of their programs in terms that politicians will find exciting, understandable, and politically worthy – hardly the environment to encourage a reduction in science hype. Despite these policy challenges, a coordinated, national, effort to improve science communication seems essential. In other countries, such as France and the United Kingdom, this has already emerged as a major policy priority.[47]

As a start, I believe that such an effort should have a number of key elements. First, funding agencies, universities, and researchers should consider the fact that science hype may not be politically necessary – at least in the context of public support. While basic science may not be as exciting as a story about the next biomedical breakthrough, the public does seem to have an appreciation for and a desire to support fundamental research. For example, one U.S. study found that 81 per cent of the public believes that '[e]ven if it brings no immediate benefits, scientific research that advances the frontiers of knowledge is necessary and should be supported by the Federal Government.'[48] Similar results have been found in other jurisdictions.[49]

Second, as noted by other commentators,[50] strategies should be developed to educate both researchers and the media on science communication. These strategies should include an ongoing reminder to both scientists and reporters to be careful not to exaggerate claims of immediate benefit and possible breakthroughs. Indeed, the report by the U.K.'s Social Issues Research Centre suggests that 'studies that appear radically to challenge existing assumptions should be handled with particular care by journalists.'[51] In addition, the education strategies should encourage researchers to communicate the benefits of basic science and the incremental nature of the advance in knowledge and reporters to seek, whenever possible, alternative points of view, especially if the researcher is claiming a significant advance. Admittedly, such reminders would be a small and relatively mild opposing force to commercialization and media interest pressures.

Third, the education of health care providers, particularly family physicians, is central. Physicians should be made aware of the risks and benefits of genetic services and the potential impact of commercial pressure on the nature of public representations. In the context of health care costs this strategy seems especially important. Primary care physicians can play a key role in educating the public on the place of genetics in health and critiquing the claims made in media representations.[52] The *Romanow Report* noted the value of educated health care providers in relation to cost control. '[T]he inflationary pressures associated with health care technologies could be better controlled through policies that influence decisions made by health care providers in their clinical encounter with patients. In other words, for health care providers to use technology effectively, they need accurate and relevant information and the right incentives for its use when they are dealing directly with patients.'[53]

Fourth, given the obvious role that the popular media play in how society frames the risks and benefits of a given technology or area of science, more research on the source, impact, and nature of media representations is clearly warranted. This should include a consideration of the long-term policy implications of the 'selling of science.'

Finally, and perhaps most importantly, the government should consider the development of a system that allows for both the independent assessment of new technologies and the communication of accurate and trustworthy information.[54] Given the growing evidence of the impact of commercial pressure on the tone and nature of science reporting both in the popular press and peer-reviewed journals, there is a pressing need for an independent source of information. The information source should also be, as much a possible, at arm's length from government and the research funding entities.

Conclusion

The involvement of industry in biomedical research is inevitable and is not, on its own, an inherently bad thing. Indeed, we live in a market economy and industry involvement in biomedical research is likely necessary to ensure the development and dissemination of useful technologies. However, there is growing evidence that the increasingly commercialized nature of the research environment is having a profound impact on the nature of biomedical research and how research results are communicated to the public. This trend could, over the long run, have an adverse impact on the public understanding of science and how new technologies are utilized. This, in turn, could affect the long-term sustainability of Canada's health care system. Indeed, the uncritical and enthusiastic reporting of new medical technologies and discoveries is often little more than inadvertent unpaid advertising. And like advertising, the result is the promotion of use. More significantly, however, this kind of science reporting could erode public trust in the research and researchers. As thoughtfully noted by Tom Wilkie: 'If science is to manage the transition from its older, academic tradition to a new style, while keeping popular assent and the popular image of science as an impartial means of getting at the truth, then the scientific community itself must recognise the importance of maintaining impartial sources of public information.'[55]

NOTES

I would like to thank Tania Bubela, Genome Canada, the Stem Cell Network and the Alberta Heritage Foundation for Medical Research. I would also like to thank the conference participants for their helpful comments. This chapter builds on the opinion paper 'Biotechnology and the Popular Press: Hype and the Selling of Science' (2004) 22 Trends in Biotechnology 337–9.

1 Robert. Steinbrook, 'Medical Journals and Medical Reporting' (2000) 342 New England J. of Med. 1668.
2 Miriam Shuchman and Micheal Wilkes, 'Medical Scientists and Health news Reporting: A Case of Miscommunication' (1997) 126 Annals of Internal Medicine 976 at 976.
3 Timothy Caulfield, 'Underwhelmed: Hyperbole, Regulatory Policy and the Genetic Revolution' (2001) 45 McGill Law Journal 437; Usher Fleising,

'In search of genohype: A content analysis of biotechnology company documents' (2001) 20:3 New Genet. and Soc. 239; and Jon Turney, 'The Public Understanding of Genetics: Where Next?' (1995) 1 Human Reproduction and Genetic Ethics 5 at 5: 'As the human genome project gathers momentum, there is wide agreement that a broad effort to improve public understanding of genetics will be needed to underpin public debate about the applications of the new genetics.'

4 See, for example, Linda Marsa, 'Medical News Requires a Skeptical Eye' *Edmonton Journal*, 14 May 2001 at A13.

5 Bryn Williams-Jones and Oonagh Corrigan, 'Rhetoric and Hype: Where's the "Ethics" in Pharmacogenomics?' (2003) 3:6 Am J. Pharmacogenomics 375 at 376.

6 See Ian Hargreaves, Justin Lewis, and Tammy Speers, *Toward a Better Map: Science, the Public and the Media* (Swindon, UK: Economic and Social Research Council, 2003); Celeste Condit, 'What Is "Public Opinion" About Genetics?' 2 Nature Rev. Genet. 811; and 'Science Communication: A National Priority, Says French Senate,' Cordis News, 14 October 2003 http://dbs.cordis.lu/fep-cgi/srchidaab?ACTION=D&SESSION= 129422005-9-164&DOC=15&TBL=EN_NEWS&RCN=EN_RCN_ID:21100& CALLER=EN_NEWS (accessed 15 September 2005): 'France's commission for culture affairs has published a report on science communication in which it states that conveying science to the masses should be made a national priority.'

7 Social Issues Research Centre (SIRC) in partnership with the Royal Society and the Royal Institution of Great Britain, *Guidelines on Science and Health Communication* (November 2001).

8 See, for example, Peter Conrad and Susan Markens. 'Constructing the "Gay Gene" in the News: Optimism and Skepticism in the US and British Press' (2001) 5 Health 373; Hargreaves, *et al.*, *supra* note 6; and Patrick Hopkins, 'Bad Copies: How Popular Media Represent Cloning as an Ethical Problem' (1998) 28:2 Hastings Center Report 6.

9 Michael Wilkes and Richard Kravitz, 'Medical Researchers and the Media: Attitudes toward Public Dissemination of Research' (1992) 268 JAMA 999 at 1000.

10 Tania Bubela and Timothy Caulfield, 'Do the Print Media "Hype" Genetic Research? A Comparison of Newspaper Stories and Peer-Reviewed Research Papers' (2004) 170 Can. Med. Assoc. J. 1399–1407.

11 See, for example, Alan Cassels, *et al.*, 'Drugs in the News: an Analysis of Canadian Newspaper Coverage of New Prescription Drugs' (2003) 168 Can. Med. Assoc. J. 1133; and Gideon Koren and Naomi Klein, 'Bias

against Negative Studies in Newspaper Reports of Medical Research'
(1991) 266 JAMA 1824, at abstract: 'The number, length, and quality of
newspaper reports on the positive study were greater than news reports
on the negative study, which suggests a bias against news reports of
studies showing no effects or no adverse effects.' Some commentators
have also noted that the inaccurate reporting of risks may also have an
adverse social impact. See, for example, Social Issues Research Centre
(SIRC), *supra* note 7 at 2: 'Information that is misleading or factually
inaccurate can cause real distress to vulnerable groups. Misleading information that provokes unfounded public reactions (e.g. reluctance to
undergo vaccination) can be said to cost lives.' See also Hopkins, *supra*
note 8 at 6. While I believe this is an important issue, a comprehensive
analysis is beyond the scope of this chapter.

12 Ray Moynihan, *et al.*, 'Coverage by the News Media of the Benefits and
Risks of Medications' (2000) 342 New England J. Med. 1645 at 1645.

13 SIRC *supra* note 7. See also, Marsa, *supra* note 4 at A13: 'It's only when
cumulative evidence points to one inexorable conclusion that medical
science feels comfortable making the connection.'

14 Ellen Tambor, *et al.*, 'Mapping the Human Genome: An Assessment of
Media Coverage and Public Reaction' (2002) 4 Genetics in Medicine 31 at
34. See also Andrew Laing, Cormex Research, 'A Report on News Media
Effects and Public Opinion Formation Regarding Biotechnology Issues'
(a study commissioned by the Canadian Biotechnology Secretariat,
Ottawa, July 2004).

15 See Timothy Caulfield, 'Sustainability and the Balancing of the Health
Care and Innovation Agendas: The Commercialization of Genetic Research'
(2003) 66 Saskatchewan Law Review 629.

16 Genome Canada, http://www.genomecanada.ca/index.htm.

17 Dorothy Nelkin, 'Beyond Risk: Reporting about Genetics in Post-Asilomar
Press' (2001) 44 Perspectives in Biology and Medicine 199 at 201. See also
Dorothy Nelkin, 'Molecular Metaphors: The Gene in Popular Discourse'
(2001) 2 Nat. Rev. Gen. 555 at 559 where she argues that the popular press
is quick to explain human disease and behaviour in biological terms. 'But
this is a leap conveyed to the public through molecular metaphor, deployed by scientists to promote their research and by the media to explain
the science of genetics.' A number of other commentators have voiced a
similar view. See, for example, Alan Petersen, 'Biofantasies: Genetics and
Medicine in the Print News Media' (2001) 52 Social Science and Medicine
1255 at 1257: 'In their effort to counter public scepticism of genetics and its
benefits, and to enhance their prestige and competitive advantage in new
fields of research, scientists have sought to gain greater control over

science news and the images that they present. They have made increasing use of public relations experts to promote favourable images of genetics.'

18 Nelkin, *ibid.* at 205.

19 See generally, *supra* note 11.

20 It is important to note that I am not saying that other, non-commercial, agendas do not play an important role in what is published in peer-reviewed journals and, in turn, the popular press. For example, there was the well-publicized case of a study, which appeared in the medical journal *Lancet*, that claimed there was a connection between childhood vaccination and autism. It later came to light that the researchers were being paid by a legal aid service 'looking into whether families could sue over the immunization.' Associated Press, 'Lancet Disowns Autism Article' (22 Feb. 2004) *Edmonton Journal* A7. Dr Richard Horton, the editor of Lancet, is reported as saying that this is a 'fatal conflict of interest' (*ibid.*).

21 Mohit Bhandari, Jason Busse, Dianne Jackowski, *et al.*, 'Association between Industry Funding and Statistically Significant Pro-Industry Findings in Medical and Surgical Randomized Trials' (2004) 170 Can. Med. Assoc. J. 477. See also, Frank van Kolfshooten, 'Can You Believe What You Read?' (2002) 416 Nature 360, at 361 where the author reports on a study that found that 'among the authors of original research papers, reviews and letters to the editor that were supportive of the drugs' use, 96% had financial relationships with the drugs' manufacturers; for publications deemed neutral or critical the figure was only 60% and 37% respectively.'

22 Tom Wilkie, 'Sources in Science: Who Can We Trust?' (1996) 347 Lancet 1308, at 1311. See also, Alan Petersen, *supra* note 17 at 1257: 'The press, like its readers, generally finds science intimidating, so editors are likely to insist on sources that have obvious credentials and credibility.'

23 *Supra* note 10 at 1400.

24 Petersen, *supra* note 17 at 1266.

25 This is a point that was also noted by Celeste Condit, 'How the Public Understands Genetics: Non-Deterministic and Non-Discriminating Interpretations of the 'Blueprint' Metaphor' (1999) 8 Public Understanding of Science 169, at 178: 'While scientists have important contributions to make, their unique world-view and interests are often over-represented in stories about scientific and technological policies.'

26 This is also consistent with the findings of the Bubela and Caulfield study, *supra* note 10, where it was found that in almost 90% of the stories, the main voice was the university, government, or hospital researcher. Only 1.3% of the newspaper stories quoted a researcher or scientist who was not an author of the peer-reviewed article.

27 David Ransohoff and Richard Ransohoff, 'Sensationalism in the Media:

When Scientists and Journalists May Be Complicit Collaborators' (2001) 4 Eff. Clin. Pract.185; and *ibid.*

28 Shuchman and Wilkes, *supra* note 2.

29 Nuffield Council on Bioethics, *Genetics and Human Behaviour: The Ethical Context* (London: Nuffield Council on Bioethics) (2002) at 236.

30 Koren and Klein, *supra* note 11 at 1826: 'The public receives much of its medical information from newspapers. If bias against reporting negative results exists, as we found in our analysis of the two studies in *JAMA*, the public is likely to receive an unbalanced picture concerning controversial health issues.'

31 Alan Petersen, *supra* note 17 at 1267 summarizes what he views to be the potential impact of the media on public attitudes as follows: 'The strong impression conveyed by these stories is that genes are the most important factor underlying disease and that science, by unlocking nature's secrets, will eventually lead to treatment, prevention or cure. By framing stories on genetics and medicine this way, the print news media are likely to exert a powerful influence on public responses to health problems. Importantly, they may lead people to overlook the importance of changing the economic, political, social, and physical environmental conditions that predispose to disease. Although it would be wrong to assume that news reports influence people's views and actions in any simple or direct way, the stories of hope and promise conveyed by many reports are likely to find a receptive audience. Such stories are deemed newsworthy precisely because they off people the promise of being able to re-make themselves anew.'

32 See, for example, Condit, *supra* note 25 where she notes that the public interpret the deterministic messages found in media stories in a much more critical and progressive fashion than is often assumed.

33 Of course, patient interest and utilization patterns are also influenced by portrayals that emphasize the seriousness of a relevant disease. As noted by Lisa Schwartz and Steven Woloshin, 'Marketing Medicine to the Public: A Reader's Guide' (2002) 287 JAMA 774 at 775: 'One way to increase demand for medical services is to promote exaggerated beliefs about disease risk and intervention benefits.' See also, Allen Buchanan, Dan Brock, Norman Daniels, and Daniel Wikler, *From Chance to Choice: Genetics and Justice* (Cambridge: Cambridge University Press, 2000) at 341: 'Given the public's lack of understanding of genetics and genetic causation, and the seriousness of disease linked to defective genes, the road to profit can lie through stimulating public fears.'

34 See, e.g., Timothy Johnson, 'Shattuck Lecture – Medicine and the Media'

(1998) 339 New England J. Med. 87. The author reports on a national poll of 2,256 Americans which found that 75% pay either a moderate or a great deal of 'attention to medical and health news reported by the media' and '[f]ifty-eight percent said they have changed their behaviour or taken some kind of action as a result of having read, seen, or heard a medical or health news story in the media.' The high degree of public interest in biomedical stories is also confirmed in the Bubela and Caulfield study, *supra* note 10, where it was found that 23% of such stories were on the first page of the newspaper. This placement indicates a perception by the editors of a good deal of public interest in stories about human genetics and health.

35 Barbara Mintzes *et al.*, 'Influences of Direct to Consumer Pharmaceutical Advertising and Patients' Requests on Prescribing Decisions' (2002) 324 Brit. Med. J. 278 at 279.

36 See, e.g., Micheal Andrykowski *et al.*, 'Hereditary Cancer Risk Notification and Testing: How Interested is the General Population?' (1997) 15 J. Clin. Oncol. 2139, found that 82% of the general population was interested in hereditary cancer risk testing.

37 Dorothy Wertz, 'Patient and Professional Views on Autonomy: A Survey in the United States and Canada' (1999) 7 Health Law Review 9, at para. 7, found that 60% of North American genetics patients surveyed thought that people are 'entitled to whatever [genetic] service they ask for if it is legal and they can pay for it out of pocket' and 69% thought that 'withholding any service is a denial of the patient's rights.'

38 Judith L. Benkendorf, *et al.*, 'Patients' Attitudes about Autonomy and Confidentiality in Genetic Testing for Breast-Ovarian Cancer Susceptibility' (1997) 73 Am. J. Med. Genet. 296 at 296. See also Timothy Caulfield, 'The Informed Gatekeeper?: A Commentary on Genetic Tests, Marketing Pressure and the Role of Primary Care Physicians' (2001) 9 Health Law Review 14.

39 See, for example, Julia. Neuberger, 'The Educated Patient: New Challenges for the Medical Profession' (2000) 247 J. Internal Med. 6 at 7 where it is argued that 'consumerism and mass communication' has begun to affect public services.'

40 Francis Giardiello, *et al.*, 'The Use and Interpretation of Commercial APC Gene Testing for Familial Adenomatous Polyposis' (1997) 20 New Engl. J. Med. 823; Alasdair Hunter *et al.*, 'Physician Knowledge and Attitudes towards Molecular Genetic (DNA) Testing of Their Patients' (1998) 53 Clin. Genet. 447; and C. James, G. Geller, Bernhardt B. *et al.*, 'Are Practicing and Future Physicians Prepared to Obtain Informed Consent? The Case of

Genetic Testing for Susceptibility to Breast Cancer' (1998) 1 Community Genetics 203.

41 See, for example, Bob Goodman, 'Do Drug Company Promotions Influence Physician Behaviour?' (2001) 174 West J. Med. 232. See also Carlos De La Cuevas, Emilio J. Sanz, and Juan A. De La Fuante, 'Variation in Antidepressant Prescribing Practice: Clinical Need or Market Influence?' (2002) 11 Pharmacoepidemiology of Drug Safety 515 at 520, where various factors that influence physician behaviour are canvassed. It was found that variation in prescribing behaviour was 'due to economic and social factors as much as to morbidity differences.'

42 Mintzes, *supra* note 35 at 278.

43 See Caulfield, *supra* note 15, where I report on a study that found Canadians believe university researchers to be highly credible. However, that credibility is degraded if there is a perceived commercial agenda. 'Most people rest their assessment of credibility on the degree to which the person or institution is perceived to be at arm's length and independent of controlling and/or funding influencers. The source of the funding seems to be the critical test.' Pollara and Earnscliffe, *Public Opinion Research into Biotechnology Issues, Third Wave* (December 2000) at 10.

44 See generally Hargreaves, *supra* note 6.

45 Public pressure and political considerations likely influenced the Ontario government's decision to fund testing for the BRCA1/2 mutations, which are associated with a predisposition to breast and ovarian cancer. Even though the clinical value of the BRCA1/2 test remains controversial, one high profile controversy resulted in a decision to fund the service. See Carolyn Abraham, 'Tenacious Woman Scores Medical Victory,' *Globe and Mail*, 27 August 1999 at A1; and Carolyn Abraham, 'Fiona's Choice: Lose Breasts or Risk Life,' *Globe and Mail*, 17 July 1998 at A1.

46 Continued hype may also cause the public to lose trust in the media. See, for example, Steinbrook, *supra* note 1 at 1670: 'Hype, however, creates unrealistic expectations and contributes to the belief that the news media cannot be trusted.'

47 See generally *supra* note 6. See also, David Adam, 'Scientists Seek Safety in Secrets of the Soundbite' (2002) 418 Nature 712, where the UK's new Science Media Centre is discussed. The centre was created in 2002 by the UK's Royal Institution 'to improve representation of science in the media.'

48 National Science Board, *Science and Engineering Indicators*, vol.1 (Arlington, VA: National Science Foundation 2002) at chap. 7, p. 2.

49 For example, see European Commission, *Candidate Countries Eurobarometer: Public Opinion in the Countries Applying for European Union*

Membership (Budapet: Gallup Organisation, 2003) at 42; and Office of Science and Technology and Wellcome Trust, *Science and the Public: A Review of Science Communication in the United Kingdom* (London: Wellcome Trust, 2000), cited *supra* note 48 at 7–14 where it was found that '72% agree that [e]ven if it brings no immediate benefits, scientific research which advances the frontiers of knowledge is necessary and should be supported by the Government.' They also cite a similar survey that was done in Japan. That survey found 80% support for basic research.

50 See, for example, SIRC, *supra* note 7.

51 *Ibid.* at 5.

52 Admittedly, placing this responsibility with primary care physicians will create further time pressures. In addition, experience has shown that it can be very difficult educating and influencing practicing physicians. Policy makers may need to adopt relatively aggressive educational strategies. See, for example, Sumit R. Majumdar, Finlay A. McAlister, and Stephen B. Soumerai, 'Synergy between Publication and Promotion: Comparing Adoption of New Evidence in Canada and the United States.' (2003) 115 Am. J. Med. 467 at 467 (abstract): 'Publication of new evidence is associated with modest changes in practice. Promotional activities appear to increase the adoption of evidence. Rather than relying on the publication of articles and creation of guidelines, those wishing to accelerate the adoption of new evidence may need to undertake more active promotion.'

53 Canada, Commission on the Future of Health Care in Canada, *Building on Values: The Future of Health Care in Canada* (Saskatoon: Commission on the Future of Health Care in Canada, 2002) at 83 (Chair: Roy Romanow).

54 Again, the importance of independent technology assessment was noted in the *Romanow Report*. Indeed, the Commission's recommendation regarding the importance of comprehensive technology assessment seems likely to be one possible strategy to help counter the utilization pressures created by marketing. *Ibid.*

55 Wilkie, *supra* note 22 at 1311.

17 Commercialized Medical Research and the Need for Regulatory Reform

TRUDO LEMMENS

Relations between academia and the pharmaceutical industry have always existed, and there has always been industry support for medical research. The growing commercialization of science in the past three decades, however, has fundamentally changed the landscape of medical research. These changes have a significant impact on health care practice itself, and they affect governmental policies related to funding of and priority setting within health care. Commercial interests increasingly determine the direction of medical research, which to a large degree determines what type of therapy will be available in the future. In addition, as I will discuss in this chapter, there are growing concerns about the impact of conflicts of interest on the integrity of the research itself. In light of the increased emphasis on evidence-based medicine, as discussed, for example, by Donna Greschner (in chapter 2), it seems particularly important to understand how financial interests may affect the quality of the evidence produced in medical research and to analyse to what extent the current regulatory framework related to research and drug development is able to deal with this threat. Recent controversies, I will argue, highlight the insufficiency of current regulatory regimes and the need for fundamental reform.

Bayh-Dole and the Commercialization of Medical Research

The enactment of the Bayh-Dole Act of 1980[1] in the United States is generally heralded as the major impetus of the increasingly commercial orientation of medical research. The Bayh-Dole Act allowed universities and researchers to obtain privately owned patents on the results of federally funded research. The goal of this legislation was to spur the development and commercialization of technology by providing incentives to universities and researchers to focus their research on marketable products. Prior to 1980 scientists, particularly basic scientists, generally frowned upon the privatization of research findings and viewed it as heresy. Arti Kaur Rai, in an article on the impact of intellectual property rights on the creation of new scientific norms, illustrates how, until the late 1970s, researchers expressed dismay at the idea of patenting path-breaking inventions. The inventers of gene-splicing, Stanley Cohen and Herbert Boyer, allowed patenting of their technique only after strong urging from Stanford University lawyers, and they set as a condition that it be licensed widely. In 1975 Nobel Prize winners Georges Köhler and Cesar Milstein considered it ethically inappropriate to patent their monoclonal antibody technique.[2] Science was largely seen to be a public calling. Research findings, according to that norm, had to be shared and made publicly accessible as soon as possible. This was often seen to be incompatible with obtaining patents, where the aim is to provide a monopoly to reward research, and where secrecy of the information that supports the patent application is considered crucial.

In the wake of Bayh-Dole this resistance quickly disappeared. Researchers have now enthusiastically joined the patent race, while several funding agencies have started encouraging, and increasingly even imposing commercial partnerships, private matching funding, and patentable outcomes as preconditions for funding. Researchers have been pushed to be as much concerned about the commercial potential of their research as about the intrinsic value of their findings. They have become part-time entrepreneurs. The number of patents obtained and the creation of start-up companies have become measures of success for governmentally funded programs. One of the ultimate goals of patenting is to promote the introduction of innovative technologies to the marketplace, and thereby to make innovations quickly accessible; nevertheless, patenting has affected the culture of sharing data. Before Bayh-Dole, hiding data was considered to be a violation of the ethical obligations inherent in research. This is not to say that it did not occur. But keeping scientific data confidential was at least perceived to be a violation of the norms of science. Bayh-Dole has normalized a culture of secrecy as a crucial component in the patent application process.

Around the same time (and likely not unrelated to this development – as defenders of Bayh-Dole like to stress) the pharmaceutical and biotechnology industry began to expand rapidly. It developed into one of the most profitable industries listed on stock exchanges. Various blockbuster drugs flooded the markets. The figures associated with the sale of drugs and their potential markets reveal the power of this booming economic sector. Pfizer's cholesterol-lowering drug Lipitor, for example, had sales of U.S.$9.2 billion in 2003;[3] the total market for this category of drugs is estimated at U.S.$92 billion.[4] The new market for the erectile dysfunction drugs is an estimated U.S.$6 billion by 2010.[5] Global sales of Glaxo-SmithKline's selective serotonin-reuptake inhibitor (SSRI) paroxetine in 2004 were U.S.$4.97 billion.[6]

With profit has come power, and the ability to use financial tools to influence the marketplace. The inherent drive for market expansion in this profitable business pushes competitors towards using all available tools to gain market share. Capturing the market for blockbuster drugs is also crucial to recover large investments in research and to compensate for failures in the developments of many other compounds. To do so, the biotech industry has extended its tentacles into all aspects of academia and society, especially those involved in the process of creating and regulating scientific knowledge and of transforming that knowledge into commercial products. The industry has attracted scientists to its ranks and created strong financial ties at all levels. Academic researchers now top up their salaries with fees or stock options, which often surpass in value their academic income, for a wide range of activities, including consultation, membership on advisory boards, and/ or membership in pharmaceutical companies' speaker bureaus. Even scientists of the U.S. National Institutes of Health (NIH) have developed paid consultancy relations with industry.[7] While financial compensation may be inappropriate to those directly involved in the approval process of new drugs, nothing prohibits industry from creating well-paid industry careers for former executives of regulatory agencies like the Food and Drug Administration (FDA) to serve as private consultants to the pharmaceutical industry.[8] A commentary in the *New England Journal of Medicine* further notes that one of the most senior administrators of the FDA previously represented tobacco and drug companies in lawsuits against the FDA.[9] One could argue that the pharmaceutical industry has thus made direct inroads into the regulatory system. Being on a company's payroll has also not prevented various experts from serving as members of influential FDA advisory panels. The line between those involved in the regulation and oversight of science and those involved in the research industry is also crossed at other levels. For example, the phenomenon of commercial research ethics boards (REBs), which review research involving human subjects in exchange for a review fee, shows how crucial regulatory components of medical research have been transformed into highly lucrative commercial ventures.[10]

In addition to traditional marketing practices, which are increasingly targeting consumers directly, pharmaceutical companies financially support those who may influence indirectly not only drug consumption but also the drug regulatory process and health care funding decisions. Much of the generous funding for consumer and advocacy groups can be explained as yet another attempt by pharmaceutical companies to gain influence in the regulatory process.[11] Benevolence and good corporate citizenship is often the official explanation for such funding, but teaming up with advocacy groups is clearly a sound business strategy. CBC's *Marketplace* reported in 2000 of a Toronto conference where drug industry experts explained how to promote sales through developing partnerships with patient groups.[12] A market report sold on the Internet states bluntly that 'the advent of abundant and well run patient advocacy groups has placed such company-patient group alliances to the top of the strategy agenda.'[13] Working with patient advocacy groups is seen as a 'prime target for sustained competitive advantage for drug companies.'[14] Barbara Mintzes mentions in a 2000 report various questionable ways in which industry has funded patient advocacy groups to promote specific products.[15] These strategic alliances are primarily useful for the promotion of sales and the creation of new markets, through stimulating disease 'awareness' among potential patient-consumers, but they also can have an impact at the research stage. Consumer groups may put pressure on governments to authorize new forms of research (for example, into stem cells) to obtain faster drug approval or to prioritize specific forms of research. In a full-page advertisement in the *New York Times*, commemorating Ronald Reagan's contributions to 'a world without Alzheimer,' the American Alzheimer's Association invites people to support 'further research into prevention and a cure [to] help ensure that our memories of Ronald Reagan live on.'[16] The advertisement, which also contains the questionable statement that 'treatments are available,' was sponsored by two producers of Alzheimer drugs: Pfizer and Eisai, both major sponsors of the Association.

Canadian Funding Agencies and Commercialization

Commercialization of medical research is an international phenomenon. The American patent approach has found its way into various international trade policies and agreements. Governments of other countries have tried to remain competitive with the United States by also implementing various commercialization strategies. Canada has been particularly keen in promoting a commercial biotechnology sector through various funding initiatives.[17] Its health-research funding agency, the Canadian Institutes of Health Research (CIHR), emphasizes in various publications that it wants to promote the fast application of research and the contribution of this research to the knowledge-based economy.[18] The CIHR does, however, embrace all areas of health research and pays particular attention to public health research and health research of no commercial interest. Other granting agencies have a much more explicit focus on commercialization. Genome Canada and the Canadian Networks of Centres for Excellence are the best examples of such initiatives. The Canadian government created Genome Canada as a Crown corporation 'dedicated to developing and implementing a national strategy in genomics and proteomics research for the benefit of Canadians.' It initially received close to $400 million from the federal government to promote large-scale genomics projects and has as its main objective 'to ensure that Canada becomes a world leader in genomics and proteomics research.'[19] A core requirement of its funding policy is that researchers have to obtain matching funds. Since Genome Canada focuses on large-scale projects, industry is the most likely source of sufficient matching funding. The potential economic outcome, that is, patentable products, is also emphasized in the evaluation of its grants. It is revealing that recently the federal budget contained a significant increase for Genome Canada – and not for the more traditional and less commercially focused CIHR.

The Canadian Networks for Centres for Excellence shares this commercialization mission with Genome Canada: It 'fosters powerful partnerships between university, government and industry [and is] aimed at turning Canadian research and entrepreneurial talent into economic and social benefits for all Canadians.'[20] This federal funding agency supports a variety of large-scale academic collaborations, some of which focus on health research. One of its more recently funded centres is the Stem Cell Network, [21] which, as requested by the agency, has a dual mandate to promote high-quality health research as well as the development of a vibrant biotechnology sector around stem cell research. To that end, the Network has set up a commercial stem cell company in which all participating institutions and researchers can become shareholders. At high-profile meetings, for example, one held in the Ontario

Legislative Building in December 2002, it has courted and been courted by all of the major pharmaceutical and biotechnology companies. This is not a unique phenomenon. Researchers and academic institutions are increasingly involved in the development of start-up companies with industry and often hold significant stock in companies that are bringing their research products to the market.[22]

The Impact on the Orientation of Medical Research

Governmental policies, consequent shifts in institutional approaches to commercialization, and developments in industry have thus blurred the lines between public and private actors in research. It has created a cozy space for interaction between industry and other 'stakeholders,' thus fulfilling a governmental desire to promote economic development through collaboration between industry and academia. Few would be opposed to the development of better health care products, but these fruits of research come at a price. The increased emphasis that governments place on the commercial outcomes and the creation of patentable products orients health research in a very specific direction. Health research inevitably focuses more on technological interventions and the use of new drugs and devices than it did before.

Promoting funding of commercializable health research is neither the only nor necessarily the best way to improve public health or to stimulate good medical research. Funding that is spent on searches for patentable genomics and stem cell products is money not available for research into preventive public health interventions. A pharmaceutical company obviously has little incentive to conduct research into, say, the social determinants of health, the health benefits of olive oil, the relation between toxic waste disposal and cancer in a community, or the relation between household chemicals and asthma. It often becomes unclear, in fact, whether improving health and health care is still the main goal of many of these new biotechnology initiatives. The flashy billboards surrounding the spectacular site of the University of Toronto's new Medical and Related Sciences (MaRS) Discovery District, for example, in which academia and new biotech ventures converge, showcase the research, biotechnological, and commercial potential of the new venture. The words 'health,' 'health care,' or 'patient care' are, surprisingly, very hard to find there. The website of MaRS is packed with terminology such as 'innovation, competitiveness and prosperity' and 'global knowledge driven economy.'[23] References to improving health and health care are conspicuously absent.

Obviously, the claim can be made that biotechnology innovation contributes to economic development and thereby also provides the economic and financial tools for other research and for improving health care. But it is noteworthy that this comes down to defending public funding of health research for the development of products and technologies, the benefits of which are only remote and indirect. The development of economic production is the focus of these investments, not health care itself. Moreover, the claim merits further scrutiny. Questions have recently been raised about the success of the significant public and private investments in the new biotechnology. In addition, the growing control over research by industry and the aggressive commercial promotion of health care products and technologies that accompany this commercialization agenda also create health risks and induce costs to the health care system. The inappropriate consumption of drugs in industrialized countries has itself become a public health concern.

The Many Faces of Commercialized Research

The commercialization of research often occurs in subtle ways. Researchers interested in improving the infrastructure of their laboratories and in hiring additional researchers may often see corporate sponsors as an easy source of funding for interesting medical research. Some pharmaceutical companies may just want to be good corporate citizens and contribute for that reason to the general promotion of health research. Both parties may often fail to reflect on the influence of corporate funding on research and on the larger impact that commercialization has on the orientation of medical research. But the courting of researchers, patients, health care workers, medical institutions, and regulators is increasingly part of aggressive, well-designed, competitive campaigns by companies trying to position themselves in the market. Direct – and preferably financial – relations with all these players are considered key. Creating ties with health care providers helps to ensure that new compounds can be rapidly steered through the drug regulatory process. The same ties are also important when it comes to marketing the drugs once they are approved.

The growing competition in the area of drug development increases the importance of establishing ties with medical researchers and physicians because of the need for research subjects. The boom in the pharmaceutical and biotechnology industries has considerably increased the number of clinical trials, thus explaining the staggering number of research subjects who currently are participants in research.[24] Perhaps it should not be surprising to anyone that industry experts identify access to research subjects as the most pressing concern for drug development, because any delay in the approval of a successful new drug can constitute a significant financial loss.[25] A company's good relations with physicians, academic researchers, and health care institutions are thus of strategic importance.

Another aspect of corporate strategy is blurring the line between the research stage and post-approval marketing of drugs. Companies can strategically use special access programs and large Phase 3 and Phase 4 trials to boost doctors' and patients' awareness of a drug and to jump-start prescription patterns. Including more subjects in such trials than are strictly needed has advantages other than increasing patients' and physicians' familiarity with the drug: it 'occupies the field' so that other sponsors may have problems finding sufficient research subjects within the same patient population to test their drugs.

Some companies have come up with interesting ways to mask marketing practices as 'educational research.' A recent study reports, for example, how a team of Canadian academic psychiatrists educated sixty-eight primary care physicians about how to diagnose depression and how to prescribe citalopram, a new antidepressant, each to ten of their patients.[26] The research, sponsored by the producers of the drug, consisted of evaluating the efficacy of these targeted educational programs in increasing diagnosis and prescription rates. The study was uniquely valuable, the authors argued, since '[u]nlike previous studies, the present study had the advantage of providing education to an audience largely unfamiliar with the use of this medication.'[27] Indeed, when the study started, the drug had just been introduced on the Canadian market.

Shifts in the Research Scene

Commercial interests have had a direct impact on the funding of academic research. As Sheldon Krimsky indicates, funding of academic research by pharmaceutical sponsors has significantly increased, particularly in most of the leading medical research centres.[28] Overall, corporate contributions to research and development in academic institutions in the United States rose by 875 per cent between 1980 and 2000.

Although other sources of funding are still more significant, the increase in industry funding has been phenomenal in many leading institutions. Krimsky reports, for example, that Duke University's industry funding, which rose by 280 per cent in the 1990s, now constitutes 31 per cent of its overall budget. In the same period, the University of Texas saw a 735 per cent increase in its private funding, compared with a 491 per cent increase at the University of California at San Francisco. And 20 per cent of the budget of the prestigious Massachussetts Institute of Technology (MIT) now comes from industry.

In addition, much more research is taking place outside academia. An increasing number of contract research organizations (CROs) conduct large numbers of clinical trials or coordinate such research undertaken in the community by primary care physicians. A report from the U.S. Office of the Inspector General (OIG) shows that the number of physicians in private practice participating in research has risen by 300 per cent.[29] As a result of the growing competition, the increased costs of doing research, and the problems of access to research subjects, clinical trials are also increasingly moving outside of the countries in which the drugs are being developed and sold. Pharmaceutical sponsors and CROs have moved many clinical trials to Africa, India, and Eastern Europe. Local governments often encourage the development of this type of industry. This may reduce some specific problems related to the competition for research subjects in North America and Western Europe, but it creates concerns about the potential exploitation of vulnerable communities. Moreover, Adriana Petryna highlights how pharmaceutical sponsors seem to appreciate 'treatment naive populations'[30] for testing new drugs, that is, populations where pharmacological treatments are the exception. Treatment naivety reduces the number of variables interfering with the research and makes it easier for a trial to show efficacy; but this, in turn, raises questions about how generalizable the research results really are. When these drugs are introduced in industrialized countries and consumed by people who are often overmedicated, they may create a host of interactions that have never been observed or anticipated.

What Are the Concerns?

Commercialization of research raises a number of concerns related to the recruitment of research subjects, particularly the risks of inappropriate recruitment practices, exploitation of impoverished research subjects, violations of informed consent, and the promotion of unnecessary drug prescription.[31] Other more structural concerns may be of even greater concern, however, since they affect the health care of not just a few people but the population at large. Manipulation of research results is possible when research is contracted out to community physicians and members of academia. Physicians and academics often get involved in industry-sponsored clinical trials as a side activity to generate extra income or as an easy way to bring in funding for their academic department. Many do not invest themselves intellectually in this type of research. While academic researchers offer greater legitimacy to a study, they are not always involved in the design of the study, do not have access to the complete data, and may do nothing more than collect and forward information about a small number of research subjects. Even when they do take a critical look at the protocol and challenge the research design or other aspects of the study, they will rarely be in a position to obtain fundamental changes to the protocol of a multicentre trial, which likely is developed by the research sponsor.

Even when a company only provides funding to conduct a study, there is potential bias. Ample empirical evidence demonstrates a statistically significant association between source of funding and research outcome. Industry-sponsored research is much more likely than noncommercially sponsored research to lead to a conclusion that a new therapy is better than the prevailing standard.[32] Although these studies do not establish a causal relationship between industry funding and an outcome that benefits the sponsors, they do raise a red flag. Sheldon Krimsky argues that 'the appearance of a conflict of interest [in these studies] provides circumstantial evidence of an influencing motivation.'[33] This appearance of bias is in and of itself a problem for medical research. As a social enterprise, medical research is largely dependent on trust: trust by researchers and research subjects that they are participating in something worthwhile, and trust that the results of the study are a reliable basis for clinical practice. Evidence of systemic bias and the lack of regulatory obligation to publicize the results of all clinical trials, which I will discuss further below, undermine the trust basis of medical research. This may in the long run affect the recruitment of research subjects, and it may also negatively affect the implementation of health care strategies based on this research.

Countervailing Forces

The view that these concerns are counterbalanced by the competing interests of other companies, by 'organized scepticism' – the culture of critique ingrained in science – and by existing regulatory regimes relies largely on the existence of a forum for scientific dialogue and for critical challenge of research findings. Commercialization has, however, also affected the environment in which these debates take place.

Shared Market Interests

First, pharmaceutical competitors often share core interests that remove any incentive to critically analyse a competitor's research. Some authors have identified, for example, how commercial interests are served by the expansion of categories of disease for which drugs or other forms of medical treatments are commercially available. Pharmaceutical companies have found ingenious ways of selling diseases to create markets for their drugs.[34] Competitors have no reason to challenge one company's claim that anxiety, shyness, premenstrual dysphoric disorder, and post-traumatic stress disorder are endemic and have to be aggressively treated with medication. On the contrary, they will stand in line to fill the shelves. Competitors may sometimes prefer not to conduct comparative studies, contenting themselves with dividing up the market. One example of study sponsored by Bristol-Myers Squibb shows, in my view, why it is naive to rely on the good will of companies to fund independent studies, in the absence of rules that force all competitors to take the same high road. In an effort to show how its cholesterol-lowering drug Pravachol was as efficient as Pfizer's Lipitor in preventing heart attacks, in 2002 Bristol-Myers Squibb funded a large comparative study. Unfortunately for that company, the study concluded that people taking Lipitor were at a 16 per cent lower risk for heart attack or death.[35] Bristol-Myers Squibb can be congratulated for sponsoring the study, but its marketing department was probably not pleased with the financial consequences. The study basically closed the door for Bristol-Myers Squibb to the lucrative market for cholesterol-lowering drugs, which is estimated at U.S.$22 billion annually. Pravachol was the company's top-selling drug in 2003, with sales of about U.S.$2.8 billion. In the absence of incentives or regulations obliging the conduct of large comparative studies and clear policies about the openness of clinical trial results, there is little reason to suppose that competitors will always fund this type of study or that unprofitable results will see the light of day. A front-page headline in the *Wall Street Journal* captures the business world's appreciation of this form of research sponsorship: 'For Bristol-Myers, Challenging Pfizer Was a Big Mistake.'[36] Had the company expected this outcome, the strategy would likely have been to continue marketing the drug without an open scientific challenge to its competitor.

Integrity of Scientific Publications

Second, there are increasing concerns about the integrity of the scientific literature, which is a crucial component of independent science. Academic journals have struggled for years with the question of how financial relations may influence the independence of the authors and the reviewers of manuscripts. Disclosure of financial interests has now become standard practice for most major academic journals, but the more stringent policies of some journals regarding the possible conflicts of interests of authors of editorials and review articles have come under stress as a result of the closer relations between academia and industry. The gold standard was always that those comparing various treatment options and making recommendations for clinical practice should have no financial relations with the producers of the products discussed or their competitors. The *New England Journal of Medicine* announced that it has had to relax this policy, as it has had trouble finding researchers without financial conflicts of interest.[37] A few established journals even continue to wrestle with basic conflict-of-interest issues. *Nature Neuroscience*, which until recently stuck stubbornly to its approach that even disclosure is not warranted, since – according to this approach – science is transparent and independent, published a review article discussing new experimental treatments for a variety of psychiatric disorders without disclosing that one of the two authors held significant financial interests in the companies producing several of the recommended products.[38] The journal subsequently refused to publish a letter by two readers who pointed out that the author in question held a patent in a product that he recommended, was a member of the scientific advisory board of the producer of another recommended product, and was the director and chairman of the Psychopharmacology Advisory Board of another company whose product received his praise. Under public pressure, created after the *New York Times* publicized this story, *Nature Neuroscience* finally revised its disclosure policy;[39] it did not, however, recognize that the significant financial interests made the review article unreliable.

Other developments are perhaps even more alarming, because they may affect the integrity of research in more subtle ways. As discussed earlier, congruent with the increasing control of the pharmaceutical industry over research is the industry's coordination of data collection, analysis, and interpretation. The results of company-sponsored research are often promoted at fancy parallel sessions of the most prestigious medical conferences and published through glossy inserts in leading medical journals. Journals have been criticized for turning their academic standing into a marketable item, particularly when company-sponsored inserts are barely distinguishable from the peer-reviewed content of the journals themselves.

More pernicious is the growing phenomenon of ghost writing. Research studies are increasingly written up and prepared for publication by medical information companies. As part of their commercial publication strategy, these companies offer nearly finished manuscripts as drafts for publications to established academics in the field, who may not have been involved in the research itself.[40] Academic authorship gives research credibility and helps to get the studies published in the most respected journals. In a recently published article in the *British Journal of Psychiatry*, David Healy and Dinah Cattell show how ghost-written articles related to sertraline, an antidepressant, were published in the most important medical journals, including the *Journal of the American Medical Association*, the *American Journal of Psychiatry*, the *Archives of General Psychiatry*, and others. The 'impact factor' – an increasingly emphasized measure of success for medical publication – of the ghost-written articles was also significantly higher than that of the other articles. The publication of these articles was part of a campaign undertaken by Current Medical Directions, one of these medical information companies. More generally, a 1998 article in the *Journal of the American Medical Association* reported that up to 11 per cent of articles published in six leading academic journals used ghost authors.[41] In the most extreme cases of ghost writing, academic authors who sign onto the studies have not seen the data, did not write the text themselves, and did not participate in the analysis. In academia, this is normally considered scientific fraud.

The normalization of secrecy in the context of the patent process has also affected the public accountability of publications and their scientific scrutiny. Scientific data are often considered proprietary and confidential, even when they are crucial to the verification of published analyses. An exchange in the journal *Toxicology* highlights the concern. Scientists complained that the authors of an article that described computer models of the structures of several human enzymes and their interactions with toxicological products had refused to provide the coordinates of the published models. Access to these models was necessary to verify the claims and reproduce the results, a crucial component of standard scientific dialogue. The authors' response to a request for access was that the rights to the models were owned by a company and were therefore proprietary information.[42] This controversy is not unique. Editorials in the *Journal of the American Medical Association* and in the *Canadian Medical Association Journal* also lament the difficulties that scientists encounter when they try to obtain information on industry-funded trials, for example, to obtain access to data or to clarify issues of trial design.[43]

Drug Regulatory Review

The proprietary nature of information is also a crucial problem for the accountability of the drug regulatory system, which fundamentally respects the confidentiality of research data. Several controversies have revealed weaknesses within the drug regulatory system, both in the United States and Canada. Drug regulatory agencies have as their official mandate the protection of public health. Over the years, however, they have yielded to significant pressure by industry and some patient advocacy groups to decrease the administrative burden of drug approval and, to some extent, protect the patents of pharmaceutical innovators.[44]

Rebecca Eisenberg notes that arising out of its regulatory role, the FDA has gained an important function in promoting innovation.[45] The regulatory regime for drugs and medical devices has de facto become an important means to obtain market exclusivity for new products and to guarantee financial returns for investors.[46] The FDA has become a crucial pillar of the patent system, a function that can bring it on a collision course with its mandate to protect the public. The role of the FDA in the patent regime, with its inherent respect for the proprietary nature of information, may undermine its accountability to the public with respect to its evaluation of drug safety and efficacy.

The FDA and Health Canada impose strict reporting obligations upon sponsors. Before commencing clinical trials, sponsors have to file an Investigational New Drug Application, with data to support the claim that research subjects will not be put at unreasonable risk. They have to keep the agencies informed of any serious and unexpected adverse events associated with the experimental treatment and any other data that suggest risks to human subjects. After testing the drug through various clinical trial stages, the applicants have to submit data supporting the efficacy and safety of the product. However, the system is largely based on self-regulation and fundamentally respects the proprietary nature of research data. As Michael Baram observes in the American context, the reporting obligations are extremely flexible and 'riddled with legalistic exceptions and deference to investigator judgment on critical matters.'[47]

Joel Lexchin points out, contrasting Health Canada and the FDA, that at least the latter gives access to more detailed data on which a decision is based.[48] When approving a product, the FDA releases a 'Summary Basis of Approval,' which includes the reviews of pharmacological and toxicological data and the comments of the FDA reviewers. In addition, third parties can request reports of the clinical trials that are submitted with a new drug application. This request is honoured within ten working days. By comparison, Health Canada does not give access to the data supporting its decisions and only gives access to the official product monograph, which contains much less information than what is made available in the United States.[49]

Disturbing insights into corporate control over the establishment of scientific evidence and deficient data disclosure to public and regulatory agencies emerge from several of the recent drug controversies. One of them is over the efficacy and potential side effects of selective serotonin-reuptake inhibitors (SSRIs). The controversy – or better controversies – surrounding SSRIs reveal much of the problems associated with corporate control over clinical research and the failure of the regulatory system, and they are therefore worth discussing in some detail.

Public hearings on the safety and efficacy of SSRIs held by regulatory agencies and evidence revealed in various lawsuits, including a lawsuit by the Attorney General of the State of New York,[50] suggest not only that the evidence supporting the use of these SSRIs in children and adolescents is extremely weak, but also that publications in the scientific literature give a different story than the data collected and analysed internally by pharmaceutical sponsors.[51] A recent British meta-analysis of published and unpublished trial data concluded that, contrary to various published studies, all but one of the analysed SSRIs had a negative benefit to risk ratio and should not be recommended for the treatment of depression in children and adolescents.[52] There is also direct evidence that companies have strategically released data, reportedly failing to disclose unfavourable results. The most disturbing case in this regard came to light in 2003, after GlaxoSmithKline applied for a licence for Paxil for the treatment of mood disorders in children. Within the full set of raw data provided to support its application, the company included two studies that became the focus of the Attorney General's lawsuit for fraud and misrepresentation.

From 1993 to 1995 a medical research division of GlaxoSmithKline conducted two large clinical trials (nos. 329 and 377) to establish the efficacy and safety of Paxil for the treatment of major depression in adolescents. A confidential memo about these studies, which was obviously not submitted to the drug regulators, states explicitly that 'the efficacy data are insufficiently robust to support a regulatory submission' and that reporting this to the regulatory authorities would be 'commercially unacceptable.'[53] In an open letter to the FDA, David Healy claims that only the positive results of Trial 329 were subsequently published, in the *Journal of the American Academy of Child and Adolescent Psychiatry*, authored by several leading academics in the field.[54] The results of the other trial were never published. The attorney general's lawsuit reveals that although the studies failed to demonstrate efficacy, and even indicated that there was an increased risk of agitation and suicidal thoughts and behaviour in children and adolescents taking Paxil, the company embarked on a campaign to promote off-label use of its drug, for example, through distributing copies of this positive publication to sales representatives.

Shortly after the raw data of these studies were submitted to the British drug regulator, it issued a warning against the use of Paxil for minors and questioned the efficacy of some of the SSRIs for the treatment of depression in minors. The Canadian Therapeutics Directorate took a similar initiative. In the United States the controversy continued, however, fed by attempts to reaffirm the safety of the drugs. Only days before the FDA hearings into the safety and efficacy of the use of SSRIs in children, a working group of the American College of Neuropsychopharmacology reported that, on the basis of the available evidence, SSRIs were safe and effective for treating children. The authors of this report, many of whom had financial relations with the producers of SSRIs, issued a caveat, however, suggesting that they had not seen the raw data. But how could that be, since, as Healy points out, three of the authors were also mentioned as authors of the article in the *Journal of the American Academy of Child and Adolescent Psychiatry* that reported the trial results?[55] How could they justify authorship without having seen and analysed the full data? These developments raise questions about the reliability and integrity of the scientific literature and about the efficacy of the drug regulatory system. An editorial in the *Lancet*, accompanying one of the meta-analyses mentioned earlier, expresses the situation well: 'The story of research into SSRI use in childhood depression is one of confusion, manipulation, and institutional failure.' This failure, according to the editors, constitutes a 'disaster' for evidence-based medical practice.[56]

The SSRI controversy also brings to light how clinical trial requirements of the regulatory agencies may be counterproductive if imposed blindly. The manufacturers of SSRIs have always rejected clinical case reports linking their products to increased suicidal ideation by referring to the absence of statistical evidence. But critics argue that clinically significant results can be obtained through small studies and clinical case reports, and that the company-sponsored trials used to support the efficacy and safety of SSRIs were not designed to detect the occurrence of suicidal ideation. The regulatory requirement of data gathering through large clinical trials offers large pharmaceutical companies much power over the gathering of information. Although these requirements are clearly intended to promote the establishment of safety and efficacy before allowing a potentially harmful product on the market, they may in the current context be manipulated for commercial purposes. Large pharmaceutical companies have the financial means to conduct the trials, and they can be selective in the type of questions they want to see answered. Once a drug is approved, there is considerable commercial pressure not to inquire further into potential side-effects, and the absence of statistical evidence can be used as a scientific shield against criticism. Not many independent organizations have the financial means to conduct these trials *in lieu* of the companies. Until a government-funded organization like, for example, the National Institutes of Health commits the time, personnel, and finances to launch a large independent study, the drug can continue to be promoted on the market.[57]

The SSRI saga also highlights another weakness of the drug regulatory system, a weakness confirmed by the recent controversy surrounding the market withdrawal of Vioxx, a blockbuster painkiller produced by Merck. In the context of both controversies, questions were raised very early on about the potential side effects of these drugs. In both cases, experts had suggested that appropriate clinical trials ought to be designed to investigate potential side effects. In 1991 in the wake of public hearings on the safety of SSRIs in adults, FDA officials even met with researchers of Eli Lilly, producer of Prozac, and they jointly developed a research design and a better clinical scale to detect the potential side effects of Prozac.[58] With respect to Vioxx, Eric J. Topol points out that he pleaded back in 2001 for appropriate clinical trials to assess cardiovascular risks associated with Vioxx.[59] None of these studies ever took place. Neither in the United States nor Canada do drug regulatory authorities have the power to impose a study once a drug has been approved, although both have monitoring programs in place. Health Canada, for example, gathers information on adverse reactions through post-marketing reporting systems that involve health professionals and consumers.[60] These adverse-reaction reporting systems can provide crucial information and have, for example, provided a basis for Health Canada to request the voluntary withdrawal of various drugs from the market.[61] The regulatory agencies do not have the authority, however, to impose additional safety studies, which has become the focus of recent criticism.[62] The system relies very much on the integrity and collaboration of the pharmaceutical sponsors and the vigilance of consumers and health professionals. It is telling that in the wake of the Vioxx controversy, Canada's Health Minister Ujjal Dosanjh expressed his frustration over the lack of cooperation from Merck and over the inability of his administration to force industry to reveal crucial data.[63] Health Canada has since taken some initiatives to improve the gathering of information after marketing. For example, Health Canada improved its Canadian Adverse Drug Reaction Monitoring Program by introducing in May 2005 an Online Query and Data Extract database, which will give the public easier access to information about adverse drug reactions.[64]

New Approaches to Promote Research Integrity

One thing that should be clear from this discussion is that the widely heralded remedy of 'disclosure' is not sufficient. Financial interests are not simply parts of the research scene that can be laid on the scale along with scientific facts. Financial interests cannot be measured and evaluated in the same way that scientific data can be. Mere disclosure of financial interests can become an empty ritual of a seemingly renewed and cleansed scientific ceremony. This is not to say that disclosure is not warranted. It can, however, provide a false sense of security. Particularly in a culture where nearly everyone has to disclose something, it becomes hard for outsiders to determine how significant these interests are. Disclosure sounds the alarm, but it does not solve the problem. And when too many alarm bells go off at the same time, no one even bothers to run away. Disclosure is often attached to an external evaluation process. Since 1998 the FDA has required that applications for the approval of a new product include information on the financial interests of the researchers involved in the supporting study.[65] But in subsequent guiding documents, the FDA has not told researchers how it will assess this information, while conveying that it remains very flexible and accommodating in imposing this requirement.[66]

A more concerned tone can be identified in a guidance document on financial conflicts of interest issued by the U.S. Department of Health and Human Services,[67] as well as in two reports on conflicts of interest made by a special task force of the Association of American Medical Colleges (AAMC).[68] These documents recognize the structural problems associated with financial conflicts of interest and offer interesting suggestions. They represent official recognition that the integrity of the research is at risk when individuals or even institutions are involved in studies related to products in which they have a financial interest. The documents rightly suggest that it may be more appropriate to have these studies conducted by other researchers and/or in another institution. The AAMC even recommends the introduction of rebuttable presumptions that financially interested individuals or institutions should not be involved in the studies in which they have such an interest.[69] But these documents are not binding, and they open the door to multiple exceptions. They rely to an inordinate degree on the work of local regulatory bodies such as REBs and conflict-of-interest committees within institutions. As discussed elsewhere, these administrative bodies are themselves affected by the conflicts of interests that they purportedly control.[70] Moreover, in Canada, they are not submitted to a coherent regulatory regime.[71]

As Sheldon Krimsky and others point out, different institutions deal very differently with conflicts of interest.[72] Institutions that more stringently implement the recommendations by the AAMC may place themselves at a competitive disadvantage, losing corporate funding and researchers. They will be under serious pressure to lower their standards and to allow their researchers to establish closer links with industry.

Many of the problems related to the commercialization of medical research are associated with studies undertaken outside academic centres. The conflicts of interest embedded in non-academic commercial research settings are endemic, and the commercial REBs invited to review the studies and potential conflicts of interest of investigators are themselves fundamentally affected by similar conflicts.[73]

Notwithstanding these concerns, the reports of the AAMC do point in the right direction and reflect a profound understanding that radical changes are needed. A comprehensive approach should be based on the fact that drug regulations, governmental patent policies, protection of human subjects, and the integrity of medical research are all fundamentally intertwined. When rules are changed in one of these areas, the impact in other areas has to be evaluated. The corporatization of medical research stimulated through changes in the patent regime has clearly affected all levels of the production, review, and use of medical knowledge. Medical research has been integrated into a highly lucrative, competitive market environment. The drug regulatory system has been adapted to accommodate a changing approach towards patents. Academic research has been significantly commercialized, and the proportion and influence of commercial research outside of academia has systematically increased. But the regulatory regimes aimed at protecting both research subjects and the public more generally have not been significantly adapted to this changing environment. Medical research functions very much within an Enron-like environment, where financial interests may create pressure to bend the rules, but nonetheless the research continues to be regulated as if it were to some extent a charitable practice with a purely humanitarian mission.

A solution has to be based on an understanding of the interactions between the various regulatory regimes and on a solid understanding of the strengths and the weaknesses of the various levels of regulation. In all of these regulatory regimes, the integrity of scientific research is relied upon. Research integrity is particularly crucial for the regulation of drugs and medical devices and for the protection of human research subjects. Drug and device regulatory agencies rely on data gained through clinical trials to assess product safety and efficacy. Health care agencies, whether private or public, decide whether to fund therapies on the basis of the results of scientific research. REBs must evaluate, relying on data provided by the sponsors and on the scientific literature and otherwise publicly accessible data, whether a research subject will be exposed to an unacceptable risk. A solid review of the scientific validity and value of a research protocol is necessary, for example, to determine whether a subject included in a trial will not be deprived of standard treatment without potential benefit. Scientific validity and value are core requirements of the research ethics review process.

All these regulatory regimes pay-lip service to the issue that conflicts of interest may affect the conduct and outcome of research. Yet none of the regimes deals sufficiently with the underlying structural causes of the demise of scientific integrity. Indeed, they have a tendency to rely on the appropriate functioning of the other regulatory regimes. The ethics guidelines and regulations dealing with REB review impose a duty to review conflicts of interest, but there is little guidance as to how REBs should measure the impact of these conflicts. Nowhere do they suggest that REBs should engage in a critical analysis of the validity of the decisions made by the drug and device regulatory agencies. REBs simply work under the presumption that published reports and approval by drug regulatory agencies are reliable benchmarks for deciding what constitutes standard treatment and what level of risk is involved.

Drug regulatory agencies, on their part, seem to rely to some extent on REBs and conflict-of-interest committees within institutions to ensure that research is conducted properly. For Canada's Therapeutic Products Directorate, REBs must 'help to ensure that conflicts of interest situations are avoided and that the health and safety of the trial subject remains the paramount concern.'[74] However, REBs are a fundamental part of the research structure that, as I demonstrate here, is affected by commercialization. Academic REBs are located within academic centres that are fundamentally influenced by the commercialization agenda. They are staffed with the same researchers who increasingly are funded by corporate sponsors. A recent survey indicated, for example, that 40 per cent of REB members in American institutions have financial relations with industry, a higher percentage than among researchers in general.[75] This in itself raises concerns about how these REB members will evaluate conflicts of interest. Various reports and publications, which cannot be discussed in detail here, have highlighted the flaws in the current REB system, both in the United States and Canada.[76] Being affected by conflicts of interest, REBs seem hardly to be the appropriate bodies to counter the pervasive structural impact of commercialization, and they have neither the mandate nor the capacity to investigate the integrity of the science on which applications for clinical trials are made. Improvements to the research ethics review system, for example, by developing a more independent and accountable system that can be legally enforced, seem an important step in the right direction.[77] But we also have to look at more fundamental structural reform of the drug regulatory regime.

Various commentators and some official reports have recommended, in the context of clinical trials, to separate those who design, conduct, and review research from those who have financial interests in the outcomes. A largely unnoticed recommendation by Roy Romanow in the Report of the Royal Commission on the Future of Health Care in Canada, for example, is that an independent National Drug Agency ought to be established in Canada.[78] This drug-testing agency would not be important only in improving the reliability of the data used to support applications for drug approval. Roy Romanow's interest in such an agency relates to its ability to conduct comparative studies that would reveal important information that is needed to make health care allocation decisions. Pharmaceutical companies currently can avoid undertaking comparative studies, preferring to use marketing tactics to gain a greater market share. A national drug-testing agency would be an important cornerstone of an evidence-based rational public health care system.

In recent books critical of corporate influence over medical research, Sheldon Krimsky[79] and Marcia Angell both recommend the establishment of a new national institute for drug testing (NIDT).[80] A company wishing to apply for approval of a new drug would negotiate an appropriate protocol with the NIDT, which would organize the clinical trial, using qualified drug assessment centres. The drug-testing procedures should be designed so that proprietary interests of drug companies would be respected, while the independence of the drug-testing agencies would ensure that no important clinical trial data remained hidden behind corporate walls.

Other less radical measures are needed immediately to tackle at least partially what one reviewer describes as 'the foremost medical research issue of our age.'[81] A potential measure for promoting the public accountability of clinical trials would be the creation of a comprehensive clinical trials register. Such a clinical trials register has already been set up by the World Health Organization (WHO) for the research that it supports.[82] In the wake of the media exposure of some of the controversies described here, several medical organizations are now also publicly calling for such a register for industry-sponsored trials. The idea itself is not new, but the public support by major medical organizations seems very much to be a response to the threat of legal action and regulatory intervention. The International Committee of Medical Journal Editors, a committee that includes the editors of twelve of the most prestigious medical journals, is now requiring the registration of clinical trials as a precondition for considering the publication of the results in one of its journals. The establishment of a clinical trials registry will certainly promote transparency and help avoid some of the more egregious examples of hiding data. But it cannot be considered a sufficient remedy to deal with the growing pressure of commercialization on the integrity of research. Indeed, a clinical trials registry cannot do the job if there are no independent researchers and drug regulators willing to and capable of putting their time and energy into scrutinizing the trials registered.

Krimsky and the AAMC, therefore, also appropriately call for a new 'culture of conscience' and a revitalization of the values of academic science. The importance of having a strong independent academic sector in medical research is, indeed, something that should be stressed in public debates about the commercialization of our universities. Most medical researchers and academics will have no problem in appreciating this as an independent value; nevertheless, it may help invoke a more utilitarian argument as formulated by Nobel Prize winner Paul Berg. In an interview with the *Atlantic Monthly*, Berg argued that the ability to conduct research without concern for immediate commercial applications is what lies behind many of the most innovative discoveries. The argument gains even more credibility in light of the fact that Berg's theoretical academic research lies behind much of the biotechnology revolution that we know today.

This cultural change cannot be achieved without some incentives. The development of a more independent, tightly regulated review sector, as well as an invigoration of traditional university values, stimulated perhaps by changes to the internal professional reward structures of academia and increased public funding, may help provide the necessary incentives. In this context, it is important to re-evaluate the existing dynamics in medical academia that may be driving medical researchers to practices such as accepting ghost-written articles as an easy way to boost their publication lists.

NOTES

This chapter is based on Trudo Lemmens, 'Leopards in the Temple: Restoring Integrity to the Commercialized Research Scene' (2004) (winter) Journal of

Law, Medicine and Ethics 641. Research for this chapter was supported by funding from Genome Canada, through the Ontario Genomics Institute; and by a fellowship from the Institute for Advanced Studies at Princeton, where I conducted much of the background research. I am grateful to Colleen Flood and to the 2003–4 members of the School of Social Science of the Institute for Advanced Studies for their useful comments on earlier versions and to Linda Hutjens and Angela Long for editorial suggestions and work on the notes.

1 Act of 12 December 1980, Pub. L. No. 96-517, s. 6(a), 94 Stat. 3015, 3019–28 (1980) (codified as amended at 35 U.S.C. ss. 200–12 (1994)).
2 Arti Kaur Rai, 'Regulating Scientific Research: Intellectual Property Rights and the Norms of Science' (1999) 94 Northwestern U. L. Rev. 77 at 93–4. Herbert Boyer set up already in 1976 the company Genentech Inc. to commercialize some of his research findings.
3 Mike McCoy, 'Bristol-Myers Study Backfires' (2004) 82:11 Chemical and Engineering News 8.
4 Ron Winslow, 'For Brystol-Myers, Challenging Pfizer Was A Big Mistake' Wall Street Journal, 9 March 2004 at 1.
5 Stuart Elliott, 'Viagra and the Battle of the Awkward Ads,' New York Times, 25 April 2004 at 3:1.
6 Editorial, 'Depressing Research' (2004) 363 Lancet 2088.
7 David Willman, 'Stealth Merger: Drug Companies and Government Medical Research' Los Angeles Times, 7 December 2003 at A1. After various media reports criticized the fact that top scientists and directors of NIH divisions were paid thousands of dollars as well as stock options for their consulting services to industry, NIH director Elias Zerhouni issued a draft of new conflict-of-interest guidelines significantly limiting the ability of NIH scientists to develop outside consultancy with industry and to have other financial relations and interests in industries that are substantially affected by NIH activities. See David Willman, 'Ex-NIH Director Now Favors Limiting Drug-Company Ties,' Los Angeles Times, 13 March 2004 at A21. For the guidelines, see Department of Health and Human Services, Supplemental Standards of Ethical Conduct and Financial Disclosure Requirements for Employees of the Department of Health and Human Services (3 February 2005) 5 CFR Parts 5501–2. The conflict-of-interest standards were submitted to a consultation process and evoked much criticism from within the National Institutes of Health. The final version of the standards, adopted in August 2005, contains more flexible and lenient rules. The argument was frequently made that the NIH would not be able to recruit top researchers if it insisted on the more stringent conflict-of-

interest rules in the original standards. For the final version of the standards, see Department of Health and Human Services, Supplemental Standards of Ethical Conduct and Financial Disclosure Requirements for Employees of the Department of Health and Human Services (31 August 2005) 5 Code of Federal Regulations Parts 5501–2; 70(168) Federal Register 51559.

8 This is not to suggest that there is anything inherently wrong with former FDA officials joining industry. But cozy relations can have an influence on regulatory oversight and enforcement. And when companies hire former senior executives from the regulatory sector, they will be in a better position to 'work the system.'

9 Susan Okie, 'What Ails the FDA?' (2005) 352 New England J. Med. 1063.

10 For a discussion, see Trudo Lemmens and Benjamin Freedman, 'Ethics Review for Sale? Conflict of Interest and Commercial Research Ethics Review Boards' (2000) 78 Milbank Quarterly 547.

11 See also the discussion of the use of patient advocacy groups as the 'third party technique' in Jocelyn Downie, chapter 18 in this volume.

12 'Promoting Drugs through Patients Advocacy Groups' 14 November 2000 http://www.cbc.ca/consumers/market/files/health/drugmarketing/ (accessed 30 May 2005).

13 F. Mills, 'Patient Groups and the Global Pharmaceutical Industry: The Growing Importance of Working Directly with the Consumer' (London: Urch Publishing, 2000), abstract at http://www.mindbranch.com/listing/product/R410-0024.html (accessed 30 May 2005).

14 *Ibid.*

15 Barbara Mintzes, *Blurring the Boundaries: New Trends in Drug Promotion* (Amsterdam: Health Action International, 1998) ch. 1. http://www.haiweb .org/pubs/blurring/blurring.intro.html.

16 *New York Times*, 11 June 2004 at A17.

17 See also Downie, chapter 18, and Tim Caulfield, chapter 16, in this volume.

18 See, e.g., Canadian Institutes for Health Research, *Revolution – CIHR: Towards a National Health Research Agenda* (Ottawa: CIHR, 2001) at 10, http://www.cihr-irsc.gc.ca/e/publications/revolution.pdf (accessed 30 May 2005); and *CIHR: Transforming Health Research in Canada*, http:// www.cihr-irsc.gc.ca/e/publications/cbj_supplement_e.pdf (accessed 30 May 2005). This publicity appeared as a supplement in the magazines Canadian Business and Actualité.

19 Geonome Canada, http://www.genomecanada.ca/GCgenomeCanada/ enBref/index.asp?l=e (accessed 6 May 2004).

20 Networks of Centres of Excellence, http://www.nce.gc.ca/about_e.htm (accessed 6 May 2004).
21 Stem Cell Networks, http://www.stemcellnetwork.ca/aboutus/overview .php (accessed 6 May 2004).
22 See Caulfield, chapter 16 in this volume, for a discussion of how research- ers themselves may often be responsible for misrepresentation of research findings in the media can be linked to this development. Researchers realize all too well the financial implications of media attention given to their inventions. They may often stand to gain significantly when stock prices of companies in which they have financial interests rise as a result of public announcements. It is interesting to mention here also that recent studies suggest that insider trading happens frequently in the context of research. See James R. Ferguson, 'Biomedical Research and Insider Trading' (Sounding Board) (1997) 337 New England J. Med. 631; C.B. Overgaard et al., 'Biotechnology Stock Prices Before Public Announce- ments: Evidence of Insider Trading?' (2000) 48 J. of Investigative Med. 118.
23 Medical and Related Sciences Discovery District, http://www.marsdd .com/am_background.html (accessed 6 May 2004).
24 Adil E. Shamoo, 'Adverse Events Reporting: The Tip of an Iceberg,' (2001) 8 Accountability in Research 197. For a very preliminary estimate of Canadian participation in research, following Shamoo's methods, see Trudo Lemmens and Paul B. Miller, 'The Human Subjects Trade: Ethical and Legal Issues Surrounding Recruitment Incentives' (2003) 31 J. Law Med. & Ethics 398.
25 Thomas Bodenheimer, 'Uneasy Alliance: Clinician Investigators and the Pharmaceutical Industry' (2000) 342 New England J. Med. 1539.
26 The journal describes itself as a 'peer-reviewed journal' of the Association of Medicine and Psychiatry that 'strives to bring together knowledge in medicine and psychiatry to improve patient care' by 'offering articles of high clinical value,' http://www.primarycarecompanion.com/ (accessed 30 May 2005).
27 Stanley Paul Kutcher et al., 'Evaluating the Impact of Educational Pro- grams on Practice Patterns of Canadian Family Physicians Interested in Depression Treatment' (2002) 4(6) Primary Care Companion Journal of Clinical Psychiatry 224 at 225.
28 See Sheldon Krimsky, Science in the Private Interest: Has the Lure of Profit Corrupted Biomedical Research (Lanhan: Rowman and Littlefield, 2003) at 79–81.
29 Department of Health and Human Services, Office of Inspector General,

Recruiting Human Subjects: Pressures in Industry-sponsored Research (Washington: author, 2000).

30 Adriana Petryna, 'Ethnic Variability: Drug Development and Globalizing Clinical Trials' (2005) 32:2 Amer. Ehnologist 183.

31 These issues have been extensively discussed elsewhere. For a discussion of problems related to the use of payment to subjects, see Trudo Lemmens and Carl Elliot, 'Guinea Pigs on the Payroll: The Ethics of Paying Healthy Subjects' (1999) 7 Accountability in Research 3 and references therein. For a discussion of the use of finder's fees to promote recruitment, see Lemmens and Miller, *supra* note 24 and references therein; and Department of Health and Human Services, Office of Inspector General, *supra* note 29.

32 See Joel Lexchin *et al.* 'Pharmaceutical Sponsorship and Research Outcome and Quality: Systemic Review,' Brit. Med. J., 326 (2003), 1167–77; and Justin E. Bekelman, Yan Li, and Cary P. Gross, 'Scope and Impact of Financial Conflicts of Interest in Biomedical Research' (2003) 289 JAMA: 463.

33 Krimsky, *supra* note 28 at 148–9.

34 See David Healy, *The Anti-Depressant Era* (Cambridge: Harvard University Press, 1997), in particular chapter 6, at 180–216. See also Carl Elliott, *Better Than Well: American Medicine Meets the American Dream* (New York: Norton, 2003) at 119–28; and James R. Brown, Funding, Objectivity and the Socialization of Medical Research' (2002) 8 Science and Engineering Ethics 295 at 303–5.

35 Christopher P. Cannon, *et al.*, 'Intensive versus Moderate Lipid Lowering with Statins After Acute Coronary Syndromes' (2004) 350 New England J. Med. 1495.

36 Winslow *supra* note 4.

37 See Jeffrey M. Drazen and Gregory D. Curfman, 'Financial Associations of Authors' (2002) 346 New England J. Med. 1901–2.

38 Charles B. Nemeroff and Michael J. Owens, 'Treatment of Mood Disorders' (2002) 5 (Suppl.) Nature Neuroscience 1068. See the discussion of the controversy in Shannon Brownlee, 'Doctors without Borders' Washington Monthly. April 2004 at 38.

39 Editorial (2003) 6 Nature Neuroscience 997.

40 Bodenheimer, *supra* note 25; David Healy and Dinah Cattell, 'Interface between Authorship, Industry and Science in the Domain of Therapeutics' (2003) 183 British J. Psychiatry 22–7; and William T. Carpenter, 'From Clinical Trial to Prescription' (2002) 59 Archives of General Psychiatry 282–5.

41 Annette Flanagin *et al.*, Prevalence of Articles with Honorary Authors and Ghost Authors in Peer-Reviewed Medical Journals (1998) 280 JAMA 222.

42 See D. Josephy, letter to the editor (2001) 156 Toxicology 171–2. As a result of the controversy, the journal changed its submission policy to include a requirement that authors agree to share the original data and materials for their publication, if so required. H.W.J. Marguardt, '"Code of conduct" – A Matter of Principle' (2001) 156 Toxicology 171.

43 See Drummond Rennie, 'Fair Conduct and Fair Reporting of Clinical Trials' (1999) 282 JAMA 1766; and Allan D. Sniderman, 'The Need for Greater Involvement of Regulatory Agencies in Assessing Adverse Drug Reactions' (2000) 162:2 Can. Med. Assoc. J. 209.

44 For a detailed analysis of the history and the developments within the FDA, see Stephen J Hiltz, *Protecting America's Health: The FDA, Business, and One Hundred Years of Regulation* (New York: Alfred Knopf, 2003).

45 Rebecca Eisenberg, 'The Robert L. Levine Distinguished Lecture Series: Patents, Product Exclusivity, and Information Dissemination: How Law Directs Biopharmaceutical Research and Development.' 2003 (72) Fordham L. Rev. 477 at 489.

46 *Ibid.* at 477.

47 Michael Baram, 'Making Clinical Trials Safer for Human Subjects' 2001 Am. J. L. & Med. 253 at 262.

48 See Joel Lexchin, 'Secrecy and the Health Protection Branch' (1998) 159 Can. Med. Assoc. J. 481 at 482–3.

49 Lexchin uses the example of his own request for access to health and safety data regarding pediatric anti-diarrheal products that were disapproved by the World Health Organization for use in children but approved for that use by Canada's Health Protection Branch – now known as Canada's Therapeutic Product Directorate. To verify the scientific basis of the decision, he wrote to various producers of the products and filed an access to information request to Health Canada, demanding further information about the clinical trials data supporting the approval. He did not receive a response. See *ibid.*

50 *AG New York v. GlaxoSmithKline*, S.C. NY, 2 June 2004.

51 E. Jane Garland, 'Facing the Evidence: Antidepressant Treatment in Children and Adolescents' (2004) 170:4 Can. Med. Assoc. J. 489.

52 Craig J. Whittington *et al.*, 'Selective Serotonin Reuptake Inhibitors in Childhood Depression: Systematic Review of Published vs Unpublished Data' (2004) 363 Lancet 1341.

53 'Seroxat/Paxil – Adolescent Depression. Position Piece on the Phase III Clinical Studies' (Oct 1998). Document obtained from David Healy.

54 David Healy, letter to Peter J. Pitts, Associate Commissioner for External Relations (19 Feb. 2004).

55 David Healy, 'Conflicting Interests: The Evolution of an Issue' (2004) 23:4 Monash Bioethics Review 8.

56 'Depressing Research' (editorial) 363 (2004) Lancet 1335.

57 Rebecca Eisenberg, e.g., discusses the large NIH-sponsored placebo-controlled study of the effects of hormone replacement therapy on risk of heart disease in post-menopausal women as an example of how large government-funded studies may uncover risks 'that the product's manufacturer had little incentive to uncover on its own.' *Supra* note 45 at 489–90.

58 See David Healy, *Let Them Eat Prozac* (Toronto: Lorimer, 2003).

59 Eric J. Topol, 'Failing the Public Health – Rofecobix, Merck, and the FDA' (2004) 351 New Engl. J. Med. 1707.

60 Canadian Adverse Drug Reaction Monitoring Program (CADRMP), *Guidelines for the Volunary Reporting of Suspected Adverse Reactions to Health Products by Health Professionals and Consumers*, http://www.hc-sc.gc.ca/hpfb-dgpsa/tpd-dpt/adr_guideline_e.html (accessed 6 April 2005).

61 See, e.g., Health Canada, Advisory 2005–17, 'Health Canada Has Asked Pfizer to Suspend Sales of Its Drug Bextra™ and Informs Canadian of New Restrictions on the Use of Celebrex®' (7 April 2005), http://hc-sc.gc.ca/english/protection/warnings/2005/2005_17.html (accessed 7 April 2005).

62 Okie, *supra* note 9 at 1064.

63 Carolyn Abraham, 'Health Minister Attacks Makers of Vioxx,' *Globe and Mail*, 25 February 2005 at A1.

64 21 C.F.R. 54 (1998).

65 See Baram, *supra* note 47 at 274.

66 Department of Health and Human Services, *Financial Relationships and Interests in Research Involving Human Subjects: Guidance for Human Subjects Protection, 2004*, 69 Federal Register 92 (12 May 2004) 26393–7.

67 Association of American Medical Colleges (AAMC), Task Force on Financial Conflicts of Interest in Clinical Research, *Protecting Subjects, Preserving Trust, Promoting Progress: Policy and Guidelines for the Oversight of Individual Financial Conflict of Interest in Human Subjects Research* (2001) at 5–6, <http://www.aamc.org/members/coitf/start.htm (accessed 7 May 2004); and AAMC, Task Force on Financial Conflict of Interest in Clinical Research, Institutional Conflict of Interest, *Protecting Subjects, Preserving Trust, Promoting Progress II: Principles and Recommendations for Oversight of an Institution's Financial Interests in Human Subjects Research* (Washington DC: AAMC, 2002).

68 AAMC (2001), *ibid.* at 16; AAMC (2002), *ibid.* at 10–11.

69 See Lemmens and Freedman, *supra* note 10.

70 I have argued that Health Canada should easily be able to introduce a coherent regulatory structure for REBs in the context of clinical trials related to drug approval. See Trudo Lemmens, 'Federal Regulation of REB Review of Clinical Trials: A Modest But Easy Step towards an Accountable REB Review Structure in Canada' (2005) 13(2–3) Health Law Review 39.

71 Krimsky, *supra* note 28 at 207–9. For an interesting overview of COI policies in U.S. institutions, see S. Van McCrary *et al.* 'A National Survey of Policies on Disclosure of Conflicts of Interest in Biomedical Research' (2000) 343 New England J. Med. 1621; and Mildred K. Cho *et al.*, 'Policies on Faculty Conflicts of Interest at US Universities' (2000) 284 JAMA 2237.

72 Lemmens and Freedman, *supra* note 10.

73 Regulations Amending the Food and Drug Regulations (102 – Clinical Trials), P.C. 2001-1042, C. Gaz. 2001.II.1116 at 1131.

74 Eric G. Campbell *et al.*, 'Characteristics of Medical School Faculty Members Serving on Institutional Review Boards: Results of a National Survey' (2003) 78 Academic Medicine 831 at 833–4.

75 See for example, Law Commission of Canada, *The Governance of Health Research Involving Human Subjects,* Michael M. MacDonald, Principal Investigator (Ottawa: Law Reform Commission of Canada, 2000); Department of Health and Human Services, Office of Inspector General, *Institutional Review Boards: A Time for Reform* (Washington: author, 1998); Committee on Assessing the System for Protecting Human Research Participants, Institute of Medicine, Daniel D. Federman, Kathi E. Hanna and Laura L. Rodriguez, eds., *Responsible Research: A Systems Approach to Protecting Research Participants* (Washington: National Academies Press, 2001); see also the discussion in Kathleen C. Glass and Trudo Lemmens, 'Research Involving Humans' in Jocelyn Downie, Timothy Caulfield, and Colleen Flood, eds., *Canadian Health Law and Policy,* 2nd ed. (Toronto: Butterworths, 2002) 459 and references therein.

76 For a discussion of the need for a legislative regime, see Duff R. Waring and Trudo Lemmens, 'Integrating Values in Risk Analysis of Biomedical Research: The Case for Regulatory and Law Reform' (2004) 54. U. Toronto L. J. 49.

77 Commission on the Future of Health Care in Canada, *Building on Values: The Future of Health Care in Canada, Final Report* (2002) http://www.hc-sc.gc.ca/english/pdf/romanow/pdfs/HCC_Final_Report.pdf (accessed 20 May 2005).

78 Krimsky, *supra* note 28 at 229.

79 Marcia Angell, *The Truth about the Pharmaceutical Industry: How They De-
    ceive Us and What to Do about It* (New York: Random House, 2004) at 244–7.
80 Shane Neilson, 'Healy and Goliath: The Creation of Psychopharmacology'
    (2004) 170 Can. Med. Assoc. J. 501.
81 Fiona Fleck, 'WHO and Science Publishers Team Up on Online Register of
    Trials' (2004) 328 Brit. Med. J. 854.
82` See Catherine De Angelis, *et al.*, 'Clinical Trials Registrations: A Statement
    from the International Committee of Medical Journal Editors' (2004) 351
    New England J. Med. 1250.

18 Grasping the Nettle: Confronting the Issue of Competing Interests and Obligations in Health Research Policy

JOCELYN DOWNIE

Health research policy has a significant, but often underappreciated, impact on access to health care in Canada. For example, when the government of Canada prohibits the creation of embryos for research, it is possible that advances in embryonic stem cell research that could potentially be relevant to the treatment of Parkinson's disease will be delayed or never realized. But perhaps the funds that would have been directed to this research will be spent on other therapeutic options that prove to be more effective and less costly to the health care system. If Health Canada lowers its requirements for the demonstration of the safety and efficacy of a new drug for the treatment of hypertension, patients with hypertension may gain quicker access to the drug, but they may also be harmed by taking what is later discovered to be an unsafe or ineffective medication. If research ethics boards (REBs) across the country refuse to approve a protocol involving the study of a new artificial heart, a transplantation option using that heart may never be developed, and people who might eventually have benefited from that heart may die of heart failure. Then again, it is possible that the decision to reject the protocol may save a number of research subjects from exposure to an ineffective device. As such, in the context of the broader discussion of access to health care in this book, it is appropriate to consider the impact of health research policy. Given space constraints and the coverage of related issues in the other chapters in this volume concerning the manufacturing of demand by the media and through the commercialization of research (in particular the preceding chapter by Trudo Lemmens), my focus is on one aspect of health research policy, namely, competing interests and obligations in the development of health research policy.

I have chosen to focus on research policy rather than practice because it has not yet received the attention it deserves and requires. I have chosen to focus on competing interests and obligations because I believe that this category is broader and less normatively loaded than its subset category 'conflicts of interest.' If you say that people are in a position of conflict of interest, it is common for them to feel criticized or attacked. However, a position of conflict of interest is not inherently a morally bad position. The moral problem arises when people are in a position of conflict of interest that requires management and they fail to engage in that management.[1] I hope that the switch to the language of 'competing interests and obligations' will enable us to identify situations in which there is a phenomenon that needs to be addressed without automatically imputing, or being taken to impute, immoral conduct on the part of the person faced with the competing interests and obligations.

I will consider competing interests and obligations as they apply to research regulators, research funders, patient advocacy groups, health care ethicists, and health law experts – all of whom have a significant role in making research policy. My objective is to raise concerns, issue a call for further research and analysis, and make the case for changes to policy and practice in this arena. This may then, among other things, have an impact on access to health care.

Research Regulators

In Canada, Health Canada (the federal Department of Health) has a mandate to protect and promote the health of Canadians. Health Canada is also responsible for the regulation of some research in Canada (specifically, clinical trials).[2] In the relatively recent past, Health Canada began to move closer to industry. For example, it began to charge companies for drug reviews necessary for the approval to market a drug in Canada. The fees for these reviews (payable by the pharmaceutical companies to Health Canada) have now reached approximately $200,000 for a new drug approval.[3] There is now, therefore, a direct and substantial financial connection between industry and the regulator. I would argue that this connection should cause us to pause as it opens up the possibility of regulatory capture.[4] Perhaps not surprisingly, it appears to have already had a disturbing effect at Health Canada as illustrated by comments made in a 1997 internal Drugs and Medical Devices Programme Quality Initiative Bulletin from the then Therapeutic Products Directorate: 'Your client is the direct recipient of your services. In many cases this is the person or company who pays for the service.'[5] The Bulletin continues:

> By adopting a client focus and service orientation, regulatory organizations can help those seeking approval to comply with regulations as easily as possible,
> - promote voluntary compliance,
> - earn goodwill from the regulated community and the public at large,
> - improve the working atmosphere for front-line staff.[6]

Despite the claim made in this bulletin that '[t]here is no conflict of interest between delivering a service to a client and functioning in a regulatory environment,' when industry is seen as 'the client' and the public is seen as 'a stakeholder,' there is good reason to be concerned about the attention being paid to the protection and promotion of the health of Canadians through the regulation of health research.[7] While charging for drug reviews does not necessarily create an unmanageable set of competing interests and obligations, it appears that in the case of Health Canada, it has created an unmanaged, or inadequately managed, one.

To its credit, Health Canada appears to have recognized the problematic potential of the drug review fees and the problems of regulatory capture – the 2003 Federal Health Protection Legislative Renewal initiative suggests the separation of the fee collection from the regulation:[8] 'For the most part, the charging of fees by government is regulated under the Financial Administration Act and the Department of Health Act. The existing legal requirements would be retained with a few technical changes. The proposed Act would require that regulatory processes for which a fee is charged be isolated from any matter relating to the collection of fees.'[9] However, it is not clear that this will solve the problem identified above. First, what does it mean to 'isolate' the regulatory processes from the collection? Second, how does this isolation eliminate the incentives to put the interests of industry above the larger public interest? The government continues to regulate the drug approval process and remains simultaneously dependent upon the income from the fees.

There is an additional concern about competing interests and obligations to be considered. That is, Health Canada may be tempted to respond to the obvious economic potential in health research by embracing a mandate to contribute to the growth of the economy. Certainly, in the corridors of power there has been a rapid and significant linkage between health research and the economy. Indeed, precisely this linkage between health research and the economy is evident in Health Canada's submission to the Government of Canada's Innovation Strategy.[10] However, I would argue that Health Canada should not embrace (or be allowed to embrace) such a competing mandate. That is, it should not have an economic mandate when the very driver of the economy that it can influence (for example, the pharmaceutical industry) is the driver that it regulates, and when the actions it can take to influence the economics in a positive direction are actions that simultaneously threaten the health protection mandate. With a dual mandate, Health Canada would have to try to both promote health and build the economy – but there is a conflict to the extent that while lower regulatory standards for research can draw more research to the country and give a positive jolt to employment, they may lead to the approval of higher risk drugs (or even what turn out to be harmful drugs).

Management of competing interests and obligations here requires that Health Canada be charged solely with protecting and promoting the health of Canadians (for example, regulating research). The battle between health interests and other interests (for example, economic ones) could then be left to the higher level of government; that is, let Health Canada and Industry Canada present their cases and let Parliament decide between them. The decisions at the intersection would then be more transparent and more democratic as the decision-makers would be more accountable to Canadians.

In this area, some hope can be found in the federal Health Protection Legislative Renewal initiative. According to the Detailed Legislative Proposal:

> The Act would stipulate clearly that its purpose is to protect the health of the people. It would also describe three underlying values that would guide health and safety decisions:
> • *health and safety should always come first*;
> • public scrutiny of government actions and public engagement in decision making will be encouraged; and
> • the Minister of Health is accountable for the administration of the Act to the people of Canada through Parliament.[11]

If the singular purpose of protecting and promoting the health of Canadians is ultimately embedded in the draft legislation, and if the draft legislation is passed, then the concern about competing interests and obligations will be at the very least reduced. However, if it is lost in the initial drafting or in the political process, then the concern will remain, and it may compromise Health Canada's ability to protect the health of Canadians.

Research Funders

Like research regulators, research funders face considerable as-yet-inadequately managed competing interests and obligations. The Canadian Institutes for Health Research (CIHR), the national public funding agency for health research), has a mandate to promote research: 'Its objective is to excel, according to internationally accepted standards of scientific excellence, in the creation of new knowledge and its translation into improved health for Canadians, more effective health services and products and a strengthened Canadian health care system.'[12] It also has a mandate to promote the commercialization of research; the Act that established the CIHR explicitly mandates 'encouraging innovation, facilitating the commercialization of health research in Canada, and promoting economic development through health research in Canada.'[13] It could also be argued that, perhaps in response to the regulatory deficit with respect to research involving humans subjects in Canada, CIHR appears to have taken on a regulatory role. For example, in its previous incarnation as the Medical Research Council of Canada and together with two other major national funding councils – the Social Sciences and Humanities Research Council (SSHRC) and the Natural Sciences and Engineering Research Council (NSERC) – CIHR set the ethics standards for research conducted at institutions receiving Council funding through authorship of the *Tri-Council Policy Statement: Ethical Conduct for Research Involving Humans* (1998) (TCPS). Moreover, Schedule 2 of the *Memorandum of Understanding* (MOU) signed between the three federal funding agencies and agency-funded institutions in 2002, clearly states that the scope of application of the TCPS extends beyond research funded by CIHR, SSHRC, and NSERC, to include all research conducted under the auspices of Tri-Agency-funded institutions.[14] The Councils also established the Interagency Panel on Research Ethics (PRE) to 'provide stewardship *by the Agencies* for the governance of research ethics policies and practices of the institutions receiving agency funding.'[15] The PRE is not independent of the Councils: its members are appointed by the Council presidents; the PRE reports to the presidents; and the membership of the PRE can include members of the agencies' governing councils or standing committees. Furthermore, its role is advisory to the agencies. The regulatory role can also be inferred from the fact that the Councils can enforce compliance with the TCPS and all other Tri-Agency research funding policies through the MOU, particularly Schedule 8[16] (that is, the Councils can withhold or withdraw funding from non-compliant institutions).

Now it might be argued that these actions represent responsible governance on the part of CIHR – the organization has been entrusted with public funds, and it has established policies and procedures for the use of those funds. However, the TCPS, PRE, and Schedule 2 of the MOU all reach beyond CIHR-funded research and beyond research that is even indirectly supported by CIHR funds. It might also be argued that these actions represent an organization stepping in and acting to protect as many research participants as it can (through a broad reading of its authority) where the entity that should be protecting them (the government) has failed to act. However, whatever the reasons for acting (and however admirable they may or may not have been), by virtue of the scope of the actions taken, it can be argued that CIHR has embraced a regulatory role in the research arena.

Genome Canada (a $300-million initiative of Industry Canada) has a mandate to promote and fund genomics research as well as a mandate to build the Canadian economy.[17] Its objectives include: '[to] encourage investment in genomics and proteomics research by others [and] create and realize economic, industrial and social benefits to Canada.'[18] As mentioned by Lemmens (chapter 17), Genome Canada has adopted a strong position in favour of commercializable research as evidenced by its matched funding requirement: 'Genome Canada will fund up to 50% of approved eligible costs for new or incremental research activities that are an integral part of the Genome Canada approved project. Applicants must assist their genome centre, which will take the lead in securing the remaining 50% of the funding from other eligible sources.'[19] It also assumes that the research it funds will have commercial potential: 'A clear commercialization process, which includes IP management and ownership, technology transfer and benefit sharing, must be defined and included in the full application.'[20] Indeed, the president and CEO of Genome Canada has actually said that 'Genome Canada is not a granting council; Genome Canada is a corporation that is investing in specific projects. It's like venture capital, but instead of having equity in the company we sponsor, we invest in projects.'[21]

Thus, we have research funding bodies with limiting or competing mandates. Genome Canada and CIHR must both promote research and build the economy. The risk here is that the two mandates, taken together, will be pursued at the expense of research without commercial potential but with significant other potential benefits for Canadians. To be more precise, while a commercialization requirement for research funded by Genome Canada or CIHR may increase Canada's economic fortunes, it may dramatically discourage and drive away conceptual and/or basic research or research directed at diseases affecting only a small subset of the country's population (usually an already disadvantaged group).[22] With the emphasis on commercialization, there is also the risk of shaping research design in a way that reduces costs for researchers and sponsors but increases risks for research participants, restricting the information that gets disclosed through confidentiality clauses in commercial research contracts, creating a positive-results bias in the published literature, and limiting access to the benefits of research as investments in research are recouped through high charges for access to the results (for example, new drugs).[23]

CIHR plays both a promotional and regulatory role in relation to a great deal of health research in Canada. This can be very difficult. For example, the TCPS takes a hotly debated position by severely restricting the use of placebos in trials for conditions for which there is a standard of care.[24] It has been argued that this policy forces researchers to design their studies using a scientifically inferior method, hence compromising the goal of 'scientific excellence.'[25] Furthermore, it has been argued that this policy may lead to research being taken out of Canada, hence compromising the goal of increased research.[26] As CIHR revisits its restrictions on the use of placebos, it must both assess the validity of these arguments and balance the potential negative consequences on research against the well-established safety concerns that ground the current TCPS position on the use of placebos.[27] This dual mandate (at the least in its current non-nuanced form, that is, without an explicit prioritization of safety) is inappropriate and, for reasons discussed below, it should not be a part of CIHR.

We must acknowledge and manage these competing mandates. With regard to management, I would argue that the regulation of research should be shifted by Parliament from CIHR to another body, and the obligation to contribute to the economy should be removed by Parliament from the mandates of CIHR and Genome Canada.[28]

First, consider the shift of the regulation of research from CIHR. This should be done because regulation is an inappropriate task given the competing interests and obligations that it creates. CIHR is, in effect, the research community (for example, the president, the heads of the institutes, and the participants in the review structures are researchers). Thus, regulation of research by CIHR is a form of self-regulation. However, the conventional arguments in support of self-regulation (as an exception to the general rule of external regulation of regulated professions or industries) do not apply in the context of CIHR.[29]

Self-regulation of professions (for example, medicine, nursing, and law) is often justified by reference to some or all of the following arguments: (1) internalization of costs – self-regulation can internalize the costs of regulation to the profession (for example, when it is paid for through membership fees and similar charges to the members instead of the state); (2) preservation of democracy and the rule of law – self-regulation protects the profession (specifically the legal profession) from interference from the state when the profession is attempting to protect individuals from the state and thereby preserves democracy and the rule of law; and (3) expertise – given the specialized body of knowledge associated with the practice of the profession in question, only the members of the profession have the expertise needed to judge the conduct of the profession. Significantly, none of these justifications apply to the health research community.

The internalization of costs argument does not apply because CIHR as the regulator consumes government – not researchers' – funds. The preservation of democracy and the rule of law argument that justifies self-regulation for lawyers obviously does not apply. Of course, the research community has scientific expertise that is needed. In addition, with the expansion of disciplines supported by CIHR, the research community increasingly has expertise in research ethics as well. However, it is not the case that only members of the research community have the expertise needed to judge the conduct of the community. The public interest, for example, is something about which the research community has no privileged knowledge or abilities. Therefore, the research community does not qualify for what can be considered the 'self-regulation exception' and so should be regulated externally.

Obviously, the research community will be needed as part of the regulatory system, and members of that community should play an important role in the system. However, the research community itself should not control the regulation.[30] Indeed, in June 2003, the Governing Council of CIHR recognized the implications of its actions in this area as outlined above and, according to the *Minutes of the Governing Council Meeting*:

> agreed that CIHR should not be taking on a regulatory role in the area of ethics review and oversight, despite the current policy vacuum in Canada on this matter. Rather, CIHR should pursue its more supportive-type role by, as examples: encouraging Health Canada to advance its research ethics governance initiative; actively supporting either new and/or existing organizations (equivalent to the Canada Council on Animal Care) to carry out review and oversight functions necessary for assuring the ethics of human research in Canada; and promoting relevant educational efforts aimed at developing a more prominent ethics culture among Canadian health researchers and institutions.[31]

It will be interesting to watch and see what steps CIHR will take to distance itself from its regulatory role in response to this Governing Council statement. It should also be noted here that, unfortunately, it is not within CIHR's power to establish an independent oversight system and so CHIR, like the rest of Canada, must wait for Parliament to act. It thus remains for Health Canada to step in, to fill the 'policy vacuum,' and to take a more active and more comprehensive role in regulating research in Canada.[32]

Second, as noted earlier, CIHR and Genome Canada are obliged by mandate to contribute to the economy. And yet, as described earlier, such an obligation may have a variety of negative consequences for the health of Canadians. My proposal to remove this obligation will be strongly opposed by political and interest groups. If these groups prevail, at least the second-best solution should be pursued. That is, the federal government should explicitly state the hierarchy of the regulatory and economic mandates, placing the protection and promotion of the health of research participants specifically and then the health of all Canadians more generally very clearly ahead of all other mandates. Furthermore, it must be recognized that in the presence of multiple mandates, the pro-economic mandate of individuals and groups within and advising the funders will probably dominate because they will have the backing of (economically and politically powerful) industry. Steps must be taken to counter-balance this. For example, representatives of those whose interests are clearly other than economic should outnumber the pro-economic mandate individuals on bodies engaged in decision-making processes that affect health care policy. Furthermore, far greater transparency must be required of these funding organizations both in terms of the disclosure of the interests of all decision-makers associated with the organizations as well as the decision-making processes themselves. For example, the Human Genetics Commission in the United Kingdom conducts all main meetings in public and places transcripts of these meetings on their website.[33]

Patient Advocacy Groups[34]

What has come to be known as 'third party technique' involves a company providing funding to an individual or group and then using the individual or group to realize the company's goals (for example, a change in a particular government policy). The extreme of this technique in the context of patient advocacy groups involves setting up artificial grassroots organizations – known as 'astroturf groups' – precisely for this purpose.[35]

There are many examples of close relationships between patient advocacy groups and industry. A brief search on the Internet for Canadian groups with significant industry connections came up with the following: the Anemia Institute for Research and Education,[36] the Arthritis Society of Canada,[37] the Cancer Advocacy Coalition,[38] the Infertility Awareness Association of Canada,[39] and the Consumer Advocare Network.[40]

A number of industry-funded patient advocacy groups have been very active in lobbying for policy development or reform that is in the interests of their industry supporters, for example, as Patti Peppin (chapter 15) discusses, relaxing restrictions on direct-to-consumer advertising (DTCA) and including specific drugs on provincial-territorial formularies. Consider the Consumer Advocare Network. According to its website, this is 'a national network of healthcare consumer organizations and individuals in Canada' with a mission 'to ensure that the Canadian healthcare system is driven by consumer needs.' Furthermore, the Consumer Advocare Network 'provides an effective voice for healthcare consumer organizations, allied groups, and individuals; promotes informed input to policy and funding decisions which support consumer priorities; and promotes consumer participation in healthcare decision making at all levels.'[41]

In a nineteen-page brief recently submitted to Health Canada, the Consumer Advocare Network called for the legalization of DTCA. A review of the brief reveals that of the twenty-four members of the Joint Working Group who prepared it, twelve were from the pharmaceutical industry or pharmaceutical marketing and/or consulting firms. Some of the other twelve were from organizations known to receive significant support from pharmaceutical companies (for example, the Canadian Arthritis Society).[42] Perhaps not surprisingly, the Network ended up lobbying for changes to legislation that better serve the pharmaceutical industry's interests.

It is instructive to explore industry's perspective on partnering with patient advocacy groups. Indeed, industry documents contain the following revealing comments on partnering:

- Industry should partner because 'input from patients' associations is increasingly sought from legislators and regulators prior to making important policy decisions.'[43]
- 'Good advocacy group relations establish positive working relationships with influential patient and professional associations that share a company's goals and that can champion a company's products'[44]
- Industry should partner because patient groups are 'influential in local, regional, federal decision-making process (participate in development of guidelines, influence drug approval).'[45]

Clearly, industry recognizes the influence that can be achieved by sponsoring patient advocacy groups.

There are a number of reasons for concern about industry support for patient advocacy groups. First, industry funding of patient advocacy groups may lead patient advocacy groups to place the interests of their funders over the interests of some or all members of their group. Second, through funding, industry influences the policy positions taken by the group but without this influence being visible to the policy-makers. Third, through funding patient advocacy groups, industry is using the groups' credibility to increase the demand and market for their drugs.[46] As noted by commentators on the issue, 'third party technique' is 'helping the drug industry separate the message from what could be seen as a self-interested messenger.'[47] Alan Cassels, a researcher and policy analyst investigating pharmaceutical practices, describes how this approach was explained to him: 'The best way to advertise is to make your promotion not look like advertising – that's what one of the presenters said ... And one of the ways you get your promotion to not look like advertising is to use ... consumer groups to speak for you.'[48]

One can easily imagine such patient advocacy groups, which now lobby around drug marketing and coverage issues, starting to lobby for policy changes with respect to the governance of research. For example, an advocacy group for people with depression might well be funded by the pharmaceutical industry and might lobby for changes to Canadian policy on placebo-controlled trials, that is, that the restriction on the use of placebos where there is a standard of care should be relaxed.

To manage the competing interests and obligations identified here, all patient advocacy groups should put in place processes to ensure accountability to their memberships for decision-making regarding policy positions. Full disclosure by patient advocacy groups and organizations and individuals associated with such groups and organizations must be required in all engagement with policy-related consultations (currently this is not required). In addition, when individuals are being considered for membership or are serving on government committees or policy-related advisory groups by virtue of their association with particular patient populations, full disclosure of any relationship with industry must be required. These latter two recommendations are particularly important and urgent given the government's increased emphasis on public consultation when making policy.

Experts in Health Care Ethics and Law

There are also reasons to be concerned about competing interests and obligations with respect to the engagement of experts in health care ethics and law in policy-making processes. I will address three of them.

First, experts in health care ethics and law are increasingly integrated into all aspects of research in Canada. Experts simultaneously sit on the committees and boards for research funding bodies (for example, CIHR), research regulators (for example, Health Canada), and research promoters (for example, Industry Canada). Health care ethics and law experts sit on governing boards, advisory boards, standing ethics committees, peer review committees, conference planning committees, planning and priorities committees, and working groups. They serve as overseers, advisers, contractors, and members, and consequently they are simultaneously (directly and indirectly) setting the research agenda, regulating research, applying for research funds, conducting research, and being regulated as researchers all at a national level. There has to date been little meaningful public discussion of the competing interests and obligations that these multiple roles create, and there have been few attempts to find ways to manage them.

A particularly acute example of this first concern comes from the fact that these experts in health care ethics and law serve simultaneously as research policy advisers and active researchers. The most significant development in this arena is the increasingly common embedding of health care ethics and law experts in scientific research projects. This directly links the prospects of initial and ongoing funding for the ethics and law components of the programs of research to the science components. Consider, for example, the embedding of health care ethics and law experts in the Stem Cell Network, which was established in March 2001, with a four-year $21.1 million grant from the Networks of Centres of Excellence. The Network has a mandate to 'investigate the immense therapeutic potential of stem cells for the treatment of diseases currently incurable by conventional approaches.'[49] Health care ethics and law experts have been and continue to be members of this Network, while remaining active in policy-making as well as in advising policy-makers on stem cell research policy. For example, these same experts were members of the CIHR Working Group ('Ad Hoc Working Group') that was developing stem cell research guidelines[50] as the application for the Stem Cell Network was being considered,[51] and they appeared as experts before the House of Commons and Senate Committees that were considering legislation related to stem cell research.[52]

Is it wise to have these people play these roles simultaneously? True, there are a limited number of health care ethics and law experts in Canada who are also very knowledgeable about stem cell research. Furthermore, there are distinct advantages to embedding such experts in the science projects – the experts contribute to the science research and the health care ethics and law research is enriched by the increased access to the scientists and their research. Arguably, the research and the research policy-making process are both improved by the embedding phenomenon. However, experts who are embedded in applications for research funds for a particular kind of scientific research or are embedded in particular instances of funded scientific research obviously have competing interests and obligations if they are concurrently providing advice to policy-makers on whether such research should be permitted and, if so, how it should be regulated.

Second, competing interests and obligations can shape what research in health care ethics and law gets done and how. Extraordinary amounts of money are available in particular areas of health research (for example, genetics and genomics research). Given the increased needs for universities to generate research funds (which manifests itself as pressure on academics to get large research grants), and given the disproportionate amount of money that is available in these areas, experts in health care ethics and law may be disproportionately drawn into them. Furthermore, because it is possible to realize a far greater financial return by participating in a large-scale science project as an ethics component than can be realized by participating in a pure ethics project, there is an added incentive to engage in research that is relevant to these large-scale projects. This shapes both the subjects researched and the way in which the research is conducted. Institutional interests in the generation of funds and personal career interests that can be realized through the maximization of research grants can compete with personal interests in other topics and the public interest in research in other arenas. For example, with so many researchers involved in genetics and genomics ethics, law, and social issues (ESLI), there are fewer available to do ESLI research in mental health or Aboriginal health.

Third, health care ethics and law experts are increasingly connected to industry as consultants, and through industry support for research projects, for research institutes, and personally through membership on industry committees or boards.[53] In 'Pharma Buys a Conscience,' Carl Elliott noted a number of such connections, for example:

- Arthur Caplan, director of the University of Pennsylvania Center for Bioethics 'consults for the drug and biotech industries, recently co-authored an article with scientists for Advanced Cell Technology, and heads a bioethics center supported by Monsanto, de Code Genetics, Millennium Pharmaceuticals, Geron Corporation, Pfizer, AstraZeneca Pharmaceuticals, E.I. du Pont de Nemours and Company, Human Genome Sciences, and the Schering-Plough Corporation.'[54]
- 'The University of Toronto houses the Sun Life Chair in Bioethics; the Stanford University Center for Biomedical Ethics has a program in genetics funded by a $1-million gift from SmithKline Beecham Corporation; the Merck Company Foundation has financed a string of international ethics centers in cities from Ankara, Turkey, to Pretoria, South Africa.'[55]
- 'A list of bioethicists reported to serve on such advisory boards [bioethics advisory boards for industry] reads like a who's who of bioethics: Nancy Dubler of Montefiore Medical, for DNA Sciences; Ronald Green of Dartmouth, for Advanced Cell Technology; Arthur Caplan of the University of Pennsylvania, for Celera Genomics and DuPont; Karen Lebacqz of the Pacific School of Religion, for Geron Corporation. Some bioethicists work pro bono while others accept fees.'[56]

At the same time, health care ethics and law experts are serving on government expert advisory committees, presenting to government committees, consulting for governments regarding policy, giving talks, and making media appearances on policy-related issues.

Engagement with industry can bring a number of significant benefits (for example, influencing industry practice in a positive direction as well as providing financial support for important research that would not be conducted without the industry support). This is not necessarily a bad thing and it does not necessarily generate untenable positions of competing interests and obligations. However, with health care ethics and law experts receiving industry support and engaging in policy-making processes, again there is reason to be concerned about the potential for visible and invisible industry influence and the purchasing of credibility. We must therefore ask how to manage the competing interests and obligations in this arena. Does it matter, for example, whether there are conditions attached to the exchange of funds? Are certain kinds of conditions acceptable and others not? Does it make a difference if the honoraria are small rather than large? Many questions remain unanswered. Yet surely they must be answered if we are to responsibly manage the many competing interests and obligations in the arena of research involving human subjects.

I believe that we must carefully consider all of the concerns above with respect to competing interests and obligations among experts in health care ethics and law. This is particularly important to do because, as a community, we have been vocal in criticizing researchers and research institutions for not recognizing and managing their competing interests and obligations. We must look at ourselves and demand reform. Reform must involve at least the following elements:

- Recognizing and using capacity (that is, knowledge and skills in health care ethics and law) that is already there so as to expand the pool of experts who are drawn upon.
- Building capacity so as to expand the pool of experts who can be drawn upon.[57]
- Conducting empirical research into the following questions: What is the extent of the phenomena described above (embedding, integration, and industry support)? Is there a correlation between positions taken by experts embedded within scientific initiatives and the interests of these initiatives? Is there a causal relationship between positions taken and embedding? Is there a homogenization due to the integration; and is there a correlation between positions taken by

experts funded by industry and industry interests? Is there a causal relationship between positions taken and industry support?[58]
- Requiring full disclosure of all engagements with policy-making processes.
- Developing and enforcing guidelines for managing *obvious* competing interests and obligations (including disclosure, but also going beyond disclosure to limits on engagement and exit, as suggested in a related context by Lemmens in chapter 17).
- Developing and enforcing guidelines for managing *complex* situations of competing interests and obligations (again including disclosure and going beyond disclosure to limits on engagement and exit).

Conclusion

Concerns about access to health care cannot be addressed in isolation from concerns about health research, and concerns about health research cannot be addressed without careful attention to policy politics, with particular attention to the impact of the increasing commercialization of research on policy politics. What treatments are available even for consideration for public funding depend upon what research is done (and not done) and how it is done. This, in turn, depends upon the regulation of research. Thus, upstream policy decisions about research have direct relevance to the downstream policy choices about funding.

We must therefore pay closer attention to the connections among research regulators and funders, patient advocacy groups, health care ethics and law experts, industry, health researchers, and policy-makers. We must both know where these connections are and recognize their influence. We must aggressively manage the competing interests and obligations that may have an influence on policy-making in the arena of research involving humans. We will then be better able to engage in the broader project of improving access to health care through better health research policy.

NOTES

The author would like to thank the following individuals for their thoughtful, critical, and constructive comments on earlier drafts of this chapter: Brad Abernethy, Françoise Baylis, Timothy Caulfield, Colleen Flood, and Patricia Kosseim.

 1 By 'manage,' I mean a process of recognizing the interests involved,
   identifying the ways in which they can (or can appear) to be in conflict,
   identifying ways of reducing or eliminating the potential harms of the
   conflicts (real or perceived), evaluating the potential harms and benefits
   of the various alternative means of reducing or eliminating the potential
   harms, and taking the steps with the most favourable harm-benefit ratio
   (these steps may include exit, disclosure, and non-participation in
   decision-making, and disclosure and non-participation in discussions
   and decisions).
 2 *Food and Drugs Act Regulations*, C.R.C., c. 870, Division 5, c. 05.016(c).
 3 Therapeutic Products Directorate, *Guidance Document on Cost Recovery
   Submission Evaluation and Fees*. www.hc-sc.gc.ca/dhp-msp/alt_formats/
   hpfb-dgpsa/pdf/prodpharma/fee_frais_guide_e.pdf (accessed 8 September 2005).
 4 The phenomenon through which the regulator, over time, comes to give
   precedence to the regulated over the larger public interest. See, for example, Kenneth Kernaghan and David Siegel, *Public Administration in
   Canada*, 4th ed. (Toronto: ITP Nelson, 1999) at 279; Marvin H. Berstein.
   Regulating Business by Independent Commission (Princeton: Princeton University Press, 1955), ch. 3; Liora Salter, 'Capture or Co-management:
   Democracy and Accountability in Regulatory Agencies,' in Greg Albo,
   David Langille, and Leo Panich, eds., *A Different Kind of State? Popular
   Power and Democratic Administration* (London: Oxford University Press,
   1993) 87–101.
 5 Health Canada Drugs and Medical Devices Programme, *Questions and
   Answers – Who Is Our Client?* (Quality Initiative Bulletin) (Ottawa: Health
   Canada, February 1997).
 6 *Ibid.*
 7 *Ibid.*
 8 Health Canada, *Health Protection Legislative Renewal: Detailed Legislative
   Proposal* (Ottawa: Health Canada, 2003) at 186, http://renewal.hc-sc.gc.ca
   (accessed 8 September 2005).
 9 *Ibid.*
10 Government of Canada, *Submission – Federal Department Report – Innovation
   and Health (Health Canada)* (Ottawa: Health Canada, 1 April 2003), http://
   innovation.gc.ca/gol/innovation/site.nsf/en/in02330.htm (accessed
   8 September 2005).
11 *Supra* note 8 at 7, emphasis added.
12 Canadian Institutes for Health Research (CIHR), *Mandate*, www.cihr-
   irsc.gc.ca/e/24418.html#3 (accessed 8 September 2005).
13 *Act to Establish the Canadian Institutes of Health Research, to Repeal the Medical*

Research Council of Canada Act, and to Make Consequential Amendments to other Acts, R.S.C. 2000, c. 6, s. 4(i).

14 Natural Sciences and Engineering Research Council of Canada (NSERC) *Memorandum of Understanding in the Management of Federal Grants and Awards* (Ottawa: NSERC, 17 July 2002) http://www.nserc.ca/institution/mou_e.htm and http://www.nserc.ca/institution/mou_sch2_e.htm (accessed 8 September 2005).

15 Interagency Advisory Panel on Research Ethics, *Governance Structure for the Tri-council Policy Statement: Ethical Conduct for Research Involving Humans* (Ottawa: Government of Canada, 1 April 2004) (emphasis added), http://pre.ethics.gc.ca/english/aboutus/termsofreference.cfm (accessed 8 September 2005).

16 NSERC, *Memorandum of Understanding*, http://www.nserc.ca/institution/mou_e.htm and http://www.nserc.ca/institution/mou_sch8_e.htm (accessed 8 September 2005).

17 Genome Canada, 'Mission and Objectives,' http://genomecanada.ca/GcgenomeCanada/enBref/mission.asp?l=e (accessed 8 September 2005).

18 *Ibid.*

19 Genome Canada, *Guidelines and Evaluation Criteria for the Competition III,* (Genome Canada, July 2004) s. 7, available at www.genomecanada.ca/GCprogrammesRecherche/CONCOURS/concoursIII/Guidelinesfinal.pdf. (accessed 8 september 2005).

20 *Ibid.* at s. 7.1.

21 'Mapping Canada's Genome: In Conversation with Genome Canada's President, Dr. Martin Godbout' (2001) Biotechnology Focus 4:5, http://www.genomecanada.ca/media/biofocus_julyaugust2001.pdf (accessed 8 September 2005).

22 Andrew Duffy, 'Rare Diseases' Troubling Questions' *Ottawa Citizen*, 21 January 2002 at 1.

23 For a discussion of the risks of commercialization, see Jocelyn Downie, 'Contemporary Health Research: A Cautionary Tale' (2003) Health Law Journal, Special Edition 1.

24 Article 7.4 Tri-Council Policy Statement, *Ethical Conduct for Research Involving Humans, 1998* (with 2000, 2002 updates). www.pre.ethics.gc.ca/english/policystatement/policystatement.cfm (accessed 8 September 2005).

25 Jurgen Fritze and Hans-Jurgen Moller, 'Design of Clinical Trials of Antidepressants: Should a Placebo Arm be Included?' (2001) 15:10 CNS Drugs 775; Franklin G. Miller and Howard Brody, 'What Makes Placebo Controlled Trials Unethical?' (2002) 2:2 Am. J. Bioeth. 3.

26 Patricia Houston, Jim Wright, and Vratislav Hadrava, '6. Regulatory
Perspective E. Recommendation: Be Consistent with International Guidelines,' in National Placebo Working Committee National Placebo Initiative,
*Final Report of the National Placebo Working Committee on the Appropriate Use
of Placebos in Clinical Trials in Canada* (July 2004) (Ottawa: Health Canada,
2004) available at www.cihr-irsc.gc.ca/e/25139.html (accessed 8 September 2005).

27 As it may do depending upon the results of the National Placebo Initiative. See www.cihr-irsc.gc.ca/e/5466.html. The National Placebo Initiative
is jointly sponsored by CIHR and Health Canada aimed at developing
recommendations that can be used by these two organizations to inform
revisions to the documents they respectively have jurisdiction over. In the
case of CIHR, the TCPS.

28 Note that I am not saying that health research should not contribute to the
economy. Rather, I am saying that contribution to the economy should not
be a mandate of CIHR and Genome Canada that they then pass on to the
research community.

29 See, for example, Ruth K. Miller, 'Individual Researcher Liability for Clini-
cal Research on Humans' (2003) 6:2 J. Biolaw Bus. 8; Daniel P. Wermeling,
'Clinical Research: Regulatory Issues' (1999) 56:(3) Am. J. Health Syst.
Pharm. 252.

30 There are, of course, other reasons for arguing that the regulatory function
should be removed from the funding councils, e.g., the fact that the funding councils' oversight is limited in its scope and can only capture research
conducted at institutions receiving council funding. However, I focus here
on only the reasons related to competing interests and obligations.

31 CIHR, *Meeting Minutes: 21st Meeting of Governing Council* (18, 19 June
2003), http://www.cihr-irsc.gc.ca/e/19817.html (accessed 8 September
2005).

32 The 2002 Speech from the Throne promised that the federal government
would 'work with provinces to implement a national system for the
governance of research involving humans, including national research
ethics and standards.' Canada, Governor General, '*The Canada We Want:
Speech from the Throne to Open the Second Session of the Thirty-Seventh Parliament of Canada, September 30, 2002,'* http://www.pco-bcp.gc.ca/sft-ddt/
hnav/hnav07_e.htm. Unless otherwise indicated, all websites referred to
below were accessed 8 September 2005. Unfortunately, no such system has
yet been implemented.

33 'HGC Business: Meetings,' http://www.hgc.gov.uk/Client/Content-
wide.asp?ContentId=145.

34 The issue of patient advocacy groups in policy-making was brought to my attention by Sharon Batt, a doctoral student in the CIHR Training Program in Health Law and Policy at Dalhousie University. 'Marching to Different Drummers: Health Advocacy Groups in Canada and Funding from the Pharmaceutical Industry,' www.hp-apsf.ca/pdf/corpFunding.pdf.

35 Sharon Batt, 'Breast Cancer Advocates and Pharmaceutical Industry Funds' (2002), http://www.bcam.qc.ca/news/advocates/html; Barbara Mintzes, 'Blurring the Boundaries: New Trends in Drug Promotion' (1998), http://www.haiweb.org.pubs/blurring/blurring.intro.html; Gordon Guyatt, 'Take Pill Ads with a Grain of Salt' *Winnipeg Free Press* (24 November 2003), http://www.hwcn.org/link/mrg/Patient.advocacy.grps.pdf.

36 Anemia Institute for Research and Education, www.anemiainstitute.org.

37 The Arthritis Society of Canada, www.arthritis.org.

38 The Cancer Advocacy Coalition, www.canceradvocacycoalition.com.

39 The Infertility Awareness Association, www.iaac.ca.

40 Consumer Advocare Network, www.consumeradvocare.org.

41 'Who We Are' and 'Mission,' *ibid.*

42 Durhane Wong-Rieger, 'A Case for Regulated Direct-to-Consumer Promotion of Prescription Drugs' (2003), http://www.consumeradvocare.org/index.php/ca/content/download/70/199/file/health_canada_proposal.pdf.

43 K. Miller, 'Patient Advocacy: Leveraging the Newest Dimension of Health Care Public Relations,' presentation to the Public Relations World Congress (2000), Public Relations Society of America, http://www.ipranet.org/workbook/page10.htm.

44 *Ibid.*

45 *Ibid.*

46 As found in a 1997 study conducted by Roper Start Worldwide, Inc. reported on by the National Health Council and cited in a 1999 report from the Attorneys General of sixteen states and the District of Columbia Corporation Counsel: 'Organizations such as the American Cancer Society or the American Diabetes Association were found to be "somewhat" or "completely believable" [as sources of medical and health news] by 93% of consumers surveyed. This level of trust is comparable to that enjoyed by such health care professionals as doctors (93%), nurses (92%) and pharmacists (92%) [whereas] 31% of those surveyed [found advertisements for medications to be] not too [or] not at all believable ... The report further noted that American consumers age 60 or over are less likely than younger consumers (for example, ages 18–29) to trust advertisements for medications, with 39% of older Americans, versus 27% of younger consumers,

saying that such advertisements are "not too" or "not at all believable." The same study noted further that Americans with greater formal education are particularly likely to identify these sources of medical information as having dubious credibility, with 43% of those with graduate degrees expressing the view that drug advertisements are "not too believable," while only 26% of those without a high school diploma express that view.' U.S., Office of New York State Attorney General Eliot Sptizer, *What's in a Nonprofit's Name? Public Trust, Profit and the Potential for Public Deception: A Preliminary Multistate Report on Corporate-Commercial/Nonprofit Product Marketing and Advertising of Commercial Products* (P.9/33) (New York: Office of New York State Attorney General Eliot Spitzer, 1999), http://www.oag.state.ny.us/press/reports/nonprofit/full_text.html.

47 Bob Burton and Andy Rowell, 'Unhealthy Spin' (2003) 326 Brit. Med. J. 1205.

48 Erica Johnson, 'Promoting Drugs through Patient Advocacy Groups' (Nov. 2000), CBC Marketplace, http://www.cbc.ca/consumers/market/files/health/drugmarketing.

49 'About Us,' http://www.stemcellnetwork.ca/aboutus/index.php.

50 '*Ad hoc* Working Group on Stem Cell Research,' http://www.cihr-irsc.gc.ca/e/2887.html.

51 http://www.stemcellnetwork.ca/aboutus/investigators.php.

52 Senate of Canada, 'Proceedings of the Standing Senate Committee on Social Affairs, Science and Technology: Issue 1 – Evidence – Meeting of February 18, 2004,' http://www.parl.gc.ca/37/3/parlbus/commbus/senate/Com-e/soci-e/01evb-e.htm?Language=E&Parl=37&Ses=3&comm_id=47; Senate of Canada, 'Proceedings of the Standing Senate Committee on Social Affairs, Science and Technology: Issue 2 – Evidence – Meeting of February 26, 2004,' http://www.parl.gc.ca/37/3/parlbus/commbus/senate/Com-e/soci-e/02evb-e.htm?Language=E&Parl=37&Ses=3&comm_id=47.

53 Carl Elliott. 'Not-so-Public Relations: How the Drug Industry is Branding Itself with Bioethics,' *Slate: Medical Examiner Online* (15 December 2003) http://slate.msn.com/id/2092442; Carl Elliott, 'Pharma Buys a Conscience.' *American Prospect* (24 September 2001) http://www.prospect.org/print/v12/17/elliott-c.html.

54 *American Prospect, ibid.*, at 1.

55 *Ibid.*, at 2.

56 *Ibid.*, at 6.

57 As a start toward this, the CIHR Training Program in Health Law and Policy has this as one of its objectives. See www.healthlawtraining.ca.

58 A comment should be made here about empirical research. Some might respond that 'there is no need for this research – we aren't influenced by our connections to, for example, the science projects and industry.' However, one must consider the studies on the influence of physician-industry contact in which doctors vigorously denied that industry contact had any influence on their prescribing patterns and yet the research demonstrated a significant influence. See, for example, Helen Prosser *et al.*, 'Influences on GPs' Decision to Prescribe New Drugs – The Importance of Who Says What' (2003) 20(1) Fam. Pract., 61; Barbara Mintzes *et al.* 'Influence of Direct to Consumer Pharmaceutical Advertising and Patients' Requests on Prescribing Decisions: Two Site Cross Sectional Survey' (2002) 324: 278 Brit. Med. J. 7332. One must also consider the more recent studies in JAMA and the British Medical Journal, which have illustrated the correlation between industry support for research and the publication of positive research results. Joel Lexchin *et al.*, 'Pharmaceutical Industry Sponsorship and Research Outcome and Quality: Systematic Review' Brit. Med. J. 326: 1167; Justine E. Bekelman *et al.*, 'Scope and Impact of Financial Conflicts of Interest in Biomedical Research: a Systematic Review' (2003) 289 JAMA 454. Our working assumption should be that correlation, causation, homogenization, and convergence exist rather than that they do not.

Conclusion

COLLEEN M. FLOOD

All countries struggle with putting limits on publicly funded health care, and Canada is no exception. This struggle is complicated by the fact that fairness must be fluid: What is fair today in terms of access will not be what is fair in twenty years' time. Changing technologies, needs, and resource levels mean that it is difficult to establish meaningful entitlements or rights that are relevant through these changing circumstances. This has particular resonance in the Canadian system of health care, as the core entitlements to hospital and physician services were laid down in the 1960s. The system is being passively privatized as other services take on greater importance, for example, drug and genetic therapies and home care. The net result is a health care system where a drug like insulin is not consistently publicly funded across Canada but, for example, annual general check-ups, for which there is no evidence of any health benefits accruing, are fully publicly funded.

Thus, the pressing challenge for Canadians is how to broaden our publicly funded system and yet narrow it at the same time. We need to expand the range of services that can attract universal first-dollar coverage to include home care and prescription drugs but simultaneously we must, in order for the system to be sustainable, weed out those services that are not truly medically necessary. We should be able to treat like medical needs alike regardless of whether the optimal therapy is a hospital service, a drug, or a genetic therapy. But of course this squarely raises the question of how we decide and who decides what services are medically necessary or, to reframe, what medical needs should be met? When resources are limited and cannot fund all 'medically necessary' services or needs, how do we prioritize?

The essays in this volume demonstrate three analytical approaches to the question of what services attract public funding. The first is to describe the existing processes for determining what is in and what is out of the publicly funded sector and what is left to the private sector or not provided at all. This is an important exercise. Without first knowing how the system really works, that is, how and when decisions are made and by whom, we cannot begin to consider how to improve it. Any reforms that do not take account of the present array of embedded relationships and incentives within the system will not work and result in unintended and perverse consequences.[1]

Surprisingly, there is little scholarship about how decisions that determine the boundaries of Medicare are actually made. All the essays in this volume contribute to a better understanding of how our system works at the present time. They demonstrate that the role of law in shaping and configuring the boundaries of Medicare is as complex as the interlocking decisions that cumulatively determine what health care is funded and for whom. Some of the essays have shown how the overarching effect of law can be to constrain what is possible. For example, the failure of Canada's *Constitution* to speak directly to the issue of Aboriginal health leads to no one level of government accepting full responsibility for the appalling state of health experienced by Aboriginal people. Legal constraints must either be challenged in law – Constance MacIntosh outlines the possible legal arguments in the case of Aboriginal peoples – or otherwise worked around to ensure better governance and accountability. Similarly, international trade agreements may constrain what is possible in domestic policy and must also either be challenged in law or otherwise worked around to ensure meaningful access to health care.

The second analytical approach used in this volume is to describe the principles that *should* guide decision-making and then examine existing decision-making processes to see whether or not such principles are applied. Here we see how complex and challenging this field is: although many principles and values are articulated there is little account of how to rank them or the values that they represent, should they conflict. Donna Greschner advocates implementation of the principle of evidence-based decision-making. Applying the best evidence would seem a sine qua non for arriving at the best possible decisions. But caution is required: such an approach may mask certain biases, for example, it may privilege randomized controlled trials at the expense of other kinds of evidence (such as that acquired by Aboriginal peoples in the use of traditional medicines). It may also discount the relevance of the severity of medical need. Sheila Wildeman argues that respect for individual autonomy should play more of a role in decision-making and that the focus should not be exclusively on health outcomes. Many of the contributors to this volume argue that the needs of the most vulnerable in society, particularly the poor, should be considered front and centre. As legal academics, their focus on the welfare of the most vulnerable puts a particular emphasis on *Charter* values. This is an important perspective. Health policy in Canada has long been dominated by economists whose work assumes the universality of a utilitarian approach and does not allow for other important Canadian values such as equality. Thus, while public health experts may prefer to examine the health of the population as a whole, economists will use that similar population base to focus on measurable health outcomes. Clinicians, meanwhile, may argue not only for future benefits but also for the relevance of medical need. All of these principles and values are reasonable – but ultimately, when in conflict, which of them should have priority?

International experience, including data from South Africa, the Netherlands, the United States (Oregon), New Zealand, and Israel, suggests that the project of determining an explicit list of principles to guide decision-making in allocating health care resources is often doomed to failure because of the apparently intractable problem of ranking those principles. Balancing competing and conflicting values would not seem such an insurmountable challenge from a legal perspective – jurists are often required do so. But political institutions – charged with making politically sensitive trade-offs between people and services – have proved either unwilling or unable to strike such a balance.

More recently, in the academic literature there has been a shift of focus to the processes of decision-making. The rationale is that fair processes can legitimate decisions. First expounded by Norman Daniels and James Sabin, this perspective has become known as 'accountability for reasonableness.'[2] It requires that decisions regarding coverage for new technologies (and other limit-setting decisions) and their rationales be publicly accessible. It also requires the existence of a 'mechanism for challenge and dispute resolution regarding limit-setting decisions, including the opportunity for revising decisions in light of further evidence or arguments.'[3]

From a legal perspective, the 'accountability for reasonableness' factors map onto our understanding of the basic requirements for procedural fairness which include a duty to provide reasons and the ability to seek review in the general courts of decisions delegated from govern-ments to administrative bodies. Thus, the focus of the third analytical approach implemented by the authors in this volume is on the pro-cesses of determining what services are publicly funded and, in par-ticular, the right of review or to appeal those decisions whether to the government itself, a specially constituted appeal body, or the general courts.

As these essays clearly demonstrate we see a vast gap between the day-to-day reality of decision-making regarding Medicare in Canada and the ideals expressed in the accountability-for-reasonableness frame-work. The principles that guide this decision-making are not transpar-ent or available for public scrutiny. Policy decisions are closed to public input. There are few formal avenues to appeal or review decisions, other than through the general courts – and the courts themselves have tended to be extremely deferential to governmental decision-making despite the failure of governments to demonstrate that fair processes have been followed. The overriding sentiment in Canadian health policy is that it is better to be secretive than open. But much can be done to fix the present system of how decisions are made in implementing Canada's health care policy.

Legal action can be taken to test the legitimacy of a decision not to fund a particular technology, this is, law can be used to establish rights to health care particularly, for example, through application of section 15 of the *Canadian Charter of Rights and Freedoms*, which guarantees equal treatment under the law. As well demonstrated in the *Eldridge* decision[4] the *Charter* can be an important mechanism to hold a govern-ment to account for discriminatory treatment (in that case a failure to fund translation services for the deaf so that they could receive the same maternity services that others did). Growing dissatisfaction and disillusionment with publicly run Medicare is resulting in an increasing number of *Charter* challenges, and some critics charge that the courts through *Charter* jurisprudence are dictating Medicare policy. Neverthe-less, the reality, as is discussed in the essays in Part I, 'Constitutional and Administrative Law Challenges,' is that the courts are very defer-ential to governmental decision-making, and they rarely overturn gov-ernmental limits. The question remains: Should courts be so deferential to governmental decision-making in light of the growing evidence that government decisions may not be guided by the best evidence but indeed by principles that no one objectively would consider meritori-ous (for example, short-term political gains from appeasing the medical profession)? The fact that the Supreme Court has chosen in the *Chaoulli*[5] decision to wade into the issue of rights to *private* health insurance underscores to an even greater extent the failure of courts to demand better accountability and performance on the part of government in managing *publicly* funded Medicare.

Much of the literature around limit-setting focuses on obvious sites of rationing, that is, health technology assessment agencies set up by government with the specific purpose of limiting the range of new technologies that are funded. Such explicit decisions are easier to subject to legal challenge than the myriad of implicit rationing decisions (for example, decisions regarding the allocation of budgets and the level of investments in research and in human resources training) that cumulatively determine what health services are publicly funded and who receives medical treatment. In Canada there has been less of a commitment to accountability and transparency in decision-making than in some other jurisdictions, for example, the United Kingdom and New Zealand, and there are fewer decision-makers who are clearly accountable for explicit limit-setting.[6] Decision-making about health care policy in Canada is often deeply embedded within central ministries of health, and it is hard to find out or obtain information about the processes.

The realpolitik of the Canadian system, however, inspired several contributors to reflect here on the legitimacy of decision-making further down the chain of publicly funded decision-making. For example, Jocelyn Downie examines conflicts of interest as experienced by research funding agencies and even on the part of health law and ethics experts. Trudo Lemmens criticizes the commercialization of research within universities. Similarly, Timothy Caulfield identifies the role of the media and the incentives facing university researchers in overhyping new genetic therapies. These are important and significant contributions to the international debate about limit-setting – a reminder that the obvious sites of explicit decision-making are only on the tip of the iceberg. There are many other important decisions made that, cumulatively, determine what happens from funding to research to commercial sale and the by-products of advertising and promotion that are directed at physicians, patients, and politicians.

Where to from here? Rudolf Klein, Professor of Social Policy, University of Bath, has said that '[t]he challenge everywhere is about how to organize and orchestrate what, for the foreseeable future, will be a continuing dialogue between politicians, professionals, and the public about the principles that should be invoked in making decisions about rationing and about how best to reconcile conflicting values and competing claims.'[7] This volume demonstrates the important and under-appreciated role of law in shaping this dialogue. It would be easy to end with a plea for further research in this field, which is obviously needed, but I would prefer to end with two specific recommendations. First, courts should take account of the processes of decision-making and hold governments accountable, wherever possible, for articulating the principles upon which health care policy decisions are made and for ensuring fair processes. This is not a recommendation that courts second-guess the substance of decisions but that courts take whatever opportunities there are for requiring decision-makers to have fair and transparent processes. Second, in recognition of the fact that only a few (usually well-resourced) individuals will be able to access the general courts to bring an action in review, Canadian provinces and territories should provide other means of redress. Canadians dissatisfied with limit-setting decisions should have an inexpensive and effective appeal route to an administrative agency. Moreover, governments should move towards devolving explicit responsibility for limit-setting away from state bureaucracies to arm's-length institutions. These institutions should be required to articulate the principles and processes that guide their decision-making. All of this may constitute an unenviable and a difficult task – but it is a necessary one.

NOTES

1 For a recent discussion, see Adam Oliver and Elias Mossialos, 'European Health Systems Reforms: Looking Backwards to See Forwards' (2005) 30:1–2 J. of Health Politics, Policy and Law 7-28 (ch. 7, p. 28). See also, Carolyn Tuohy, *Accidental Logics: The Dynamics of Change in the Health Care Arena in the United Stated, Britain, and Canada* (New York: Oxford University Press, 1999).

2 Norman Daniels and James Sabin, 'The Ethics of Accountability in Managed Care Reform' (1998) 17:5 Health Affairs 50 at 57.

3 *Ibid.* at 57.

4 *Eldridge v. British Columbia (Attorney General)*, [1997] 3 S.C.R. 624.

5 *Chaoulli v. Quebec (Attorney General)* 2005 SCC 35. See also Colleen M. Flood, Kent Roach, and Lorne Sossin, Access to Care, *Access to Justice: The Legal*

Debate Over Private Health Insurance (University of Toronto Press, October 2005).

6 In the United Kingdom and New Zealand there are many more bodies, devolved from central government, that are charged with resource allocation decision-making. For example, the U.K., Primary Care Trusts and Regional Health Authorities and the New Zealand District Health Authorities.

7 Rudolf Klein, 'Puzzling out Priorities' (1998) 317 Brit. Med. J. 959.

Contributors

Adalsteinn D. Brown Department of Health Policy, Management, and Evaluation, University of Toronto

Timothy Caulfield Canada Research Chair in Health Law and Policy, Professor, Faculty of Law and Faculty of Medicine and Dentistry, Health Law Institute, University of Alberta

Niteesh K. Choudhry Brigham and Women's Hospital and Harvard Medical School, Boston, Department of Medicine, University of Toronto

Sujit Choudhry Faculty of Law, and Joint Centre for Bioethics, University of Toronto

Rebecca J. Cook Professor, Faculty of Law, University of Toronto

Michelle Dagnino LLB Candidate 2006, Osgoode Hall Law School, Toronto

André den Exter Radboud University, Faculty of Law, Department of International and European Law

Jocelyn Downie Canada Research Chair in Health Law and Policy; Director, Health Law Institute at Dalhousie University

Joanna N. Erdman JD, Faculty of Law, University of Toronto

Colleen M. Flood Canada Research Chair in Health Law and Policy, Associate Professor, Faculty of Law, University of Toronto

Lisa Forman SJD Candidate, Faculty of Law, University of Toronto

Donna Greschner Professor, University of La Verne College of Law, California

Martha Jackman Professor, Faculty of Law, University of Ottawa

Robert P. Kouri Professor, Faculty of Law, University of Sherbrooke

Janesca Kydd JD, Faculty of Law, University of Toronto

Trudo Lemmens Associate Professor, Faculty of Law, University of Toronto

Constance MacIntosh Assistant Professor, Dalhousie University

Roxanne Mykitiuk Associate Professor, Osgoode Hall Law School, Toronto

Patricia Peppin Professor, Faculty of Law, Queens University

Sanda Rodgers Professor, Faculty of Law, University of Ottawa

Richard S. Saver Assistant Professor of Law, Health Law and Policy Institute, University of Houston Law Center

Mark Stabile Associate Professor, Department of Economics, University of Toronto

Carolyn Tuohy Professor, Department of Political Science, University of Toronto

Sheila Wildeman Assistant Professor, Dalhousie University